Ācārya Vāgbhaṭa's

Aṣṭāṅga Hṛdayam

The Essence of Āyurveda

Volume 1

Chapters I to IV

Dr Sanjay Pisharodi

Description of the cover

The picture on the cover is a Dhanvantari yantra. Yantras are great cosmic conductors of energy, worshiped for harmony, prosperity, success, good health, yoga and meditation. Yantras consist of a series of geometric patterns. The eyes and mind are concentrated at the center of the yantra to achieve higher levels of consciousness.

ISBN: 9352583639
ISBN 13: 978-9352583638

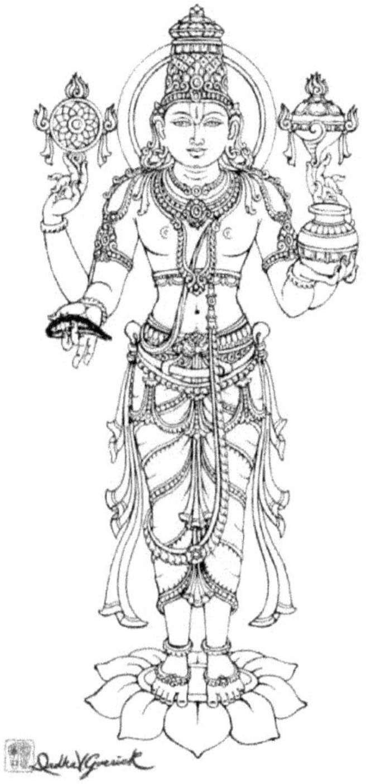

namāmi dhanvantarim ādi devam
surāsurair vandita pāda padmam
loke jarāruk bhaya mṛtyu nāśam
dhātāramīśam vividhauṣadhīnām

śrīkṛṣṇa caitanya prabhu nityānanda
śrī advaita gadādhar śrīvāsādi gaura bhakta vṛnda

hare kṛṣṇa hare kṛṣṇa kṛṣṇa kṛṣṇa hare hare
hare rāma hare rāma rāma rāma hare hare

Prayers

samsāra dāvānalalīḍha loka
trāṇāya kāruṇya ghanāghanatvam
prāptasya kalyāṇa guṇārṇavasya
vande guroḥ śrī caraṇāravindam

I offer my respects unto the lotus feet of my spiritual master whose mercy is like the rain cloud from the benevolent ocean that extinguishes the blazing forest fire of material existence.

om ajñāna timirāndhasya jñānāñjana śalākayā
cakṣur unmīlitam yena tasmai śrī gurave namaḥ

I offer my respects to my spiritual master who applied the salve of knowledge with the *śalāka* (an applicator) and opened my eyes from the darkness of ignorance.

caturmukha samārambhām
vāgbhaṭācārya madhyamām
asmad-ācārya paryantam
vande guru-paramparām

Beginning with Lord *Brahma*, *Vāgbhaṭa ācārya* in the middle and up to the contemporary *ācāryas*, I offer my respects to the all the *gurus* in the disciplic line.

Reviews by experts:

"Ashtanga Hridyam is one of the three great ancient classics of Ayurveda and among these, perhaps the most comprehensive and easy to understand. Dr Sanjay Pisharodi has provided an excellent new English version of the text that includes the Sanskrit, transliteration, translation and a lucid commentary that makes this Ayurvedic classic accessible in all of its depth and detail. I regard it as the best version of Ashtanga Hridaya available. All serious students of Ayurveda, East and West, can benefit from studying the book and keeping it as an important reference guide."

Dr. David Frawley (Paṇḍita Vāmadeva Śāstri)
Padma Bhūṣaṇ (3rd highest civilian award) in 2015 by the President of India
Director, American Institute of Vedic Studies
Advisor, National Ayurvedic Medical Association (NAMA) & Association of Ayurveda Professionals of North America (AAPNA), USA
Master Educator at The Chopra Center
Advisor at Kerala Ayurveda Academy
Founder and first president of American Council of Vedic Astrology

"Though among Ayurveda's brhat trayi Astanga Hrdayam is today the most actively consulted and employed of the three, a translation of this work by Vagbhata (whose name literally means "Language Expert") worthy of its author has long sadly been lacking. At long last this lacuna has been filled, with this effort which is written in clear English and contains in addition traditional commentaries. All serious students of Ayurveda will

find this rendition of great benefit, a book which is likely to actively benefit the spread of the Science of Life to all who require it."

Dr. Robert E Svoboda

First westerner to complete the BAMS degree from India
Advisor, National Ayurvedic Medical Association, USA
Author Ayurveda section in Encyclopaedia Britannica 2000
Adjunct faculty at the Ayurvedic Institute, Dinacarya Institute and Bastyr University

Svadhyaya (self study) of the Astanga Hridaya is a continuous exercise that an aspiring physician has to engage with to get established in the Ayurvedic thought process and to apply it in clinical practice. This process can be compared with repeated diving into the ocean to collect precious gems that lie on the ocean floor. Every time, the diver comes up with new discoveries and in a similar manner, the diligent student of the Astanga Hridaya is able to discover many layers of meanings and principles of Ayurveda through the constant svadhyaya. Dr. Sanjay's verse by verse, word by word translation and interpretation of the Astanga Hridaya is a good example of harvest that can be reaped through Svadhyaya. I am sure this work will serve as a stimulation for aspirants of Ayurveda to engage in a deeper study of the text.

Dr. Ram Manohar

Research Director at Amrita School of Ayurveda
Director and Chief Scientific Officer at AVP Research Foundation

This book is dedicated to

my respected spiritual master,
His Holiness Śrīla Rādhānāth Swāmi Maharāja;

my respected teachers, who are constantly inspiring and helping me understand the sacred science of *Āyurveda*;

and all the sincere seekers, students, and practitioners of *Āyurveda* in the past, present and future.

Acknowledgments

I am eternally grateful to my spiritual master, Śrila Rādhānāth Swami Maharāja, for helping me develop deep appreciation for and faith in the teachings of the *Vedas* and showing me how to practically live by them. I also sincerely thank all my teachers for giving me their precious time, inspiring and guiding me in my study of *Āyurveda*. I am thankful to Padmashree Dr Krishna Kumarji for his infectious enthusiasm in organizing so many unique educational programs, Late Padmashree Dr. K Rajagopalan, Late Professor C. R. Agniveś, Dr. K. Murali , Dr. Sasikumar Nechiyil , Dr. Ram Manohar, Dr. S. Gopakumar, Dr. K. Jayarajan and Vaidya M. Prasād, Dr Radhakrishnan and Dr V. C. Deep Chandran who taught me at the National Research Institute of Pañcakarma and many others. Without their kindness I could never have begun to understand the mysteries of *Āyurveda*. I thank all my friends and colleagues who encouraged me on my path, Chitra Eder Turley, who helped with the proofreading of this book and made many suggestions for its improvement. Especially grateful to Dr. Robert Svoboda, Dr. David Frawley (Pundit Vāmadeva Śāstri) and Dr. Ram Manohar for their reviews on this book. I extend a special word of gratitude to Professor Kenneth Zysk at the University of Copenhagen who was kind enough to share many of the commentaries of the *ācāryas* with me. I thank my dear friend Daniel Laflor who is more like a brother to me, and has expertly designed the cover for this book and the photograph on the cover. I would like to thank Umesh Modak for the artistic rendition of the Dhanvantari Yantra and title font. I am deeply indebted to my parents, Balakrishna Pisharodi and Jayalakshmi Pisharodi, for their kindness and support at all times in life. Last, but not the least, I extend my special feelings of love and gratitude to my dear wife, Dr. Swati Vasava, who is the wind beneath my wings, sacrificing more than words can say, helping immensely behind the scene, and patiently tolerating my absence and supporting me in unlimited ways while I continued studying and writing, unable to give sufficient time to the family—and Navkishori, my little angel, who deserves so much more of my time. Thank you all.

Sanskrit transliteration symbols:

Vowels

Devanāgarī	Transcription	
अ	A	A
आ	Ā	Ā
इ	I	I
ई	Ī	Ī
उ	U	U
ऊ	Ū	Ū
ऋ	ṛ	Ṛ
ॠ	ṝ	Ṝ
ऌ	ḷ	Ḷ
ॡ	ḹ	Ḹ
ए	E	E
ऐ	Ai	Ai
ओ	O	O
औ	Au	Au
अं	ṃ	Ṃ
अः	ḥ	Ḥ
अऽ	'	

Consonants

क	च	ट	त	प
k K	c C	ṭ Ṭ	t T	p P
ख	छ	ठ	थ	फ
kh Kh	ch Ch	ṭh Ṭh	th Th	ph Ph
ग	ज	ड	द	ब
g G	j J	ḍ Ḍ	d D	b B
घ	झ	ढ	ध	भ
gh Gh	jh Jh	ḍh Ḍh	dh Dh	bh Bh
ङ	ञ	ण	न	म
ṅ Ṅ	ñ Ñ	ṇ Ṇ	n N	m M
ह	य	र	ल	व
h H	y Y	r R	l L	v V
	श	ष	स	
	ś Ś	ṣ Ṣ	s S	

Contents

Introduction

OM ŚRĪ GURUBHYOḤ NAMAḤ

OM DHANVANTARAYE NAMAḤ

Avighnam astu

Āyurveda is a subsidiary section of the *Vedic* literature (*upaveda*) that deals with the concepts of health and wellness with respect to prevention and cure. It is also sometimes referred to as the fifth *veda* (*Pañcam Veda*). According to modern historians, it is at least forty-five hundred years old, and as per *Vedic* historians, it is an eternal science that manifested at the beginning of the creation of the cosmos (refer AH Sū. 1.3, "*brahmā smṛtvā...*").

We are a part of the cosmos

We are all a part of nature and affected in many ways by internal and external environments. The *Vedic* aphorism *"yathā pinḍe tathā brahmāṇḍe"* or "*puruṣoḥ ayam loka sammitaḥ*" means "as is the human body, so is the cosmos." The ancient seers of *Āyurveda* have studied this relationship, understood it, and explained these unchanging fundamental concepts in their writings. The concepts have been passed down the generations, helping people enjoy good health and prosperity. There is a continuous circulation of energy around us, both within the body and without, which accounts for all regular physiological changes such as eating and sleeping. It is the same with the universe as well. The concepts of energy flow in the body and the universe are very simple, but their applications are multifarious.

Importance of *Aṣṭāṅga Hṛdayam*

The *Aṣṭāṅga Hṛdayam*, (known as *Bṛhat Trayi* along with *Caraka Samhita* and *Suśruta Samhita*) is one of the three major textbooks of *Āyurveda*. *Aṣṭāṅga Hṛdayam*, compiled around the seventh century AD, is an essential extract of all the *Āyurvedic* literature that existed during that time and has become accepted as the main pillar of *Āyurvedic* practice, especially in the Indian state of Kerala (known as the cradle of *Āyurveda*) today. It contains all essential information from all the important books of *Āyurveda*, written in a beautiful poetic meter which can be sung and memorized easily. It was a common traditional practice for all the *vaidya*s (physicians) of Kerala to memorize the 7000 odd verses of the *Aṣṭāṅga Hṛdayam*. The *Aṣṭāṅga Hṛdayam* is written with the intention of making it a practical clinician's handbook, keeping the essence in focus and elaborate philosophical discussions to a minimum with practical aspects given predominance, unlike in the *Caraka Samhita* and *Suśruta Samhita*[1]. It specifically collates scattered information from all the existing textbooks and *Āyurvedic* literature of its time and presents the concepts in a systematic manner for easier study and comprehension.

Āyurveda and subsidiary *Vedic* literature

Since *Āyurveda* is a part of the *Vedic* literature, it liberally borrows from all sections of the *Vedas*, such as astrology, astronomy, and philosophy. Some concepts may not be

---

[1] This does not mean that Caraka Samhita and Suśruta Samhita are unimportant.

explained in detail in the *Āyurvedic* texts due to the expectation that the student would already be familiar with other *Vedic* literatures and will correlate the information appropriately. In this book I have quoted contextually from some of these literatures. *Bhagavad Gīta* is an ancient philosophical treatise of India that summarizes the entire gamut of *Vedic* philosophy in about seven hundred verses divided into eighteen chapters. It is a part of the *Mahābharata,* which is a historical account of the world written about five thousand years ago. I have extracted some sections from *Bhagavad Gīta* to correlate and explain some of the concepts of *Āyurveda*.

The logic of the *vaidya* is most important

The ancient *Āyurvedic* texts are written in such an open manner as to help develop the thinking patterns of students and enable them to handle any situation related to health and wellness. Instead of giving rigid protocols and diagnoses or names of diseases, the text is liberal enough to say that the names of diseases are not important but understanding the underlying pathology is. There is no rigid method to treat any disease, but the physician is advised to closely observe the progressing pathology and treat accordingly. So one who has a comprehensive understanding of the entire text can take the principles and apply them in variegated ways he or she feels suitable. This is called *yukti.* It is this *yukti* (logical thinking) of the *vaidya* that stands supreme in *Āyurveda*. But to be able to do this, one has to have a thorough understanding of the principles. For this one should study the ancient texts. These texts clearly explain the eternal principles that do not change. Their applications, however, may change.

How I decided to work on the *Aṣṭāṅga Hṛdayam*

After studying *Āyurveda* at some of the academies in India and the West, I still found myself not confident enough to help people who came to me for guidance. I was not feeling fully rooted in the ancient tradition from where *Āyurveda* originates. So I decided to foray into studying the *Sanskṛt* texts containing the timeless wisdom. When I started looking into the ancient texts of *Āyurveda*, *Caraka Samhita* and *Suśruta Samhita* seemed the obvious choices initially. While reading the *Caraka Samhita*, I realized that the concepts, though brilliant, were scattered all over the book. I wanted something more concise, structured and focused on practice. This is when a teacher advised me to study the *Aṣṭāṅga Hṛdayam*. It was nothing short of a blessing. Every verse in the *Aṣṭāṅga Hṛdayam* spoke to me so clearly. The flow was very logical. Within no time I was able to understand the essential concepts of *Āyurveda* and put them into practice. I was convinced that this is the book for the beginner student. I also noticed that the *Aṣṭāṅga Hṛdayam* is the book that has the maximum number of commentaries by previous *ācāryas*, which adds to its richness. I was fortunately able to study all these writings because of the ability to understand *Sanskṛt* (due to my training for 8 years as a student in a *vedic* monastery) and the local language of Kerala (*Malayalam* which is my mother tongue) in which many of the commentaries were written, along with the many seminars and classes that I attended (almost all in Malayalam) and the kindness of the experienced teachers and practitioners who graciously allowed me much of their time. While I was at the academy in the USA, my co-students often asked me to recommend a translation of the *Aṣṭāṅga Hṛdayam* for them to study. But honestly, I did not feel comfortable recommending the existing translations because I felt that they did not cater specifically to the needs of international students. And thus I began to think, "What if I could find a way to share this treasure with everyone out there?" So my writings that initially started as personal notes of my studies with many teachers and books began to take the shape of a book.

Purpose of this book

When I asked myself, "What is the best way that I can serve the science[2] of *Āyurveda*?" the answer came to my heart clearly, like a flash: by being a transparent medium to carry the message of the sages to the students in an authentic way. Hence, I have taken up this work despite feeling unqualified. It is my firm faith that my readers will overlook the faults in my presentation and accept the message.

Although there exist some English translations of the ancient texts, written by eminent scholars, the impression I have is that they do not sufficiently connect the student with the ancient lineage of *Āyurveda*.

---

[2] The definition of science being the study of cause and effect

Āyurveda is becoming popular all over the world, with several books being written by professionals and amateur authors or practitioners. I have a deep appreciation for their efforts. At the same time, I also have concerns that in the effort of making the science relevant for present times, these books may have compromised the core conceptual understanding and application in favour of correlating the science with modern medicine. I also found that many of the new-age books lacked complete references for what is mentioned in the book. This prevents the student from going to the source to explore further. It is also unclear whether the conclusions are those of the ancient sages or opinions of the present author. This was summarized beautifully by a swamiji I met recently who is also a *Vaidya.* He said "Most of the modern books have a lot of information but the soul is missing." Then one will ask "What is the soul of *Āyurveda*?" The soul of all *vedic* sciences is "*dharma*". It is primarily meant to learn how to conduct ourselves according to the principles of *dharma.* Diagnosing and treating diseases is a secondary purpose.

Two things could happen due to the lack of references:

1. The information is selectively and incompletely presented.
2. When the authors express their personal opinions without clearly mentioning so, the student might accept them as the absolute word of the *śāstra.*

There are specific requirements to be fulfilled for any book to be accepted as *śāstra.* Others can be accepted only as opinions or observations.

The study and practice of *Āyurveda* is spreading all over the globe rapidly. At this juncture, it is of utmost importance that the concepts of this science be understood in its full authenticity and actuality by students everywhere. Correct conceptual understanding is critical. If a wrong or incomplete concept is propagated, it eventually snowballs into a catastrophic misunderstanding that is difficult to rectify. A clear understanding of the concepts can be accomplished by giving students a connection to the unbroken tradition from the roots.

Due to various reasons, through the annals of time, *Āyurveda* has been practiced in different ways in different places all over the world and will continue to be so in the future. This is natural and recommended as well. This book series is an attempt to give *Āyurvedic* students access to the original ancient texts along with their explanations by *Āyurveda's* exalted teachers of the past. By understanding the concepts clearly, the students will be empowered to translate the same concepts into practices that suit their own cultures and environments.

Status of *Āyurveda* in the world

In India there is often a tendency for the general populace to look down upon *Āyurvedic* medicine, which reflects on the confidence of students to practice the same with dignity. This outlook has led to many trained *Āyurvedic* doctors practicing Western medicine, with incomplete training in the latter, after having studied *Āyurveda* for more than five years. There is a great need to instill confidence in the practitioners of *Āyurveda* through educational, social, administrative and political initiatives and create opportunities for *Āyurveda* to progress shoulder to shoulder with its Western counterpart.

In the modern world, quite often *Āyurvedic concepts are* explained by force fitting them into the concepts of Western medical anatomy, physiology, and pathology without using the authentic explanations from ancient texts. This creates confusion. Both systems have their own unique ways of classifiying and understanding the functioning of the body. Mixing them together would not be a good idea to understand either one. The *ācāryas* have given us a specific methodology to study *Āyurveda*.

Students who try to apply such a westernized understanding of *Āyurveda* to a clinical setting experience confusion and failure to adequately understand, diagnose and treat different disease conditions. This can result in loss of confidence and faith in the science. Proper application of the science is possible only if the concepts are understood in an authentic manner, which will ensure demonstrable results on application.

Is there the need for a commentary?

I asked myself, "What is the need for my commentary when the *ācāryas* have already commented?" The *ācāryas* had written the commentaries during a time when many of the basic concepts were commonplace in the culture and lifestyle of the people; it was taken for granted that they were understood by all, and the *ācāryas* expected their students to have a basic understanding of several *Vedic* concepts, which cannot be done in the present day since many of us have a mixed culture having moved far away from pure traditions. Times have changed, and we are not as familiar with the tenets of *Vedic* life and culture. So I have chipped in to fill that gap as much as possible and help students better understand what the *ācārya* is trying to convey. If two *ācāryas* have repeated the same point, repetition is avoided in the book.

At certain times there are instances where the *ācāryas* differ among themselves in opinion. This is only an apparent contradiction. We cannot imitate them and concoct our own opinions, because we are not at that level. One of the aspects of studying *Āyurveda* is that students should be able to harmonize the apparent contradictory opinions of the *ācāryas* and apply it as appropriate to the given circumstance. The *ācāryas* usually do not contradict in terms of principle but in terms of application only.

I see my role only as a bridge trying to connect you, the student, with *Vāgbhaṭa,* the author of *Aṣṭāṅga Hṛdayam,* and the great teachers who have written the commentaries. It is my great desire that this knowledge should be available, as it is, without any distortion for the benefit of students and *Āyurveda.*

Commentaries used in writing this book

The commentaries used are as follows:

1. *Sarvāṅgasundara*, by *Aruṇadutta*

2. *Āyurvedarasāyana*, by *Hemādri*
3. *Vākyapradīpika*, by *Parameśvardās*
4. *Hṛdayabodhika*, by *Sridas Paṇḍita*
5. *Aruṇodaya*, by *Govindan Vaidyar*
6. *Bhāvaprakāśa*, by *Kaikkulangara Ramavāriyar*

While studying the *Aṣṭāṅga Hṛdayam*, I noticed that the wonderful commentaries written by the *ācāryas* were hardly studied by students. I found them to be very useful in clarifying my concepts and have thus included them in this book. The whereabouts of the lives of these great teachers are shrouded in a lot of controversy, and the exact period they lived in is also not clear. But their writings are timeless.

The translations of these commentaries have never been available to international students, and now, for the first time, they are being made available. This will help them attain a deeper understanding of the subject. The views of the ancient commentators have been included without changing or distorting them. As a result, some of the comments may appear irrelevant or unpalatable to the modern student, but I have still kept them as they are.

Āyurveda is a science that has been passed down from master to disciple for thousands of years. The methodology of study has changed over the course of time. It used to be passed down in an unbroken oral tradition from *guru* to disciple, wherein the student lived with the teacher closely, observing him or her and being observed (*gurukula* system). Later the educational system was changed to a university style as we see today. The modern university style education has a disadvantage in that the student does not get as much personal attention of the *guru* and vice versa compared to the traditional *gurukula* system.

The knowledge of *Āyurveda* has been recorded in *Sanskṛt,* which is a very cryptic but versatile language. As with any other medical science, *Āyurveda* also has a huge compendium of medical terminologies. *Sanskṛt* is a language in which each word can have multiple meanings according to context. Hence, translation into another language becomes a challenge.

Moreover *Āyurveda* has its own special meanings for certain terms that can also vary with context within the subject. The greatest challenge for me in writing this book has been to remain loyal to the authenticity of these terms. However, I would like to say that some of the fundamental concepts in *Āyurveda* (e.g., *āma, agni, snāyu, koṣṭha*) have such broad connotations that it is not possible to restrict the translation to either one word or a few words, although for reasons of convention, I have translated or described them in one or two words in some places in the book. These terms will require elaboration and deeper study by the student. This is a different subject called *padārtha vijñānam* (knowledge of terminologies).

If I am successful in igniting the spirit of deeper study in the minds of the students, I will consider my effort successful. I want to invite all students of *Āyurveda* to study the classical textbooks deeply. Study should not be restricted to notes and memorization that help to pass exams. The spirit and practice of *Āyurveda* should be kept vibrant, updated, authentic, and alive in our heads, hearts, and hands.

I once again hope that you will forgive my audacity in considering myself qualified to write this book. Your suggestions, debates, and criticisms are most welcome.
Aṣṭāṅga Hṛdayam is like a vast ocean and I have made a humble effort to pick out a few gems with the help of my gurus. May this book serve as a beginning to inspire us to dive deeper into an authentic study of the limitless ocean of *Āyurveda*.

I pray to *Srila Gurudev*, all the *ācāryas,* saintly persons, teachers, the Supreme Lord, and my beloved readers for blessings upon this insignificant endeavor.

Dr Sanjay Pisharodi

How to study this book

The presentation

In this book each of the verses is presented in *Devanāgari* as well as in English transliteration. The format adopted in this book will help the student to read the original *Sanskṛt* verse and appreciate it, despite not having complete knowledge of *Sanskṛt* (*Devanāgari*) script. After each verse you will find a word-for-word translation of the verse. The word-for-word translation is followed by a translation of the verse and commentary. In the commentary there are two sections—my own insights from studies with experienced *Āyurvedic* physicians on the subject matter and the commentaries of the *ācāryas*.

One word—many meanings

When we try to understand a *Sanskṛt* word in a verse, we should be mentally prepared to accept the various meanings of the word and choose the best one for the given context. At times more than one meaning may be applicable, or the author may have used a specific word to convey multiple meanings. These aspects must be kept in mind. As the student progresses, he or she could discover deeper, broader, and multiple understandings for the same word as well. Sometimes you may find more than one translation for a word in the word-for-word section, and even another one in the translation. This is not an error. It is only to help expand your thinking, reveal the wide range of meanings that a word in *Sanskṛt* can cover, and help you look at the verse from different viewpoints.

Combination of many words into one word

Sanskṛt is a language where words are often combined together. This is called *sandhi.* The junction of the two words will sound different when they merge. In cases where they are located at the end of a quartet or half verse, the words have been split in the English transliteration to enable easy reading/recitation for Western students. In cases where they have not been split, you will see the separation in the word-for-word translation. The conjunction is kept as it is in the *Sanskṛt* version.

Conceptual understanding

Sometimes the literal translation of the *Sanskṛt* word is not enough to understand the concept, because the translated word in English may have a different conceptual understanding although the word is the same. For example, when you say *cough* in modern medicine, it indicates a pathology in a particular system. But in *Āyurveda* the word *kāsa* indicates a systemic pathology that can affect all the organs of the body and even be a cause of death. It may be treated by giving an enema. So when you say *cough* in *Āyurveda*, it implies something different from the *cough* of modern medicine. Another example is *āyu*, which can be translated as longevity. But in *Āyurveda* it includes the body, senses, mind, soul, and the realization that life flows like a river from one body to the next. *Longevity* in English might just mean a long life-span or staying alive.

Contextual understanding

I have translated the words into meanings that can fit the particular context, but suffice to say that it is not necessarily the only meaning of the word. For one who is a serious student of *Āyurveda*, it will be fascinating to enter into the deeper meanings of these words. The deeper meanings of the words are a doorway to understanding various applications of the concepts. I have only tried to scratch the surface and awaken the curiosity of the student, while a huge body of knowledge lies hidden and unexplored in the pages of these ancient texts.

Each word in a verse is very significant and can have multiple meanings. The translations of the words and text have been, at times, contextual rather than literary to make more practical sense to a student of *Āyurveda*. However, this does not mean that there cannot be other meanings to the words. What is expressed here is simply one possible understanding.

Encouraging the use of *Sanskṛt* words

In many instances I have deliberately used the *Sanskṛt* words in the commentary, so the student can become more familiar with the *Sanskṛt* terminology. The meanings of some *Sanskṛt* words have been repeated in order to increase the familiarity and also because the meanings of the same words may change according to context. *Sanskṛt* words that are part of the original verse and translated in the word-for-word section may not be translated again in the commentaries. Please refer to the word-for-word section.

In the commentary I have avoided unnecessarily repeating the English translation of a word after it has been done once or twice in the beginning. This is in order to encourage the student to become familiar with the *Sanskṛt* word. But in the word-for-word section, the translation will be repeated wherever a word appears. I hope that it will inspire the students to take up a parallel study of *Sanskṛt* as well.

Understanding the same concept from different angles

The *ācāryas* have tried to explain the same concepts from different angles so that we can grasp the full gamut of the principles and applications. It is possible that you will find the verses explained slightly differently in different places. When something is defined or described in one part of the text, it need not be the only understanding about it. So avoid fixing your mind on one description exclusively.

Key to solving the mystery of the *Aṣṭāṅga Hṛdayam*

The key is to understand the thought process behind the flow of the text. Understanding this will also help to solve the mystery of *Āyurveda*. There is a philosophical chain of thought in the *Aṣṭāṅga Hṛdayam* between the *sthānas* (sections) of the book, the chapters in the *sthānas*, the verses in the chapters, and the concepts within the verses. There is a unique reason why a verse is placed in a particular *sthāna*, chapter and a particular part of the chapter. Each of the verses is also interconnected to several other parts of the book. Understanding this thought process or flow and its purpose will help you establish the interconnections and flow of the discussion in *Aṣṭāṅga Hṛdayam*.

While reading the commentary you may come across concepts or words that have not been explained before in the text. Do not get disturbed by it. It is the nature of the ancient literature and the *ācāryas* as well to comment by connecting the verses to concepts that are ahead or behind. This helps to develop a networked thinking pattern and interconnect all the concepts in different ways across different parts of the text. These concepts will be explained in the book.

During the ancient days, the students went through a rigorous study of literature, poetry and the science of logical thinking (*tarka*). This taught them how to think and analyse. Most of the *Āyurvedic* texts are written in a poetic style description of the scientific concepts. This is also due to the reason that subtle concepts can be better expressed in poetry than in prose. Each word in the verse is selected very carefully indicating a clear logical concept.

Important steps to study a classical text

When you study a classical text, try to think of the following items:

- Why is this chapter placed in this part of the book?
- What is its relation with the preceding and succeeding chapters?
- What is its relation with other sections of the book?
- Why is this verse placed in this position of the chapter?
- What is its relation with the preceding and succeeding verses?
- Why is this word placed in this part of the verse?

- What is the relation of this word with the other words in the verse?
- In which other contexts, does the same word appear in the book?
- Why is this particular word chosen over the other synonyms of the same word?
- What is the BIG picture of the section or the chapter or the section?
- What is the written obvious message in the verse?
- Which are the unwritten words in the verse? If you can read the unwritten lines, you have actually understood the text. Every verse is a puzzle that the ācāryas have left for us to solve. We have to learn to connect the dots.
- ...these are just a few suggestions and I am sure there are more ways.

Expanding from the core

The *Aṣṭāṅga Hṛdayam* is written in such a way that the first chapter covers all the basic concepts of *Āyurveda*. Then the first section, called *Sūtra sthāna*, covers the concepts explained in chapter 1 more elaborately. The remaining sections describe the same concepts in further detail.

Conclusion

The method of study to be adopted has been explained by *Suśruta* in SS Sū. 4.5, "Every word, part of the verse and the full verse of all the chapters should be explained by the teacher and understood by the students."

May the divine blessings of Lord *Dhanvantari* descend upon us, the light of *Āyurveda* always shine in our hearts, and enable us to achieve all the perfections of human life! I wish you all the very best. *Om tat sat.*

Chapter 1

आयुष्कामीयम्

Āyuṣkāmīyam

The Quest for Longevity

Summary of the chapter

This chapter contains the gist of the entire *Aṣṭāṅga Hṛdayam*. It describes all the concepts, to be elaborated further in the book, in a coded form. At the end of the chapter is the index of the whole book divided into sections. The name of this chapter indicates the purpose of *Āyurveda,* which is described in the second verse of the chapter. This title is apt since this chapter is the summary of the entire book.

Sections in the chapter

I. Invocation and appearance of *Āyurveda*—1 to 6a

II. *Doṣas*: location, time, *agni*, *koṣṭḥa*, *prakṛti*, and *guṇa*—6b to 12a

III. Imbalances: what is imbalanced; how to correct—12b to 18

IV. Concept of disease—19 to 21b

V. Assessment—22a to 24a

VI. Treatments—24b to 29b

VII. Prognosis—30 to 35a

VIII. Index of the whole book—35b to 48½

Key *Sanskṛt* words in this chapter

doṣa, dhātu, mala, agni, rāga, krodha, moha, āyuḥ, prakṛti, vāyuḥ, vāta, pitta, kapha, hṛd, nābhi, koṣṭha, guṇa, dūṣya, rasa, rakta, māmsa, medas, asthi, majja, śukra, sannipāta, vṛddhi, kṣaya, uṣṇa, śīta, vipāka, kāla, artha, karma, hīna, ati, mithyā, ārogya, roga, nija, āgantu, rajas, tamas, darśana, sparśana, praśna, jāṅghalam, ānūpam, sādhāraṇam, bheṣaja, śodhana, śamana, vasti, vireka, vamana, manas, bhiṣak, dravya, upasthātā, rogī, susādhya, kṛcchra sādhya, yāpya, anupakrama

Maṅgalācaraṇaṁ (Invocation)

रागादिरोगान् सततानुषक्तानशेषकायप्रसृतानशेषान्
औत्सुक्यमोहारतिदान् जघान योऽपूर्ववैद्याय नमोऽस्तुतस्मैः ॥१॥

rāgādi-rogān satatānuṣaktān-
aśeṣa-kāya-prasṛtān-aśeṣān
autsukya-mohāratidān jaghāna
yo'pūrva-vaidyāya namo'stu-tasmai //1//

rāgādi – all the qualities accompanying attachment (*kāma, krodha, lobha, mada, mātsarya*, etc.), color, music; *rogān* – to the diseases; *satata* – always; *anuṣakta* – closely associated with; *aśeṣa* – limitless, totally; *kāya* – body; *prasṛtān* – issuing from, spreading (derived from *prasāra*); *aśeṣān* – limitless; *autsukya* – anxieties; *moha* – delusion; *arati* – not having any interest, restlessness; *dān* – that which produces; *jaghāna* – has destroyed, eradicated; *yaḥ* – who; *apūrva* – rare, never seen before (signifying greatness); *vaidyāya* – unto the physician; *namaḥ astu* – let there be obeisances; *tasmai* – unto him

Translation

Obeisances unto that unique and rare (uncomparable) physician who has completely eliminated limitless diseases that are closely and constantly associated with the body, spreading all over the body and mind, perpetually causing anxiety, confusion, and restlessness. These diseases include attachment (and aversion) and their various transformations, which are an integral aspect of all living beings.

Commentary

The opening verse is an invocation, namely, an invocation for auspiciousness. It is called *mangalācaraṇa* in *Sanskṛt*. It is tradition to begin a book in this manner.

The components of an invocation are as follows:

1. *Āśīrvād* (blessings or benefits of studying the book)
2. *Namaskār* (Greetings and offering of respects to one and all)
3. *Vastu nirdeśa* (Statement of purpose of the book)

The words *unique and rare physician* indicates the almighty Lord, who is the only one who can completely cure *rāga* (attachment) and its transformations, such as greed, vanity, and ignorance.

Many questions are addressed in this invocation verse.

1. What is the root cause of disease?
2. Where does it come from?
3. What are the symptoms of the root cause?

4. How can we get rid of it?
5. Who will help us to do it?
6. How should we approach such a person?

What is *rāgādi*? Literally it means attachment and everything that follows. What are the things that follow? It is explained by *Vāgbhaṭa* himself in the *Aṣṭāṅga Hṛdayam* (AH Sū. 4.24),[1] "Greed, jealousy, hatred, envy are the *rāgādis.*" In the *Bhagavad Gīta* 2.64,[2] it is explained that one who is freed from attachment and aversion and is sense controlled will achieve the highest destination. Attachment and aversion are the two ends of the spectrum of the human mind; *rāga* is attachment and *dveṣa* is aversion.

In simpler words, attachment and aversion, the only two causes of disease, can be explained as follows:

1. I am attached to something, but I am unable to obtain it (*rāga*).
2. I am averse to something, but I am being forced to accept it (*dveṣa*).

The first word, *rāgādi*, is very significant. It is described here as the initial trigger of disease, and all other diseases follow it. The word *ādi* also means "the initial starting point." Attachment and aversion by themselves are not bad, but misdirected attachment is the beginning of all suffering or disease. Attachment to the right things and aversion from the wrong things is the doorway to liberation from suffering. Thus, the only way to become free from all diseases is to become free from *misdirected* attachment. Attachment grows like a banyan tree, with multiple branches and roots. Once we become entwined and entangled within this tree of attachment, it is difficult to ascertain where it all started. That banyan tree, along with its branches, represents all our attachments and aversions. The process of freeing ourselves from it is described beautifully in the *Bhagavad Gīta* 15.1–4.[3] With firmness and perseverance, one should thoroughly cut down this tree from its root with the weapons of knowledge and detachment.

Through this verse *Vāgbhaṭa* conveys the message that the foremost thing for a student of *Āyurveda* is to develop the right mental attitude. With such an attitude, knowledge will manifest naturally. In other words, if the mind-set is not right in the beginning, one may miss the essence of *Āyurveda*. There has to be a positive transformation of the mind through all the processes of gathering information.

***Āyurvedarasāyana* of *Hemādri*:** Respects unto Lord *Gaṇeśa*. Respects also unto the four-handed Lord *Viṣṇu* who bestowed freedom from old age and death to the gods in the heavens with the nectar obtained by churning the ocean of milk using the mountain as a churning rod, kept on the back of Lord *Kūrma*, the divine turtle incarnation of the Lord.

The commentary by *Hemādri* bestows the reader with all the four perfections (*dharma, artha, kāma, mokṣa*), which fulfill all desires in life (*catur varga cintāmaṇi*). The blessing to have a long and healthy life is also given. The commentary is being written in line with the teachings of *Caraka, Suśruta, Hārita*, and other great teachers.

Desiring to explain *Āyurveda*, *Vāgbhaṭācārya* prays to his sacred deity in the first verse. The words *apūrva vaidya* denote the deity. The word *apūrva* indicates wonderful powers of one who can quell all the diseases beginning with *jvara* (loosely translated as agitation, inflammation, or fevers). According to *Āyurveda*, *jvara* is a pathology that is the beginning and end of all diseases, and one who knows how to treat *jvara* can cure any disease. Being tormented by many diseases (viz., the *rāgādis*[4]), the pure consciousness becomes colored by *rajas* and *tamas,* which are the roots of lust, anger, and so on.

The words *satata anuṣakta* indicate that symptoms of inflammation are inseparable from the body and mind at all times. They are spread all over and situated internally and externally, manifesting as many diseases in various stages. According to the adherents of the above doctrine of *satata anuṣakta*, the subtle forms of *jvara* are called anxiety, delusion, and restlessness (*autsukya, moha, arati*).

- *Autsukya*: action without thinking
- *Moha*: inability to think properly
- *Arati*: unhappiness

These are acting on all living entities at all times, giving them trouble (*kleśa*). Hence, diseases are called *rāgādi roga*. The word *jaghāna* indicates liberation from, or destruction of suffering, not the destruction of the self.

Note: You will note that at times the same word has been explained by different gurus in ways more than one. The student has to take all the different meanings and harmonize them to get an all-around understanding of the concept.

The purpose of the entire book (or rather the entire science of *Āyurveda*) is mentioned in the next verse as "the quest for longevity."

***Sarvāṅgasundara* of *Aruṇadutta*:** The word *rāgādi* denotes the totality of all diseases. The word *ādi* denotes aversion or hatred, greed, and so on (*dveṣa*, *lobha*, etc.) In general, whatever causes pain is called *roga*.

Aruṇadutta compares life to the phenomenon of "a pot of ghee hanging above and dripping slowly into a slowly burning fire." Ghee is falling drop by drop into the fire keeping it alive. As long as ghee continues to drop into the fire, the fire will keep burning. This analogy is very insightful and significant. Fire is the *agni* in the body and ghee represents the *ojas*. According to the philosophy of *Āyurveda*, the healthy state of the body is called *śītam snigdham āgneyam*, meaning "cool, unctuous, and inflammable." This can also be understood from the analogy of a burning ghee lamp. The ghee is cool and unctuous, but it is being slowly used up by the burning flame, which is the flame of life. A perfect balance is required between the ghee and fire to keep the flame going. If too much ghee falls in, the fire will go off. If the fire burns too big, the ghee will get spoilt or exhausted quickly. The ghee represents the *soma* energy and the fire represents the *agni* energy. All phenomena of life are controlled and balanced interactions between the *soma* and *agni* energies. In the universe the *soma* and *agni* energies are represented by the moon and sun, respectively.

Aśeṣa kāya prasṛtān aśeṣān has two aspects with respect to human life—(1) being all pervasive in the body and (2) being present in the body from the time of birth until death—which are included in this phrase. The words *aśeṣa kāya* also mean that all species of life are included in this description and not just human beings. So that gives three different meanings to the same phrase. Note how one phrase can convey so much information.

Some of the words in the verse are explained as follows:

- *Satatānuṣaktaḥ*: will be inseparable from and present in the body up to the point of death and pass on to the next body after death
- *Aśeṣa kāya*: all living beings include humans, animals, and plants (elephants, horses, snakes, etc.) and all species of life
- *Autsukya*, *moha*, *arati*: three important symptoms seen from the beginning to the end of life
- *Autsukya*: anxiety due to desire for sense objects

- *Moha*: not aware of what is to be done or not to be done
- *Arati*: instability or unsteadiness
- *Apūrva vaidya*: one who is able to differentiate, diagnose, and cure all diseases

The purpose of this tantra (see below for definition) is explained from many different angles:

- *Caraka* says that the purpose of this tantra is to bring about balance of body tissues (*dhātu sāmyata*—Sū. 1.52);
- the study of the *tantra* is to be done by *pātha* (recitation), *avabodha* (understanding), and *anuṣṭhāna* (practice);
- for attaining the four *puruṣārthas* (goals of life) of *dharma* (unchanging quality of anything), *artha* (wealth, prosperity), *kāma* (desires), and *mokṣa* (liberation);
- to explain the three sections of *Āyurveda*: etiology (*hetu*), symptoms (*liṅga*), and treatment (*auṣadha*);
- to explain the nature of relationships (*sambandha*), how to act in that relationship (*abhidheya*), and the result of such action (*prayojana*).

Definition of *tantra*: In an *Āyurvedic* context, the word *tantra* denotes that this is practical advice meant for maintaining *āyu* (CS Sū. 30.70) by its application and not just an intellectual exercise. *Āyurvedic* knowledge is referred to as *tantra*, because it is meant for practical application.

***Aruṇodaya* by Govindan *vaidya*:** The first verse is called *mangalācaraṇa*, meaning that which invokes auspiciousness.

Vāgbhaṭa has offered his prayers for the unobstructed completion of the writing of the book. He also offers prayers for students to be able to complete studying the book. *Apūrva vaidya* is worshipped here and it means the primeval *vaidya*. Ordinary *vaidyas* are capable of curing physical diseases like *jvara*, and so on, but the *apūrva vaidya* can cure both physical and psychological ailments of the entire body-mind complex.

- *Satatānuṣaktān* indicates that diseases continue to follow us from the time of birth up to the point of death.
- *Aśeṣa kaya prasṛtān* indicates that it is not only applicable to human beings but all living beings.
- *Jaghāna*, in this context, indicates that not only has the *apūrva vaidya* eliminated all such diseases in the past but has also revealed the technique by which others students can do the same in the future as well.

Any science created by human beings will also contain the defects of human beings. But a medical science needs to be perfect, and hence, the *vaidya*s should perform their duties in full spiritual consciousness.

***Vākyapradīpika*:** *Rāgādis* are transformations of the mind. *Rāga* is the starting point of *dveṣa*. The word *tasmai* is being told for the purpose of attaining all fame. An *apūrva vaidya* is supposed to be famous and respected everywhere. The word *vaidya* means "one who knows." For one who is afflicted with material disease, the only real cure is to attain the feet of the Supreme Lord. Here the words *apūrva vaidya* indicate *Mahādeva* or *Lord Śiva*. The word *astu* denotes heartfelt *namaskār* (obeisances) with mind, body, and words, which bestow divine blessings upon the work being performed and assure completion. Unless the *namaskār* is performed, it is impossible to attain *kārya samāpti* (completion of the purpose).

Rāgādis are transformations of the mind. *Rāga* is the beginning point of *dveṣa, lobha*, and all other transformations. The *rāgādis* are not the causes but are themselves identified as diseases, because they cause pain to the body and mind. The afflictions of the body and mind are closely connected in a way similar to how the heat of the pot is related to the heat of the hot ghee inside it.

Rāga is a transformation of the mind which:

- is connected to the essence of the living entity;
- makes the material world function;
- is the cause of all ignorance;
- is not manifested in childhood like the fragrance in a flower bud (but manifests as we grow);
- becomes gradually manifest under favorable circumstances; and
- causes *tāpa* (inflammation) of the body and mind if *karma* (activities) are not correct.

Dveṣa is the intense attitude of wanting to *destroy* another person using all of one's resources. Ignorance is the cause of all suffering. The word *aśeṣa* indicates that if *rāgādis* are removed, all ignorance will be completely eradicated and knowledge will manifest.

The word *jaghāna* means to eradicate something to such an extent that it will never recur. The word *anu* indicates that the *rāgādis* are following each other, that is, when *rāga* is gone, *dveṣa* will manifest; when *dveṣa* is gone, *lobha* will manifest, and so on. This does not mean that the *rāgādis* should manifest in the same linear pattern all the time. *Anu* also signifies that the *rāgādis* follow the person from one body to the next. *Autsukya* is the mental anxiety resulting from inability to attain the things desired by the mind, causing the body to become emaciated.

The students of any science should have clarity concerning its content, meaning, and purpose from the very beginning of their study. Those who study the science without understanding the content, meaning, and purpose will be unable to effectively put the teachings into practice. Here the *upāya-upeya* (plan-purpose) relationship is explained. *Upāya* is the science and *upeya* are life-span, *dharma, artha, kāma*, and *mokṣa*. The science of *Āyurveda* consists of three parts: *hetu* (causes), *linga* (symptoms), and *auṣadha* (medicine/treatment). All the three are put together in this invocation.

AH Sū. Prose verse 1

Name of chapter and blessings of the sages

अथात आयुष्कामीयमध्यायं व्याख्यास्यामः

इति ह स्माहुरात्रेयादयो महर्षयः ॥ *गद्य सूत्रम्* १ ॥

athāta āyuṣkāmīyam-adhyāyaṁ vyākhyāsyāmaḥ
iti ha smāhur-ātreyādayo maharṣayaḥ // prose 1//

athāta – therefore; *āyuṣkāmīyam* – quest for longevity; *adhyāyaṁ* – chapter; *vyākhyāsyāmaḥ* – will describe; *iti* – this; *ha sma-āhur* – as spoken by; *ātreyādayo* – Ātreya *rṣi* and others; *maharṣayaḥ* – the sages

Translation

Therefore as advised/spoken by the great hermit *Ātreya* and the group of sages is described the chapter on the quest for longevity.

Commentary

The three implications of using the word *atha* are

1. auspiciousness, indicating that this work will be uninterrupted till completion and accepted by all those who read and study this book;
2. the subject that is about to be narrated (i.e., *Āyurveda*); and
3. willingness of the disciple to learn and the teacher to teach.

Āyu means "something that which is going on continuously." This is very significant to note. The *Vedic* concept of life is not linear. Time is cyclical and so is life. It indicates that the body may come to an end, but life still continues in another shape or form. As opposed to this, modern medical science, due to a lack of understanding of the concept of soul (*ātma*), considers birth as the beginning and death as the end of life.

Sma indicates past tense, which means that this knowledge already existed in the past. We may note that *Vāgbhaṭa* is not taking any credit for this. One should not take knowledge from the *śāstra* and present it as if it is created out of one's own intelligence. This is called plagiarism, which is condemned today and was done so in the past as well.

Here we notice the humility of *Vāgbhaṭa* who is following in the footsteps of the great sages. This is called the *parampara* or disciplic succession. The liberated sages are free from the influence of passion and ignorance, and thus, the knowledge that emanates from them is pure and free from the four human defects.[5] This is called as *āptavacana* (words of the perfected beings who are free of any faults) which is one of the four ways of acquiring knowledge.[6] Thus, what is narrated herein is not a figment of imagination or the concoction of *Vāgbhaṭa* but rather a sacred body of knowledge that has been handed down carefully from generation to generation through the bona fide disciplic succession.

Here *Vāgbhaṭa* does not say, "I will narrate according to my intelligence." One should not write books to express one's own conceived opinions without supportive statements from *śāstra* (ancient texts).

In many of the modern books written today, we find the author's own opinions predominating without any reference to *śāstra*. This is not the correct method of learning according to the *Vedic* system. One should faithfully represent the *ācāryas* in an unadulterated manner and that is how knowledge is passed down from one generation to the next without distortion.

There are two *paramparas* (disciplic lines) in *Āyurveda*: *ātreya* and *dhanvantari*. *Ātreyādaya* includes both of them.

Note: The knowledge of ***Ā****yurveda* as it came down the line, at some point of time, got divided into two: the medical and surgical branches. The medical branch was further developed by the students in the line of *Ātreya*. The surgical branch was developed by the students in the line of *Suśruta*. Since then these two *paramparas* have coexisted.

The first lesson to the student from the *mangalācaraṇam* was to develop the right attitude. The second lesson for the student is that one should have faith in the words of the great *ācāryas* and should faithfully represent them everywhere.

***Sarvāṅgasundara*:** The word *ha* indicates compassion. This work is not composed out of a desire for profit but out of compassion for the suffering humanity. By saying that he is following the teachings of *ātreya ṛsi*; *Vāgbhaṭa* means that he will not concoct anything on his own, but only present the knowledge as it is, faithfully, in a way that is relevant to the time (*yugānurūpa*) and arranged in a suitable order (*krama-mātra*) as handed down by the great sages.

The plural form is used in the description of *āyu*. This is because the word *āyu* includes body, sense organs, mind, and soul (refer CS Sū. 1.42, "*śarīrendriya...*"). *Āyu* is also qualified by the words *nityaga*, which means "that which keeps flowing continuously" and *anubandha*, which means that "it is connected from one life to another."

***Vākyapradīpika*:** The words *om* and *atha* originated from Lord *Brahma* at the beginning of creation and invoke auspiciousness. Usually *om* is used in the *Vedas* and *atha* is used in the *śāstras*. It means "let there be auspiciousness in the life of those who study this *śāstra*." The word *atha* means "therefore." Since the disciple has the qualification of attentive hearing, good behavior, cleanliness, and so on, *therefore* all auspiciousness will manifest, and *dharma, artha, kāma and mokṣa* will be obtained.

The word *vyākhyāsyāmaḥ* indicates that the *guru* should explain each of the concepts of this science till the disciple understands the meaning completely. The words *ha smā* mean that the explanations given in the book are not the figments of anyone's wild imagination. They are coming from proper scientific observation, inference, and authoritative sources.

The word *maharṣayaḥ* is significant. It is a combination of two words. *Mahā* means "great" and *ṛṣi* comes from the word *ṛṣati* that means "to move." *Ṛṣi* is one who has understood the movement or changes occurring in the universe. This means that a *śāstra* is the compilation of the knowledge and realization of many *ṛṣis*. This also means that students should try to free themselves (move away) from the *rāgādis* in order to assimilate the knowledge of *Āyurveda*.

What is the purpose of this knowledge that is being carefully passed down the disciplic line?

AH Sū. 1.2

Purpose of *Āyurveda*

आयुःकामायमानेन धर्मार्थसुखसाधनम् ।
आयुर्वेदोपदेशेषु विधेयः परमादरः॥ २॥

āyuḥ-kāmayamānena dharmārtha-sukha-sādhanam
āyurvedopadeśeṣu vidheyaḥ paramādaraḥ //2//

āyuṣ – long life; *kāmayamānena* – since it causes the desire; *dharma* – virtue, duty; *artha* – wealth; *sukha* – happiness; *sādhanam* – goal; *āyurveda upadeśeṣu* – in the teachings of *āyurveda*; *vidheyaḥ* – practiced, applied; *paramādaraḥ* – with great care and respect

Translation

One who desires a long life in order to attain virtue, wealth, and happiness should very respectfully apply oneself to (study, understand, implement, and advocate) the teachings of *Āyurveda*.

Commentary

In the very first word, the purpose of *Āyurveda* is clarified. *Āyuḥ kāma* means 'desiring a long life'. Whenever there is a discussion, four items should be clarified.

1. What is the topic? (āyurvedopadeśam)
2. Who is the person qualified to learn it? (āyuḥ kami)
3. What is the method of learning it? (vidheya paramādaraḥ)

4. What is the result of learning it? (dharma, artha, sukha)

This is described in Vedic parlance as *sambandha, abhidheya and prayojana.*

Sambandha refers to the components and their relationship with each other

Abhidheya refers to the process of establishing that relationship

Prayojana refers to the result of establishing that relationship

Note that *mokṣa* is not mentioned here. Only *dharma, artha* and *sukha* are mentioned. There are several interpretations to this. One is that the author is making it clear that this is primarily not a *mokṣa śāstra* (a book specifically meant to attain liberation). Another is that, by following the tenets of *dharma, artha* and *sukha, mokṣa* will be automatically obtained.

Sarvāṅgasundara: The knowledge of *Āyurveda* includes *prakṛti-jñāna, rasāyana, dūta, ariṣṭa*, and so on (knowledge of nature, rejuvenation, signs of messenger, signs of death—these are different topics that will be discussed later). *Āyurveda* is a *tantra* (knowledge meant for application). The word *paramādaraḥ* indicates that one should engage in continuous *pāṭha, avabodha, anuṣṭhāna* (recite, contemplate, and practice the science) of the book. The word *āyurvedopadeśeṣu* used here is a plural form that indicates that it has been compiled from multiple sources including accessory sciences as well (e.g., *jyotiṣa* and *vāstu*).

Why should one follow *Āyurveda*? For the sake of a long life. Why does one need a long life? To obtain *dharma*, *artha,* and *sukha* (ethics, wealth, and happiness). The connotation of *dharma* is *ghriyate loko anena iti dharma*, meaning "that which is faultless and people should adhere to."

There are two types of *sukha*: *tadāttvikam* and *ātyantikam*. *Tadāttvikam* is described as *kriyāt kālāntara asthāyitvāt sukha avabhāsam*, meaning that it is a temporary experience lost with the passage of time. It is not *paramārtha*[7] *sukham*, meaning spiritual pleasure, whereas *ātyantika sukha* as explained in CS Sū. 1.28 - 37 is permanent *mokṣa* or liberation, where there is no suffering anymore. That which is a means to attain these is called *dharmārthasukha sādhanam*.

Hṛdayabodhika: At the very outset, it is being mentioned that this science is meant for one who is desirous of a long life. *Āyurveda* should be approached with utmost respect. To respect *Āyurveda* means to make the effort to recite, contemplate, and practice the science (*pāṭha, avabodha, anuṣṭhāna*).

But is the purpose of *Āyurveda* to just have a long life? No. There are many trees that live more than one thousand years, but generally trees do not have the capacity to achieve *mokṣa*. The purpose of desiring a long life is mentioned next. It is futile to live a long life devoid of *dharma*. In other words, it is better to die immediately than to go on living by compromising *dharma*. It is *dharma* that upholds the sanity of each person in the society and the progressive life toward liberation. Deviation from the principles of *dharma* is the root cause of anxiety, illusion, restlessness, and every other disease. This is the verdict of all the sections of the *Vedas* including *Āyurveda*. So *Āyurveda* must only be understood, practiced, and advocated in accordance with the principles of *dharma*. In AH Sū. 2.20, it is stated *sukhaṁ ca na vinā dharmāt tasmād dharma-paro bhavet*, which means that without dharma there cannot be any happiness in life. (So everytime there is *autsukya*, *moha*, or *arati*—the three basic diseases arising out of *rāgādis*—it is worth contemplating the following: "What principle of *dharma* did I break to cause this suffering upon myself?")

Thus it is of utmost importance for every person to understand their *dharma*. Understanding our *dharma* essentially means asking ourselves, "What is the real essence of my existence?"; finding the answer to that question; and performing every thought, word, and action with that understanding. Literally *dharma* means "to not deviate from a position of stability." Everything is most stable in its natural state. *Dharma* is the natural state of every thing and every person.

Dharma is defined as the inherent characteristic of something that can never be separated from it. It is the "natural state of existence." For example the *dharma* of water is to be wet, fire is to be hot, air is to be dry, and so on. According to this definition, we can say that the *dharma* of every living being is "to serve," because there is no living being who is not serving someone knowingly or unknowingly. Thus a healthy service attitude, devoid of selfish intentions, is the foundation of a healthy and happy life. The essence of *dharma* has been explained in a very practical manner in the *subhāṣitam* where it is said *śrūyatām dharma-sarvasvam śrutvācaiva vicāryatām, ātmane* which means 'Do not do unto others what you do not want others to do unto you.'

The four goals of human life (*puruṣārtha*) are indicated. They are *dharma* (virtue), *artha* (wealth), *kāma* (fulfillment of desires), and *mokṣa* (liberation). The word *sukha* here denotes both *kāma* and *mokṣa*.

In this verse the word *sukha* and *dharma* specifically refer to "one's personal *sukha* and *dharma*" as opposed to the concept of *dharma* used in AH 2.20, which means social *dharma* in that context.

The word *vidheya* indicates that *Āyurveda* cannot be learned by philosophical armchair discussions alone; practical application is essential. The methodology of achieving a complete understanding of the subject is by reading or hearing, introspecting and thinking deeply about the subject, applying it practically in one's own life as well as in the lives of others, and teaching it.[8]

Every student of *Āyurveda* needs to be a good listener. This is the first step. *Ākānksha* (eagerness), *yogyata* (qualification), and *sannidhi* (presence of mind) are the three qualities of a good listener.

Aruṇodaya: For achieving the *puruṣārthas (dharma, artha, kāma*, and *mokṣa*), one requires *āyus* (long life-span), and in order to have *āyus*, *ārogya* (good health) is a prerequisite. The word *upadeśa* indicates that *Āyurveda* is a science that is to be understood through the medium of receiving instruction from the *gurus* in a disciplic succession in addition to reading books. Studying from books alone cannot compensate for learning from a living master.

> It is wonderful that *Āyurveda* helps to achieve all this. How did this science come into being?

AH Sū. 1.3

Advent of Āyurveda

ब्रह्मा स्मृत्वायुषोवेदं प्रजापतिमजिग्रहत् ।
सोऽश्विनौ तौ सहस्राक्षं सोऽत्रिपुत्रादिकान्मुनीन् ॥ ३ ॥
तेऽग्निवेशादिकांस्ते तु पृथक् तन्त्राणि तेनिरे ।

brahmā smṛtvāyuṣo-vedaṁ prajāpatim-ajigrahat
so'śvinau tau sahasrākṣaṁ so'tri-putrādikān-munīn //3//
te'gniveśādikāṁste tu pṛthak tantrāṇi tenire //4a//

brahmā – Lord Brahma; *smṛtvā* – having recollected; *āyuṣo-vedaṁ* – the science of longevity (*āyurveda*); *prajāpatim* – unto *Dakṣa Prajāpati*; *ajigrahat* – given; *saḥ* – he (*Prajāpati*); *aśvinau* – to the *aśvini kumāras*; *tau* – two of them; *sahasrākṣaṁ* – unto Lord *Indra*; *saḥ* – he (Indra); *atri-putrādikān* – unto the son of *Atri muni* and others; *munīn* – unto the sages; *te* – they (the sages); *agniveśādikān* – to *Agniveśa* and others; te – they (referring to *Agniveśa* and others); *tu* – indeed; *pṛthak* – discretely, separately; *tantrāṇi* – all the *tantrās*; *tenire* – spread, propagated

Translation

Lord *Brahma* recollected the science of *Āyurveda* and delivered it to *Prajāpati Dakṣa*. He in turn taught the twin brothers, *Aśvini Kumāras*, who imparted the same to King *Indra*. King *Indra* passed it down to the great sages like the son of sage *Atri* and others, who later taught *Agniveśa* and other sages. They then composed their own separate treatises, which were propagated all around the world.

Commentary

Vedic concept of time revolves around a cyclical quartet: *satya yuga, treta yuga, dvāpar yuga*, and *kali yuga*. The change of *yugas* is determined by the change of the predominating quality *(guṇa)*. The first in the cycle, *satya yuga*, is predominated by *sattva guṇa*, which is the purest of the three and hence witnesses little occurrence of disease. With the passage of time, predominance of *rajas* and *tamas* gradually increase, and diseases begin to manifest in the mind. The initial symptoms are *autsukya, moha*, and *arati* arising from *rāgādi* as mentioned in the invocation verse. Interestingly these three are also the symptoms of the end of life.

Noticing this, the sages commissioned *Bharadvāj muni* (son of sage *Bṛhaspati)* and one of the *saptarṣis* (seven great sages) to approach the heavenly realms, learn *Āyurveda* from King *Indra* (king of the demigods), and bring the knowledge down to the earthly realm. This was then passed down in a disciplic chain. After the great sage *Agniveśa,* the single body of the science of *Āyurveda* was divided into multiple parts called *tantrās* (aphorismic texts) and propagated everywhere.

The word *recollected* is significant and indicates that the science of *Āyurveda* was already existing before Lord *Brahma,* the first living being in the universe according to *Vedic* literature. The fundamental principles of nature are eternal and not manufactured by any person. They were existing in the past, are existing now, and will continue to exist in the future. For example, the law of gravity was always there, even before Newton discovered it. But due to the influence of time, they become manifest or unmanifest. These universal principles were revealed in the *Vedas* and further elaborated by the sages.

Another question that may be asked is this: "Where did Lord *Brahma* get this knowledge from? Who was there before Lord *Brahma* to teach him?" The answer to this question can be obtained from the fifth chapter of *Brahma Samhita* (BS), composed by Lord *Brahma* himself. (BS Ch. 5.22–28). It is explained there that Lord *Brahma* was initiated in all knowledge, from within his heart, by the Supreme Lord Himself at the beginning of creation.

This verse is the description of a disciplic lineage (*parampara*) beginning from Lord *Brahma.* He explained the science of

Āyurveda to his son *Prajāpati Dakṣa* who gave it to the twins, *Aśvini Kumaras*, the physicians of the demigods. The demigods are the administrators of the cosmos. The *Aśvini Kumaras* explained it to *sahasrākṣa*, meaning one who has a thousand eyes, or better known as *Indra* who later explained it to *Bharadvāja* muni. This knowledge was transmitted down through the son of *Atri muni* (son of *Atri* is called *Ātreya)* to *Agniveśa* and has been passed down in disciplic succession since then. In due course of time, the lineage appeared to have broken, and the knowledge seemed to have been lost. But we can rest assured that *Āyurveda* is eternal and all the principles and teachings are also eternal. They are never lost. If we qualify ourselves to receive this knowledge, the *vidya* will automatically become manifest to us.

The term *sahasrākṣa* (thousand eyes) also indicates that one should keep one's "eyes" (i.e., senses and mind) wide open to receive this knowledge. It is also explained that five hundred pairs of eyes mean that he was able to analyse a given topic or situation from five hundred different view points or angles. The word *tantra* indicates that this knowledge is especially meant for practical application and should be experienced directly or indirectly. Only by that method can the knowledge be understood properly and not just by theoretical debates.

***Sarvāṅgasundara*:** The fact that Lord *Brahma* remembered the science but did not compose it indicates that this science is eternal. The word *prajāpati* indicates *gati* (movement), *buddhi* (intellect), and *karma samjñā* (ability to perform an action, etc.). *Ātreya* had six disciples who wrote their own treatises. They are referred to here as *agniveśādi*. They are *Agniveśa, Bhela, Jātūkarṇa, Parāśara, Hārīta, and Kṣārapāṇi*. Many of these treatises are lost today. *Caraka Samhita* is a redacted version of *Agniveśa Samhita*.

When all these *ācāryas* have already written so many books, what was the need to write the *Aṣṭāṅga Hṛdayam*?

AH Sū. 1.4

Why was the *Aṣṭāṅga Hṛdayam* written?

तेभ्योऽतिविप्रकीर्णेभ्यः प्रायः सारतरोच्चयः॥४॥

क्रियतेऽष्टाङ्गहृदयं नातिसंक्षेपविस्तरम् ।

tebhyo'ti-viprakīrṇebhyaḥ prāyaḥ sārataroccayaḥ //4//

kriyate'ṣṭāṅga-hṛdayam nāti-saṅkṣepa-vistaram

tebhyo – for the people; *ati* – too much (various sources); *viprakīrṇebhyaḥ* – from the scattered (tantrās in previous verse); *prāyaḥ* – mostly; *sāratara* – the better parts of the essence; *uccayaḥ* – is spoken; *kriyate* – is composed; *aṣṭāṅga-hṛdayam* – this book *aṣṭāṅga hṛdayam*; *nāti* – not too much; *saṅkṣepa* – concise; *vistaram* – expansive

Translation

For the benefit of the people, the essence of the science, which was scattered in the form of several *tantras*, is now being presented, in the form of *Aṣṭāṅga Hṛdayaṁ*, which is neither too expansive nor too concise.

Commentary

Aṣṭāṅga Hṛdayam (written in about seventh century AD) is a systematic review of all the *Āyurvedic* literature that existed at that time. It appears that all the knowledge of *Āyurveda* scattered in different books at various locations was collated just as how we have the Cochrane Reviews today.

sārataroccayaḥ indicates that ācārya admits that this book contains only the essence and not detail. Some of the detailed explanations have been omitted and the essence has been kept intact.

One may ask, what is the need for a condensed version to be written? An argument can be raised that condensed versions may discourage people from studying the elaborate versions, since they will look for shortcuts. The *Vedic* understanding indicates that with the passage of time, the capacity of people to grasp intricate, multidimensional subject matter is becoming less and less. In fact today we see that one of the major reasons for confusion leading to unhealthy mental patterns is the information overload through media and the Internet, which leave people dazed, confused, and engaging in futile debates with each other.

The *Srimad Bhagavātam* 12.2.1[9] describes the deterioration of the ability to comprehend complex information in the present time

tataścānudinam dharma satyam śaucam kṣamā dayā
kālena balinā rājan nāṅkṣatyāyur balam smṛtiḥ
The word *smṛtiḥ* in this verse is noteworthy. It means that the memory power of people in general will decrease with the passage of time. Thus they will not be competent to process a large amount of information to come to the right conclusion and only confusion will prevail. To avoid this situation, the *Aṣṭāṅga Hṛdayam* was composed where the student/ reader is led to the right conclusions in a simple, systematic manner.

Note: Religion, truthfulness, cleanliness, tolerance, mercy, duration of life, physical strength, and memory will all diminish day by day because of the powerful influence of the age of Kali.

In due course, many books, expressing several different opinions of various physicians came to be written. Contradictory opinions were causing confusions about the conclusions. Hence, to dispel these confusions, such a work was necessary and was composed by *Vāgbhaṭa*. *Viprakīrṇebhyaḥ* means "from all the scattered branches" (*tantrās*)" mentioned in the previous verse 4a or, in others words, the scattered opinions.
The word *sārataroccayaḥ* is very significant, which means that the essence or conclusion is extracted and presented here. So it is a relieving reassurance that if we just study this one book, we will not miss out on any of the essential aspects of *Āyurveda*.

There are different levels of information indicated by the words *sāra, sāratara, sāratama*, and so on, which are nothing but adjectives of different superlative degrees.

Sarvāṅgasundara: *Hṛdaya* (heart) is the most important organ in the body. In the case of the failure of any other organ except the heart, life can still go on. . If the heart stops working life cannot exist in the body anymore. Hence this book is given this name, since it contains the core or essence of *Āyurveda*. It has not been made too concise, in which case a high level of background knowledge will be required to understand it and those who are less intelligent would not be able to understand. It is not made too expansive because it would then become too difficult to study.

It was explained that the knowledge of *Āyurveda* was scattered all over, in different books, and *ācārya Vāgbhaṭa* organized it systematically. How is it organized?

AH Sū. 1.5

Eight branches of *Āyurveda*

कायबालग्रहोर्ध्वाङ्गशल्यदंष्ट्राजरावृषान् ॥५॥
अष्टावङ्गानि तस्याहुश्चिकित्सा येषु संश्रिताः ।

kāya-bāla-grahordhvānga-śalya-daṁṣṭrā-jarā-vṛṣāṅ //5//
aṣṭāvaṅgāni tasyāhuś-cikitsā yeṣu saṁśritāḥ

kāya - internal medicine; *bāla* – pediatrics, gynecology and obstetrics; *graha* – psychiatry, medical astrology, spirits;

ūṛdhvānga – upper part of body (head, neck and face); *śalyā* – surgery; *daṁṣtra* – toxicology; *jarā* – rejuvenation and geriatrics (*rasāyana*); *vrṣān* – aphrodisiacs, virility, fertility, dealing with procreation and health of reproductive system; *aṣṭa* – eight; *aṅgāni* – parts; *tasya* – of them; *āhus* – it is said; *cikitṣa* – treatment/ management of diseases; *eṣu* – among them (the eight branches mentioned above); *saṁśritāḥ* – completely depends upon

Translation

The management of diseases is completely dependent upon the eight branches (limbs) of *Āyurveda*, which are said to be general medicine, pediatrics (including gynecology and obstetrics), psychiatry and medical astrology, diseases of the head and neck (above the clavicle), surgery, toxicology, rejuvenation, and virility.

Note: We find that the word *graha* is used here to describe a branch of *Āyurveda*. In *Vedic* astrology, the planets are also called *graha*. The word *graha* means "that which seizes," meaning that this branch of *Āyurveda* studies the influence of planets on the human body, which is the science of medical astrology.

Commentary

This again demonstrates the action taken by *Vāgbhaṭa* and other *ācāryas* to facilitate easy understanding. Division of a subject into various parts is helpful for easy comprehension and application. During the *Vedic* period, the science of *Āyurveda* was not divided into many branches and specialities. Later it was divided and subdivided. And these days we have specializations and super specializations in each branch. During earlier days this was not required, as people were quite capable of studying and processing large amounts of information.

Similar is the case with the *Vedas*, which was originally one and was later divided into four by *Vedavyāsa ṛṣi* for the sake of the people. The *Aṣṭāṅga Hṛdayam* will deal with the eight branches of *Āyurveda* one by one.

Bhāvaprakāśa: Since the heart is the most important of all the organs in the body, this book is named *Aṣṭāṅga Hṛdayam* (*hṛdayam* means heart). *Kāya* is the body where the *dhātus* are fully formed. *Bāla* (a child's body) is the body where the *dhātus* are not fully formed. *Graha* represents the spirits or energies that affect *bāla* (the child).

How did the eight branches come to be?

The term *Kāya* includes *avastha* (stage of life), *avayava* (organs), *sattva* (mind), *samparka* (contact from external environment), and *śīrṇa* (decay) of *śarīra*.

- *Avastha*: *Bālya avastha* is dealt with in *bāla cikitsa*. *Jarā avastha* is dealt with in *rasāyana cikitsa*.
- *Avayava*: *Ūrdvāṅga* (in *Śārīra sthāna* the root (*mūla)* of the body is described to be the head). So head is given more importance than the other body parts. All the five sense organs are present on the head. Thus there is *ūrdhvāṅga* or *śālākya cikitsa to deal with the head and shoulders.*

- *Sattva* means mind. *Graha cikitsa* is the branch of *Āyurveda* that deals with prevention and treatment of mental abnormalities.
- *Samparka*: *śastra*, *viṣa* (foreign bodies and poisons) are two types of external threats to the body. The branch of *Āyurveda* that deals with *samparka* is *śalya cikitsa* and *viṣa cikitsa.*
- *Śīrṇa* means withering away or decaying. *Rasāyana* is the branch of *Āyurveda* to prevent or slow down the decaying process of the body.
- Finally there is a need to reproduce and continue the species by producing another body before the previous one dies. *Vājīkaraṇa* is the branch of *Āyurveda* that deals with virility.

Therefore, we can see that the eight divisions of *Āyurveda* make sure that your *sarīra* (body), *indriya* (senses), and *sattva* (mind) are protected internally during all stages of life and from external attack by *śalya* (foreign body) and *viṣa* (poison, toxins). And while the protection is going on, reproduction takes place, which is the branch called *vājīkaraṇa*. Death is dealt with in *Kāya cikitsa.*

Bāla cikitsa starts before childbirth or rather even before the child is conceived. All the arrangements are first made to protect the health of the child in the womb before conceiving. Thus all treatments of the mother and women in general (gynecology and obstetrics) are described under *bala cikitsa*, since a healthy mother is a primary prerequisite for a healthy child.

In the present day, we see elaborate planning to avoid conception through contraceptive pills and other methods. In many cases conception is a result of failed contraception. On the contrary, in *Āyurveda* we see elaborate planning for the purpose of conception. It is interesting that the health of the female gender is explained in relation to pregnancy indicating this as one of the very significant contributions of a female in the best interests of the larger society.

Āyurveda divides women's health into three stages:

1. before pregnancy;
2. during pregnancy; and
3. after pregnancy.

Each of the stages is covered in different sections of *Āyurveda*. For example, Menopausal stage is covered under rejuvenation and geriatrics. A species would survive the onslaughts of nature only if it is able to bring forth a healthy future generation. There was a very systematic and elaborate process being followed to ensure the health of the next generation. This is why it is said in the *Vedas*[10] that if the women are not cared for, nourished, and protected, the entire civilization will perish.

Āyurveda is nicely organized into eight branches. What is the essence of the knowledge presented in all these eight branches?

AH Sū. 1.6

Three *doṣas* maintain and destroy the body

वायुः पित्तं कफश्चेति त्रयो दोषाः समासतः॥६॥
विकृताऽविकृता देहं घ्नन्ति ते वर्तयन्ति च ।

vāyu pittaṁ kaphaśceti trayo doṣāḥ samāsataḥ //6//
vikṛtā 'vikṛtāḥ dehaṁ ghnanti te vartayanti ca

vāyu pittaṁ kaphaśceti – of *vāta, pitta* and *kapha*; *iti* – referring to something that has already been said; *trayo doṣāḥ* – the three *doṣās*; *samāsataḥ* – in brief (meaning that detail will come later); *vikṛtā* – imbalance (disease); *avikṛtāḥ* – without imbalance (health); *dehaṁ* – body; *ghnanti te* – they destroy; *vartayanti ca* – and maintain

Translation

In short, *vāta*, *pitta* and *kapha* are the three *doṣas* responsible for destroying and maintaining the body in their vitiated and balanced states respectively.

Commentary

The word *samāsataḥ* means "in short." This indicates that there are various descriptions of health and disease possible, and all those can be summarized into interactions of these three *doṣas*. There can be many perspectives. *Āyurveda* is a flexible science open to opinions and discussions. It does not inhibit free thinking or force us to accept concepts without logical understanding.

Vikṛtā'vikṛtā deham refers to the body that constantly undergoes balance and imbalance.

The concept of three *doṣas* is a very unique contribution of *Āyurveda*. Rather than just a physical understanding, the *doṣa* concept indicates a functional bioenergetic level of the working of the human body. It is an amazing fact that every single physiological or pathological transformation in the body can be understood using these three concepts only.

The *tridoṣic* theory ensures that there will never be an instance where we are unable to understand the cause of an illness unlike in modern medicine where we have idiopathic illnesses. It is also understood that as long as the *doṣas* are kept in balance, there is no chance of developing any disease. There could have been many theories about the number of *doṣas*, but here it has been conclusively stated to be three in number.

A question could arise "Why should it be three? Why not four?" This is because there are only two opposing energies in the world – *agni* and *soma* – and the third energy is to control and facilitate the functioning of the two opposing energies. This is also to illustrate that *Āyurveda* is a science with mathematical precision.

Why are the most important pillars of the body called *doṣa* (faults)? This is explained in *Bhāva Prakāśa* – *doṣa* is the only thing in the body that can vitiate others. Hence they are called *doṣā*. They can get vitiated by themselves and then vitiate other aspects of the body – *dhātu, srotas* and *mala*.

Why are the *doṣas* not fighting with each other? *Madhukośa* says – only by the grace of daiva (Lord).

Sarvāṅgasundara: The meaning of the word '*doṣa*' is that it has the ability to vitiate the *dhātus*. There is no fourth *doṣa*. The *doṣas* are divided into three depending on their actions or functions (*nirdeśe kartavye yadeṣām pṛthak vibhaktyā*). The functional aspect is more important (*pradhānatvāt*).

Similar to the *doṣas rakta* (blood) also has a location, symptoms, functions, vitiation, treatment of the *doṣas* is also *rakta*. Hence sometimes *rakta* is also considered as a *doṣa*. It is also spread all over the body. Its symptom is that it is colored reddish like a lotus or *indragopa* insect. Its function is production and maintenance of body (*dehasya utpatti sthiti*). Its vitiation is called *visarpa*, *plīha* and so on. The specific treatment for *rakta* vitiation is blood letting (*sirāvyadha*).

Another opinion is that only the *vātādis* (*tridoṣās* are called *vātādis*) are called *doṣa* and not the *rasādis* (*dhātus* are called *rasādis*). The *vātādis* are independent (*svatantra*). This is because *doṣa* is defined as that which vitiates. *Rasādis* are *paratantra* (dependent on something else) in nature. *Rasādis* are vitiated by the *doṣās* and hence called *dūṣya*. Hence *rakta* is a *dūṣya* and not *doṣa*. It is the *vātādis* that always vitiate the *rasādis* and not viceversa.

The *vātādis* also have the ability to vitiate each other. In the case of *pāṇḍu* disease, *pitta* is found to be vitiated by *kapha*. It is a *pitta* predominant disease and vitiates *kapha, tvak, rakta, māmsa. Vāta doṣa* has the ability to vitiate both the other *doṣas*.

There are only three types of *prakṛtis* – *vāta prakṛti*, *pitta prakṛti* and *kapha prakṛti*. There is nothing called *rakta prakṛti*. Hence *Ācārya Vāgbhaṭa* has divided *jvara* and all other diseases according to the *vātādis*. Hence there is *vāta jvara*, *pitta jvara* and *kapha jvara* but no *rakta* jvara.

The diseases originating from *rakta* vitiation like *visarpa* and *plīhā* are explained using the logic of *ghṛta dagdha* (burning of ghee). The fire for the burning of ghee is present within the ghee itself though we cannot see it. In the same way the *raktaja* diseases are caused by the *vātādis* which are present in the *rakta* itself but conventionally called *raktaja* disease.

Some indication of *rakta* as a *doṣa* may be seen in a disease like *kuṣṭha*. It is only in the form of a *samjña* and not as *anugata*. Hence it is *dūṣya* in this situation too. If *rakta* can be called *doṣā* here, then *purīṣa* can also be called *doṣa*.

From another point of view, *āma* can also be called *doṣa* because it is the cause of disease as described by *Caraka*. Thus in essence we can conclude that only the *vātādis* can be called *doṣas* and not *rakta*. And then they combine in unlimited ways, aggravate, deplete (*tāratamya parikalpanayā*) and so on.

vikṛtā means changing its *svabhāva* (own nature). This breaks down the body. The word *deha* indicates that it is a living body that we are talking about. When *vikṛti* takes place, it becomes difficult to stay alive. The duty of the *Vaidya* is to keep the doṣas in *prakṛti avastha* (their natural state).

Āyurvedarasāyana: This verse describes two *doṣa avasthas* (*doṣa* state) - *vikṛta* and *avikṛta*. The first one destroys the body and second maintains the body.

Bhāvaprakāśa: *Vāta* is the first of the *doṣas* mentioned, and in keeping with the *Vedic* writing it should be understood that *vāta* is the most important of the three. *Pitta* is mentioned second, meaning that it is more important than *kapha*. Importance is allocated depending on the *doṣa*, which has the greatest tendency to get vitiated, thus needing more attention. *Kapha* is the most stable of the three *doṣas*. Since they are mentioned individually, it is to be understood that they are also individually important.

How are the *doṣas* related to the human body in terms of space and time?

AH Sū. 1.7

The predominant locations of three *doṣas* in the body

Predominant *doṣa* periods related to age, day, night, and digestion

ते व्यापिनोऽपि हृन्नाभ्योरधोमध्योर्ध्वसंश्रयाः॥७॥

वयोऽहोरात्रिभुक्तानां तेऽन्तमध्यादिगाः क्रमात् ।

te vyāpino'pi hṛnnābhyor-adho-madhyordhva-saṁśrayāḥ //7//

vayo'ho-rātri-bhuktānāṁ te'nta-madhyādigāḥ kramāt

te – those (three *doṣas* mentioned above); *vyāpinaḥ* – are spreading all over at all times; *api* – although, yet; *hṛn* (hṛd) – heart; *nābhyo* – umbilicus; *adho* – lower; *madhya* – middle; *ūrdhva* – top; *samśrayāḥ* – residing, sheltered; *vayah* – age, life; *aho* – day; *rātri* – night; *bhuktānām* – food that is already eaten (i.e. being digested); *te* – that; *anta* – end; *madhya* – middle; *ādi* – beginning; gāḥ – going (in that order); *kramāt* – in systematic order, respectively

Translation

The three *doṣas* are spread all over the body at all times. Yet they are sheltered in the area below the umbilicus (primary location of *vāta*), between the umbilicus and the heart (primary location of *pitta*) and above the heart (primary location of *kapha*), in that order. The end, middle, and beginning of (each of the following) life, day, night, and digestion of food are predominantly influenced by the *tridoṣas*, in the same order (i.e., *vāta, pitta, and kapha*).

Commentary

The first line describes the division based on location (topographical classification), and the second line describes division based on time (temporal classification).

With regard to topography, although the three *doṣa*s are spread all over the body at all times, they can be classified as predominantly located in the lower, middle, and upper part of the body—*adho madhyordhva saṁśrayāḥ*.

1. Lower: beginning below the level of the umbilicus to the bottom of the feet—*vāta*
2. Middle: between the heart and umbilicus—*pitta*
3. Upper: beginning above the level of the heart up to the top of the head—*kapha*

   (in the order as given in AH Sū 1.6, i.e., *vāta*, *pitta*, *kapha*)

And with regard to the temporal aspect, age, day, night, and digestion are used for classification. The *doṣas* predominate during the following times: *vāta* phase in the end, *pitta* phase in the middle, and *kapha* phase in the beginning—*te anta-madhya-ādi-gāḥ kramāt.*

Note: *Kapha* is predominant in the first phase of life (childhood), *pitta* in the second (youth), and *vāta* in the third (old age). The first phase of the day (morning) is predominantly *kapha*, second phase (around midday) is *pitta*, and third phase (evening) is *vāta*. The first phase of the night (late evening) is *kapha*, second phase (around midnight) is *pitta*, and the third phase (early morning hours) is *vāta*. Among the three phases of digestion[11] described in *Āyurveda* (before digestion begins, while digestion is going on, after digestion is completed), the first phase is predominantly *kapha*, second is *pitta*, and third is *vāta*.

The word *vyāpino'pi* indicates that the *doṣa*s are everywhere in the body as well as the universe. Nothing happens without the involvement of *doṣa*s. Here a division of the body according to the *doṣa* predominance is described. The influence of the *doṣa*s on the *agni* (digestive fire), *koṣṭha* (alimentary canal), and *prakṛti* (body constitution) are described in future verses.

The reason why our body is described as beginning from the lower side is due to its description as *ūrdhvamlulamadhaḥ śākham ṛṣayaḥ puruṣam viduḥ*, meaning that the human being is described by the sages to be like a tree having the roots above and branches below. In that case the upper part of the body, which is *kapha* predominant, is represented by the root; the lower part of the body, which is *vāta* predominant, is represented by the branches of the tree, widely spreading everywhere like *vāta*; the central part of the body is represented by the trunk of the tree (*pitta*), which assists the branches in spreading everywhere just as *pitta* assists *vāta* in spreading.

From this description of location, one can also understand that it is easy for *vāta* to influence *pitta* than *kapha*, because *pitta* is close-by and vice versa. *Pitta*, at the same time, is situated in the middle of *vāta* and *kapha*. Thus, the location of *pitta* can be influenced equally by *vāta* or *kapha*, causing disturbances.

An example of the clinical application of the understanding of this verse is that children are naturally more susceptible to *kapha* vitiation. Hence, a *kapha* disease in childhood is relatively difficult to cure due to the similarity.

If a symptom is aggravated more during the morning, it is *kapha* predominant; a symptom aggravated during the middle of the day is *pitta* predominant; and a symptom aggravated during the end of the day is *vāta* predominant. The principle holds true for nighttime as well. (e.g., pain in the case of *gulma*).

The digestion is one of the most important aspects that is analyzed by an *Āyurvedic* physician—in a *kapha* predominant imbalance, there is a delay in initiating the digestion, and the difficulty is experienced soon after the meal. In a *pitta* predominant imbalance, there is difficulty experienced while the digestion is occurring. In a *vāta* imbalance, the difficulty is experienced some time after the meal is over or when the digestion reaches the final stage.

Note: *Gulma* is a type of abdominal mass or space-occupying lesion that can be produced due to any of the three *doṣas*. We will study about *gulma* in pathology (*Nidāna sthāna*).

Chapter 12 of the *Aṣṭāṅga Hṛdayam* is a more detailed description of the sites of the three *doṣas*. Thus we can understand that there can be finer and finer descriptions of the locations of the three *doṣas*, that is, the whole body being divided into three, and those three divisions again being divided, and so on. This description is more a functional division of the body rather than a structural one.

The *doṣas* are present everywhere in the creation in the living and non living beings. What is it that makes them function so harmoniously inside the living body to maintain life? It is *agni* that makes the *doṣās* function optimally. What are the various ways in which *agni* exists in the body?

AH Sū. 1.8

Four types of fires (*agni*)

तैर्भवेद्विषमस्तीक्ष्णो मन्दश्चाग्निः समैः समः॥८॥

tair-bhaved-viṣamas-tīkṣṇo mandaś-cāgniḥ samai samaḥ //8//

tair – due to those (three *doṣas*); *bhaved* – becomes; *viṣamas* – irregular or erratic; *tīkṣṇo* – sharp, quick & intense; *manda* – dull, poor, inadequate; *ca* – and; *agni* – digestive and metabolic fire; *samai* – that in which all the *doṣa*s are balanced; *samaḥ* – is known as balanced digestive fire

Translation

Of the digestive fires, the (four) types are unpredictably irregular, intensely sharp, inadequately slow, and balanced.

Commentary

This is the first place in *Aṣṭāṅga Hṛdayam* that *Vāgbhaṭa* is introducing the very important concept of *agni*. According to *Āyurveda*, *agni* is the fire principle responsible for all kinds of transformation. Nothing can change from one form to another without the action of *agni*. All the digestive, metabolic, and biochemical reactions in the body are under the purview of *agni*. Some textbooks even say that *Āyurvedic* treatments are nothing but restoring the *agni* to its normalcy and *Āyurvedic* lifestyle is nothing but protecting the *agni*.

The symptoms of the four types of digestive fires and their clinical applications are as follows:

1. Irregular or erratic fire—bloating and flatulence
2. Intense fire—burning sensation and thirst
3. Dull fire—heaviness and lassitude, taking a long time to digest
4. Balanced fire—feeling of lightness, energetic, absence of the above symptoms

Bhāvaprakāśa: We should also understand that *vāta pitta* aggravation causes the *agni* to become *tīkṣṇa*, while *vāta kapha* aggravation causes the *agni* to become *manda*. Though it is not clearly said here, since it is mentioned elsewhere that *vāta* has a *yogavāhi* (combining with another *doṣa* to enhance the property of the *doṣa* it combines with) property, this logic is valid. When there is *kapha pitta* aggravation, the *agni* can logically be either *tīkṣṇa* or *manda*. Since *vāta* has the property of *cala* (movement) and *yogavāhi*, it can combine with either *kapha* to enhance its *manda* quality or with *pitta* to enhance its *tīkṣṇa* quality. This is why it is called *viṣama* (difficult).

During an *Āyurvedic* consultation, it is most important to analyze the status of the *agni* of a client. It is often said that *agni* of the body is that which maintains health. All treatments in *Āyurveda* are directed mainly toward correcting the *agni*. This is why a *vaidya* always asks about the appetite and digestion of the client during a consultation. This also indicates the structure of the *Aṣṭāṅga Hṛdayam* as a clinician's textbook. *Vāghbhaṭa* mentions *tridoṣa* first, *kāla* (time) and *deśa* (place) are second, and *agni* is third in the order of importance to note during a consultation.

Suśruta Samhita Sū. 35.27 explains *"jaṭharo bhagavān-agnir-īśvaro annasya pācakaḥ,"* which means that the *agni* in our body is the Supreme Lord Himself and He digests all the foodstuff. So when we deal with *agni*, we must remember that we are dealing with the Supreme Lord. What a divine meditation for a *vaidya*! Lord *Kṛṣṇa* also says the same thing in *Bhagavad Gīta* 15.14, "*aham vaiśvānaro bhūtvā prāṇinām dehamāśritaḥ.*"

Where does *agni* perform all these actions? It is in the *koṣṭha.*

AH Sū. 1.9a

Three types of channels: *koṣthas*

कोष्ठः क्रूरो मृदुर्मध्यो मध्यः स्यात्तैः समैरपि ॥९॥

koṣṭhaḥ krūro mṛdur-madhyo madhyaḥ syāttaiḥ samair-api

koṣṭhaḥ – lumen, digestive tract; *krūra* – cruel (meaning hard and dry - of *vāta*); *mṛdu* – soft (of *pitta*); *madhyaḥ* - medium or moderate (of *kapha*); *syāt* – that; *taiḥ* – of those; *samair* – of balanced (*doṣas)*; *api* – also

Translation

The (three) types of digestive tracts are dry, soft, and moderate. Balanced *doṣa* also has moderate *koṣṭha*.

Commentary

The *agni* is responsible for the digestion and metabolism of food. After the digestion and metabolism are over, the nutrition has to be circulated to different parts of the body, and the waste has to be excreted. For this purpose, the understanding of *koṣṭha* (channels in the body) is important.

On a gross level, the *koṣṭha*, which literally means lumen, is described as the gastrointestinal tract. This is known as the central lumen of the body. Clinically one can collectively assess the status of the lumen of every single channel (*srotas*) in the body by assessing the status of the central lumen (gastrointestinal tract).

Vāta prakṛti will have *krūra koṣṭha* (the dry type). *Krūra koṣṭha* is called so, because it is very "cruel" on the person, making him or her constipated. *Pitta prakṛti* will have *mṛdu koṣṭha*. Balanced *doṣa (sama)* and *kapha* predominance will both have *madhyaḥ koṣṭha.*

There are two types of *madhya koṣṭhas* described here: – one represents *kapha madhya* and another represents *samyak madhya*. *Kapha madhya* will have a regular bowel movement daily. But *tridoṣa (samyak madhya)* will get a bowel movement at the ***same time*** every day. This is the difference.

The concept of *koṣṭha* is "one of the very important" foundational concepts in *Āyurveda*. Basically *koṣṭha*, in a gross sense, means a lumen surrounded by walls. All transformations (e.g., digestion), movements (e.g., circulation) or metabolic reactions (eg. glycolysis, Kreb's cycle) happen in the *koṣṭha*. The concept extends from macroscopic to microscopic or from gross to subtle levels of understanding. Generally *koṣṭha* refers to the gastrointestinal tract but can also be used to describe any other lumen or metabolic pathway in the body.

Each of these types corresponds to one of the three *doṣa* predominances, and the fourth one, to the balanced *doṣa* state. The gastrointestinal tract being the largest *koṣṭha* in the body gives us an idea of how all the other *koṣṭhas* in the body of the person are working.

Type of koṣṭha	*Doṣa*	Symptoms
Krūra	*Vāta*	Dry stools, constipation
Mṛdu	*Pitta*	Loose stools
Madhyama	*Kapha*	Medium consistency, for example, like a banana
Madhyama	*Sama*	Medium consistency

Bhāvaprakāśa: *Krūra koṣṭha* (also known as *kaṭhina koṣṭha*) in a person is identified by the difficulty to induce purgation in spite of taking a moderate dose of purgatives. *Krūra koṣṭha* is predominant in *vāta*. It means that such persons will require a higher dose of purgatives than the other types if purgation is to be induced.

Mṛdu koṣṭha is identified by the ease to induce purgation in spite of using a very small dose of purgative and is predominant in *pitta*.

Sama koṣṭha is identified by the fact that it is neither difficult nor easy to induce purgation. This means that the purgative will produce an expected level of purgation in a moderate dose.

The *koṣṭha* in which it is neither difficult nor easy to induce purgation is understood to be predominant in *kapha*, which causes *madhyama koṣṭha*.

These are all relative measurements that have to be judged according to the acumen of the *vaidya*. The only clinical diagnostic procedure recommended in *Āyurveda* is to administer milk at bedtime and observe the reactions described above.

Why does the *sama doṣa* assume the *madhyama* state of *koṣṭha*?

In *sama doṣa* avastha, all *doṣa*s are equal in strength. *Vāta* is not strong enough to overcome *pitta* and cause *krūra koṣṭha. Pitta* is not strong enough to overcome *vāta* and cause *mṛdu koṣṭha*. In this condition, *kapha* takes the opportunity to cause *madhyama koṣṭha*.

What is the difference between the *madhyama* state of *koṣṭha* in *kapha* and *sama doṣa*s?

Both are same in action but different in results. The *madhyama koṣṭha* due to *kapha* predominance causes ease of *vamana* (therapeutic emesis). The *madhyama* due to *sama doṣa* causes ease of *virecana* (therapeutic purgation). In the case of *kapha madhyama koṣṭha*, the stool will show increase of *kapha* (mucoid stool), and in the case of *sama madhyama koṣṭha*, stools will be healthy.

When the *agni* interacts with the *doṣas*, many effects occur which give rise to life in a specific combination. What are these combinations?

AH Sū. 1.9b–10

***Prakṛtiḥ* (Individual body constitution)**

शुक्रार्तवस्थैर्जन्मादौ विषेणेव विषक्रिमेः॥९॥
तैश्च तिस्रः प्रकृतयो हीनमध्योत्तमाः पृथक्।
समधातुः समस्तासु श्रेष्ठा निन्द्या द्विदोषजाः॥१०॥

śukrārtava-sthair-janmādau viṣeṇeva viṣakrimeḥ //9//
taiśca tisraḥ prakṛtayo hīna-madhyottamāḥ pṛthak
samadhātuḥ samastāsu śreṣṭhā nindyā dvidoṣajāḥ //10//

śukra – semen; ārtava – ovum; *sthair* – firmly situated in the; *janmādau* – at the time of conception; *viṣeṇeva* – just as (their own) poison is; *viṣakrimeḥ* – (not poisonous) for poisonous insects, worms, microbes (originate); *taiśca* – from them and; *tisraḥ* – three types of; *prakṛtayo* – of constitution; *hīna* – inferior; *madhya* – medium; *uttamāḥ* – superior; *pṛthak* – discrete, separate (single *doṣa*); *samadhātuḥ* – balanced tissues;

samastāsu – combined, put together; *śreṣṭhā* – best *nindyā* – abhorred; *dvidoṣajāḥ* – born of combination of two *doṣas*

Translation

In the beginning, at the time of conception, that is, at the union of the sperm and ovum, the constitution (*prakṛti*) of a living being is formed. *Prakṛti* is like the poison of the poisonous creatures (i.e., which does not cause them any harm). There are three separate single *doṣa* predominant constitutions: inferior, medium, and superior, in that order. There is one constitution in which all the three *doṣa*s are balanced. The other (three) constitutions in which two *doṣa*s are predominant are abhorred.

Commentary

The body is composed of three *doṣa*s. How do all the three *doṣa*s exist together in the body? This verse describes how the *doṣas* exist together.

Definition of *prakṛti*

prakṛtir nāma janma maraṇāntarāla bhāvini garbhāvakrānti samaye

svakāraṇa udreka-janita nirvikāriṇi doṣa sthiti

—*nṛsimha bhāṣyam*, 2000 BC

Prakṛti is a state of *tridoṣa* that is dominant in a person between his birth and death. It is self-manifested (*sva kāraṇa udreka*) at the time of conception. *Prakṛti* will never cause any disease on its own and will remain unchanged throughout the life of an individual.

One may ask, "*Samadhātu* (tri-*doṣa*) and *dvidoṣaja (*dual *doṣa) prakṛtis* are mentioned here. But where is *eka doṣa (*single *doṣa) prakṛti* mentioned?"

Three single *prakṛti (eka doṣaja)* types

The answer is indicated by the term *tisraḥ*—meaning the three types—indicating the three constitutions, which are *vāta*, *pitta*, and *kapha* predominant types. They are called *hīna* (poor constitution, *vāta*), *madhyama* (moderate constitution, *pitta*), and uttama (best constitution, *kapha*). Of the single *doṣa* constitutions, *vāta* is the weakest, and *kapha* is the strongest.

Three dual *prakṛti (dvidoṣaja)* types

The dual constitutions are *vāta-pitta, vāta-kapha* and *pitta-kapha.* They are the weakest of the three groups (i.e., single, dual, and tri *doṣa* constitutions), always have a greater tendency to become imbalanced, and are more difficult to restore into balance.

One *tridosic prakṛti* type

Tridoṣic prakṛti (vāta-pitta-kapha) is the strongest, *ekadoṣa prakṛti* is medium, and *dvidoṣa*ja prakṛti is the weakest type. Thus there are broadly seven different *prakṛti* types as mentioned above.

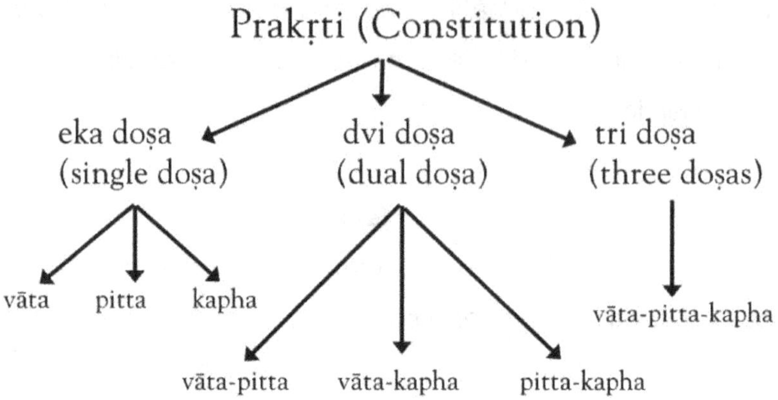

There are two types of *doṣic* increase that can take place.

1. One is due to the aggravation of *doṣas* in the sperm and ovum of the parents, which form the constitution of the baby. However, just as the poison of a poisonous creature will never kill the creature (*viṣeṇeva viṣa krime*), the *prakṛti* of a baby will never harm the baby but will only cause some physiological changes in the fetus.
2. If the increase in the *doṣa*s occurs due to the changes taking place in the womb of the mother, that is, changes in the body of the mother due to wrong diet or lifestyle, it is called *vikṛti*, which can cause destruction or malformation of the embryo.

Note

Prakṛti is the body constitution determined at the time of conception and which never changes till the point of death. It never causes any harm to the person.

Vikṛti are the changes in the body that occur due to internal or external factors.

Note: Change in physiology does not mean that *prakṛti* is changed. It means that the physiological transformations are occurring according to unchanging *prakṛti.* Earlier in the commentary, we already defined *prakṛti* as that which does not change from the point of conception to death. Always remember that *prakṛti* and *vikṛti* are concepts of changes happening in the body. Some people mistakenly think that *prakṛti* is health and *vikṛti* is disease. This is wrong. *Vikṛti* is what is seen at any given moment. *Prakṛti* is what was determined at the time of conception. That is a more fitting understanding. *Vikṛti* is *not* the opposite of *prakṛti.* It is not essential that *vikṛti* should always cause a disease. But disease is always caused by *vikṛti.*

The *doṣas* combine in these special ways. It is explained that most of these combinations are unstable. How can we stabilize them? For that one must first understand the qualities of the individual *doṣas.*

Qualities of three *doṣas* 11–12

AH Sū. 1.11

Qualities of *vāta*

तत्र रूक्षो लघुः शीतः खरः सूक्ष्मश्चलोऽनिलः॥ ११ ॥

tatra rūkṣo laghu śītaḥ kharaḥ sūkṣmaś-calo 'nilaḥ

tatra – of that; *rūkṣa* – dry; *laghu* – light; *śītaḥ* – cold; *kharaḥ* – rough; *sūkṣma* – subtle; *calaḥ* – that which initiates movement; *anilaḥ* – *vāta*

Translation

Among them, *vāta* is dry, light, cold, rough, subtle, and initiates all processes i.e. movements or transformations.

Commentary

After describing how the *doṣa*s exist in combination, let us look more closely at each of them.

The word *tatra* indicates "defining something." So here *Vāgbhaṭa* is going to define *vāta*. The *sūkṣma* guṇa indicates *srota pracāritvāt*, meaning "ability to move through the *srotas*."

Calaḥ, meaning "that which initiates movement" is significant. It is through the quality of *cala* that *vāta* is connected to the nervous system of the body, since it is the nervous system that provides the stimulus for movement.

There is a reason why the qualities of *vāta* are described in this particular order in the verse above. As far as *vāta* is concerned, the quality that is most predominant is *rūkṣa* (dry). Hence, the quality that is most potent in the treatment of *vāta* aggravation is *snigdha* (unctuous). The quality that is second most predominant is *laghu*, and hence, in the treatment of *vāta*, the quality of *guru* (heavy) is very important. So most of the *vāta* balancing treatments are *snigdha* and *guru*. Similarly, the other qualities of *vāta* mentioned in the verse above follow in the same order of importance.

According to the *Caraka Samhita, vāta* is not different from the Supreme Lord. It should be borne in mind that when we are dealing with *vāta*, we are actually interacting directly with the Supreme Lord. We should be very respectful.

Six qualities of *vāta* are mentioned here. What about the other four – *manda, sāndra, mṛdu, viśada* – with respect to verse AH Sū 1.18? These are the questions of a thoughtful mind.

AH Sū. 1.11 (contd.)

Qualities of *pitta*

पित्तं सस्नेहतीक्ष्णोष्णं लघु विस्रं सरं द्रवम् ॥११॥

pittaṁ sasneha tīkṣṇoṣṇaṁ laghu visraṁ saraṁ dravaṁ //11//

pittaṁ – *pitta*; *sa-sneha* – a little oily (accompanied by oily quality); *tīkṣṇa* – sharp, quick; *uṣṇaṁ* – hot; *laghu* – light; *visraṁ* – foul smelling; *saraṁ* – moving; *dravaṁ* – fluid

Translation

Pitta is a little oily, sharp, hot, light, foul smelling, mobile, and fluid.

Commentary

Seven qualities of *pitta* are enumerated here. *Sarvāṅgasundara* explains that *sasneham* indicates a little oiliness accompanies *pitta* (*īṣāt sneham*). *Tīkṣṇa* indicates *śīghra* or the quality of quick and speedy action. *Visram* indicates foul smell similar to that of undigested fish (*matsyāma gandhi*). *Saram* indicates the tendency to spread above and below without staying static and helps in moving the bowels.

Pitta and *vāta* are both described as mobile. The difference is that *vāta* is the initiating force and *pitta* is the executing force. All movement requires a little lubrication, and this is why there is a little oiliness associated with *pitta*.

When we look at the order in which the *guṇas* of *pitta* are enumerated here, it is interesting. The basic nature of *pitta* is to burn or digest. For burning, the first thing that is required is fuel but an excess supply of fuel can cause the fire to extinguish (hence *sa-sneha*), the fuel should be inflammable (*tīkṣṇa*), then it will catch fire (*uṣṇa*). As the burning goes on, the fuel is consumed and it becomes *laghu*. There is release of metabolic by products causing a strong odor (*visram*). If it keeps burning for long time, it can cause *dravya* or *dhātus* to melt and flow away.

Make a note of the fact that *vāta* is described as *calaḥ* and *pitta* is described as *saram*. What is the difference?
Kapha is described as *snigdha* while *pitta* is *sasneha*. What is the difference between *sasneha* and *snigdha*? *Sasneha* means that it is being accompanied by a little unctuousness. *Snigdha* means it is completely unctuous.

The four remaining qualities in the list with respect to AH Sū 1.18 are *slakṣṇa, mṛdu, sūkṣma and viśada.*

AH Sū. 1.12

Qualities of *kapha*

स्निग्धः शीतो गुरुर्मन्दः श्लक्ष्णो मृत्स्नः स्थिरः कफः॥१२॥

snigdhaḥ śīto gurur mandaḥ ślakṣṇo mṛtsnaḥ sthiraḥ kaphaḥ

snigdhaḥ – unctuous; *śīto* – cold; *guru* – heavy; *mandaḥ* – slow; *ślakṣṇo* – fine, smooth, slippery; *mṛtsnaḥ* – sticky like glue; *sthiraḥ* – stable; *kaphaḥ* – *kapha*

Translation

Kapha is unctuous, cold, heavy, slow, smooth or slimy, sticky and stable.

Commentary

Seven qualities of *kapha* have been enumerated here.

Ślakṣṇa is the opposite of *paruṣa. Paruṣa* means hard, stiff, harsh, rough, uneven, severe and so on. So *slakṣṇa* must be soft, flexible, gentle, smooth, even, and so on.

Mṛtsnaḥ is described as "*mṛdyamānaḥ* (delicate and tender), *aṅguli grāhi* (that which can be understood by touching with the finger), *picchila guṇa yukta* (associated with slimy quality), and *cakacakāyamāna* (shining or glistening)."

The order in which the qualities are enumerated here is significant because the quality that is most important for balancing *kapha* is *rūkṣa* (dryness), and the second most important quality is *uṣṇa* (heat).

Unlike some of the common translations of the *tridoṣas*, the *Aṣṭāṅga Hṛdayam* gives a more complex understanding about the *doṣas*. It is important to note that *vāta* is not just air or wind, *pitta* is not just fire or bile, and *kapha* is not just mucus. The *doṣas* are a manifestation of a conglomeration of qualities as mentioned above. These qualities correspond to specific functions, which will be explained in AH. Sū 1.18. Understanding the qualities of the three *doṣas* and their multifarious functions in the body comprise the foundation of all diet and lifestyle recommendations, diagnoses, and treatments in *Āyurveda*.

Other textbooks describe a few more properties for *vāta* and *kapha*:

- for *vāta—viśada* (clear), *amūrta* (formless), *anavasthita* (fluctuating), *śīghra* (swift), *paruṣa* (rugged), *avyakta* (subtle), *tiryak gata* (lateral movement), *acintya vīrya* (inconceivable potency), *yogavāhi* (enhances the qualities of other *doṣa*s), *asamghāta* (noncompactness)
- for *kapha—mṛdu* (soft), *madhura*, *picchila* (*mṛtsna*), *bala* (strength), *varṇa* (complexion), *sāndra* (density), *sthimita* (stillness), *accha* (clear)

Understanding the qualities and actions of the three *doṣa*s forms the basis for understanding all the physiological and pathological transformations occurring in the body. It is extremely important for diagnosis and treatment. The actions of the qualities have been enumerated in verse 18 of this chapter. The actions of the *doṣa*s will be described in more detail in chapters 11 and 12 of the sūtra sthāna of the Aṣṭāṅga Hṛdayam.

The qualities that have been left out with respect to AH Sū 1.18 are *sāndra*, *mṛdu*, *sūkṣma*, *viśada*.

What is the difference between *mṛtsna* and *picchila*? The quality of *picchila* is included within *mṛtsna*.

Apart from functioning individually, they also function in combinations.

AH Sū. 1.12 (contd.)

Types of imbalances

संसर्गः सन्निपातश्च तद्द्वित्रिक्षयकोपतः॥१२॥

samsargaḥ sannipātaśca tad-dvi-tri-kṣaya-kopataḥ //12//

samsargaḥ – called by the name *samsarga*; *sannipātaśca* – and called by the name *sannipāta*; *ca* – and; *tad* – that; *dvi* – two (*doṣās*); *tri* – three (*doṣās*); *kṣaya* – decrease; *kopataḥ* – aggravation

Translation

Involvement of two *doṣas* is called *samsargaḥ* and of three *doṣas* is called *sannipātaḥ*. There can be either increase or decrease of each of the *doṣas* in this combination.

Commentary

When two *doṣas* are involved in the disease, it is called *samsargaḥ* and when three *doṣas* are involved it is called *sannipātaḥ*. There can be two possibilities in each of these cases:

increase or decrease. This increase or decrease can occur in either of the *doṣas* or both the *doṣa*s involved.

What about single *doṣa* involvement in disease? The word *tad* indicates each of the *doṣa*s individually. *Vāta* is usually involved in every disease. Without *vāta*, either of the other two *doṣas, kapha* and *pitta*, cannot move from their sites to other places. So in one sense, there are essentially only two types of disease combinations: *samsarga* and *sannipāta.*

Practically in most cases, there is involvement of two or more *doṣa*s in the disease process. It is only in the very initial stages (the *sañcaya* stage) of the disease that you find single *doṣa* involvement.

Āyurvedarasāyana: The definition of *samsarga* is given by *Hemādri*, "*avastha viśiṣṭa samyoga nimittam doṣa samjna dvayam*," which means "specifically based on the state of two *doṣas* (aggravated or depleted) and the existence of a cause for their combining resulting in both of them mixing together." This is called *samsarga.* This occurs when two *doṣas* are aggravated or depleted or if one of the *doṣas* is aggravated and the other is depleted. When the same happens with three *doṣas*, it is called *sannipāta.* The different ways in which the *doṣas* can combine are explained in chapter 12: *doṣabehdiyam.*

What is the substrata on which the *doṣās* carry out their functions?

AH Sū. 1.13

Seven *dhātūs* (also known as *dūṣyas*)

रसासृङ्मांसमेदोऽस्थिमज्जशुक्राणि धातवः॥ १ ३॥

rasāsṛṇg-māṁsa-medo-'sthi majja-śukrāni dhātavaḥ

rasa – lymphatic tissue; *asṛk* – blood tissue; *māṁsa* – muscle tissue; *medas* – adipose tissue; *asthi* – bone or skeletal tissue; *majja* – marrow or nerve tissue; *śukrāni* – reproductive tissue; *dhātavaḥ* – the support of the body

Translation

Those that support the body are lymph, blood, muscle, fat, bone, marrow, and reproductive tissues.

Commentary

After having described the invisible *doṣa*s in the body, *ācārya Vāgbhaṭa* next describes the visible *dhātu*s. All the physical organs or parts of the body are dependent on these seven *dhātu*s.

Sometimes the word *dhātu* is translated as body tissue. This is all right in the gross sense. As we go into finer or subtler levels, this may not hold true (e.g., on a cellular level). *Dhātus* are present on every level—the whole body, every system of the body, every organ, and even in every cell.

Dhātus are the medium through which the *doṣas* express themselves. The *dhātu* originates from the word *dhāraṇa*, which means "to hold or support." The concept of *dhātu* has to be understood very carefully in order to be able to recognize imbalances. This is because it is the *dhātu*s in which imbalances manifest.

Āyurveda is primarily a functional science, and thus, the concept of *dhātu* should be understood in a functional manner. Although the *dhātus* have been named according to certain structures in the body, actually the intention is to represent a certain function. Thus we understand that though the *dhātus* have been translated as certain tissues in western medicine, the concept is obviously much broader from the functional perspective than what they represent in modern medicine. The *dhātus* can also be understood as the principle that holds all the organs together. It is not just the tissue but it is the holding power behind the tissues and organs. These are some of the deeper ways to understand the concept of *dhātu*. Each *dhātu* also transforms in a sequence to the next *dhātu*.

The function of the *dhātu*s are as follows (AH Sū. 11.4).

Dhātu	**Main function**	**Additional comments**
Rasa	*Prīṇana*	*Tṛptikara, tarpaka* (satisfying, nourishing) CS 1.207
Rakta	*Jīvana*	*Prāṇa-dhāraṇa-kriya* (upholds the *prāṇa*) CS 1.108

Māmsa	*Lepana*	*Pradeha ālepaśca* (forming a protective layer over the body), *rakta pitta prasāda* (alleviates *rakta pitta)*, *snaihika* (unctuousness), *nirvāpaṇa* (alleviating), *prasādana* (pleasing), *stambhana* (arresting), *vilāyana* (dissolving), *pācana* (digesting), *pīḍana* (pressuring), *śodhana* (cleansing), *ropaṇa* (healing), *varṇakara* (giving complexion)
Medas	*Snehana* (unctuousness)	*Snaigdhyam* (providing unctuousness), *śleṣmakarma svekam* (kapha type of actions), *deha mārdavakaram* (softening of the body), *anila hananam* (reduces vāta), *malasanga nāśanam* (relieves constipation), upholds the *prāṇa*
Asthi	*Dhāraṇa* (support)	*Stambhana karma* (arresting or fixation), *indriyāṇām dhāraṇa śakti* (ability of the senses to grasp and hold information), *jñānasya buddhau dhāraṇa* (ability of the intellect to retain knowledge), *bala dānam* (giving strength)

Majja	*Pūraṇa* (filling)	*Santarpaṇam* (nourishing), *bharaṇam* (occupying)
Śukra	*Garbhotpāda*	

In order to properly understand the *dhātu*s, we need to understand the deeper meaning of their respective functions—how their functions are interdependent and how they manifest in the body. For example, "What are the symptoms of *prīṇanam, jīvanam*, and so on?"

And please keep in mind that though the functions enumerated above are predominantly performed by the specific *dhātu* mentioned, the other *dhātus* can also have a direct or indirect role in accomplishing each of these functions. Overlapping is also possible. In *Vedic* understanding, the word "predominant" is very important. There are no tight compartments, and the function of a *dhātu* may be understood by what it predominantly does, though it may subdominantly carry out the functions of other *dhātus* as well.

An example to understand that difference between the concepts is as follows:

According to āyurveda, asthi is what gives support of the body (dhāraṇa) and also responsible for movement while māmsa serves only to create a layer (lepana). But western anatomy ascribes the function of movement to muscle tissue.

We can see here that fat is an essential component of the body. If only *medas* becomes excessive or depleted, that is a problem. One should not try to remove all the adipose tissue from one's body in the name of beauty. It will lead to imbalance. Similarly, we should understand the principle of exclusivity versus interdependence in relation to all the other *dhātus* as well.

Another important point about the *dhātus*

Of all the *dhātus* in the body, *rakta* is considered the most vital for maintaining life. Hence, in the event of a depletion, all the other *dhātus* will try to contribute in an effort to prevent any further depletion of *rakta dhātu.* If *rakta dhātu* gets depleted, it atomatically means that all the other *dhātus* are definitely affected.

When there is nourishment of the *dhātus*, *mala* is produced. What are they?

AH Sū. 1.13 (contd.)

Three *malās*

सप्त दूष्याः मला मूत्रशकृत्स्वेदादयोऽपि च ॥१३॥

sapta dūṣyāḥ malāḥ mūtra-śakṛt-svedādayo'pi ca //13//

sapta – seven; *dūṣyaḥ* – those which are vitiated (i.e. *dhātus*); *malāḥ* – waste (of the *dhātus*); *mūtra* – urine; *śakṛt* – faeces; *sveda* – sweat; *ādayoḥ* – and others; *api* – also ; *ca* – and

Translation

Each of these seven (*dhātus*) can get vitiated. The waste products, which are feces, urine, sweat, and others can also get vitiated (by *doṣa*s).

Commentary

Since the *dhātus* and *malas* can get vitiated by the *doṣas*, they are also known as *dūṣyas*, meaning those which can get vitiated. An important point to note is that *dūṣyas* will not vitiate on their own, unless the *doṣas* vitiate them. Until now, *Vāgbhaṭa ācārya* has been describing the *Āyurvedic* concept of the human body. We should understand the *Āyurvedic* concept of the human body independent of modern anatomical or physiological concepts. Otherwise we run the risk of getting confused when both the concepts do not match.

Sarvāṅgasundara: The *dhātu*s are called so, because they support and uphold the body. They are also called *dūṣyas*, because they get vitiated by the *doṣas*. *Vāta*, *pitta*, and *kapha* are called *doṣas*, because they have a tendency to vitiate the *dhātu*s. *Malāḥ* refers to the wastes arising from the digestive tract as well as metabolic waste products arising from all the body tissues. There are three principal waste products: feces, urine, and sweat. Many other (auxiliary or secondary) waste products are formed in different parts of the body as indicated by the words *ādayo'pi ca*, meaning "and so on."

Everything has a function in the body, including *waste* matter. The concept of *waste* in *Āyurveda* is different from what is understood by the term in conventional medicine. This will be described later in chapter 11. Hence, it is important that one should not eliminate all the waste from the body at once. Some amount of waste should be retained in the body for the sake of the functions they perform. *Āyurveda* explains that in the case of certain diseases where the strength of the body is severely depleted, it is the waste that provides strength and holds the body up. An example is that of carbon dioxide, which is a waste product but needs to be retained in the body in small amounts to maintain the acid-base balance of the body.

After describing the components, now he describes how to bring the *Āyurvedic* concepts of the human body that we discussed so far, into practical application.

AH Sū. 1.14

Increase and decrease of *doṣa*

वृद्धिः समानैः सर्वेषां विपरीतैर्विपर्ययः॥१४।

vṛddhiḥ samānaiḥ sarveṣāṁ viparītair-viparyayaḥ

vṛddhiḥ – increase; *samānaiḥ* – similar qualities; *sarveṣāṁ* – of them all (i.e. *dhātus* & *malas*); *viparītair* – opposites; *viparyayaḥ* – do the reverse (i.e. reduce)

Translation

Similar qualities cause an increase (i.e., of the *doṣas, dūṣyas*, and *malas* having similar qualities*)*. Opposite qualities cause the reverse (i.e., decrease of *doṣas, dūṣyas*, and *malas* having the opposite qualities).

Commentary

This is the fundamental rule that governs the interaction between the different internal components of the body as well as with the external environment. There are one or more of three basic factors in any interaction – *guṇa* (attributes)*, dravya* (substances) and *karma* (activity). Each of these can interact in two different ways – *sāmānya* (similar or general) and *viśeṣa* (opposite or special). In this way we have six different *padārthas* (substances). This is being illustrated here.

Food *(āhāra),* medicine (*auṣadha*) and poisons (*viṣa*) are categorized under *dravyas* which *Vāgbhaṭa* will begin to describe in the forthcoming chapters. This is why he is beginning the concept of *dravya* here.

The qualities of each of the three *doṣas* have been described earlier. Any food or lifestyle activity that increases these qualities will aggravate the respective *doṣa*. For example, excessive movement will aggravate *vāta*, and excessive heat will aggravate *pitta*. Similarly, anything that has an opposite quality will have the opposite effect. For example, stillness and meditation will pacify and calm the *vāta*. This is the fundamental principle of all *Āyurvedic* treatments, nutrition, and lifestyle recommendations.

Sarvāṅgasundara: There are two aspects to understand *vṛddhi* and *kshaya*: *sāmānya* (generalized) and *viśeṣa* (specialized). *Sāmānya* and *viśeṣa* types can again be divided as occurring in three ways—*dravya* (substance), *guṇa* (quality), and *karma* (action).

Some examples of *vṛddhi* and *ksaya* caused by *dravya*

- *Rakta* will be nourished fastest with blood (e.g., blood transfusion) because both have got similarity in terms of having water *mahabhuta* (*bhūta sāmānya*).
- Muscle tissue will be nourished fastest with meat (meat soup for *māmsa kṣaya*).
- Bone is nourished with tender bones (soup or broth made of tender bones nourish *asthi kṣaya*).
- *Majja* is nourished by *majja* (goat's brain is used in multiple sclerosis).
- *Kapha* is increased by cow milk.
- *Śukra* is nourished by ghee, which is made from milk (*dravya sāmānya*).
- *Saumya dhātu*s of the body are nourished by herbs like *jīvanti* (*Leptadenia reticulata*) and *kākoli* (*Fritilleria roylei*) are cooling in nature (*somātmaka*) and provide *sneha* (unctuousness), *bala* (strength), and *ojas* (vitality).
- *Buddhi* (intellect), *medha* (brain substance), and *agni* are nourished by *marīca* (black pepper), *pañcakola* (mixture

of five digestive herbs), *bhallātaka* (marking nut), and so on, as they are heating in nature.

Some examples of *vṛddhi* and *kṣaya* caused by similarity and differences in *guṇas*

Each substance has an elemental predisposition.

- *Moca* (banana), *coca* (jackfruit), *kharjūra* (dates) are *pārthiva* (have more of the earth element).
- *Kapha* is increased by dates, banana, and jackfruit, because they share the *śīta* and *snigdha guṇa* (*guṇa sāmānya*).

These substances have tendency to increase *kapha*, which means that the qualities of *guru*, *snigdha, śīta*, and so on will increase. Thus, it is possible to cause *vṛddhi* and *ksaya* by causing an increase or decrease in the *guṇas*.

Some examples of *vṛddhi* and *ksaya* caused by *karma*

- This is called *karma sāmānya (*similarity in action*)* There are three types of *karmas*: physical (activities such as running and swimming nourish the body), verbal (speaking, reading, singing, and the like nourish our speech), and mental (thinking nourishes the mind).

Different emotions like *kāma*, *krodha*, *bhaya*, and *śoka* can increase when there is a cause for them to increase, and this is called *vṛddhi* of mind.

- General heating causes an increase of *krodha,* envy and so on resulting in an increase in *pitta*.

- Activities like sleeping, laziness, lying in bed for a long time, and so on increase the *sthairya guṇa* and thus increase *kapha*; the opposite causes *kṣaya*.

Āyurvedarasāyana: There are two causes for disease: internal and external. The external causes are described in the commentary above. They can be divided into two: cause for increase and cause for decrease.

The similarity between the *doṣas* and *dhātus* are described in AH. Sū. 11.26, "*tartrāsthāni....*" The *rasa, māmsa, medas, majja*, and *śukra* are similar to *kapha*; *asthi* is related reciprocally to *vāta*; and *rakta* is similar to *pitta*. It means that those substances which increase *kapha* will also increase the *dhātus* which have similarity to *kapha*, and so on.

Bhāvaprakāśa: The same is true with *dhātu*, *mala*, and *guṇa*. *Māmsa* increases *māmsa*. Since the milk of purebred cows that are happy and raised in a natural environment, grazing in open fields, has the same quality as *ojas*, drinking cow's milk increases *ojas*. This is *guṇa sāmya hetu*. Running increases *vāta*. This is *kriyā sāmya hetu*.

> Study Tip: From AH. Sū 1.14 to 18 is the unique methodology by which *Āyurveda* studies and categorizes all the substances in the universe. This helps to determine the utility of a substance as well.

Now, that you know what the *doṣas* are, where they act and how they increase and decrease, you are ready to understand the factors that cause their increase and decrease. Food is a basic need of the living organism. How does food cause variation in *doṣā*? This brings in the concept of *rasa*.

AH Sū. 1.14–15

Six tastes enumerated

रसाःस्वाद्वम्ललवणतिक्तोषणकषायकाः॥१४॥
षड् द्रव्यमाश्रितास्ते च यथापूर्वंबलावहाः॥१५॥

rasāḥ svādvamla-lavaṇa-tiktoṣaṇa-kaṣāyakāḥ //14//
ṣaḍ dravyam-āśritāste ca yathā-pūrvaṁ-balāvahāḥ

rasāḥ – tastes; *svādu* – sweet; *amla* – sour; *lavaṇa* – salty; *tikta* – bitter; *uṣṇa* – pungent; *kaṣāya* – astringent; *ṣaḍ* – six; *dravyam* – substances; *āśritāste* – (their properties) depend upon; *ca* – and; *yathāpūrvam* – in the preceding order, the first half of the list; *balāvahaḥ* – providing strength (strengthening)

Translation

The tastes are six in number and they are sweet, sour, salty, bitter, pungent, and astringent. The tastes are dependent on substances (for their expression). The strengthening effect of the tastes mentioned here decreases in the ascending order.

Commentary

This is the point where *Vāgbhaṭa* slowly enters into the concept of *dravya*. The concept of *rasa* is very broad but for the simplicity of understanding we shall take the aspect of taste. The six primary tastes are enumerated here.

The second important concept introduced here is *dravya* . The properties of substances depend on their taste. The *rasas* (tastes) are dependent on *dravyas* (substances) for their *karma* (action). *Rasa*s do not have any *karma* (action). Only *dravya* has *karma.* So for *rasa* to perform *karma*, they have to depend on *dravya. Dravya* is the field of action. There are nine dravyas enumerated in *Caraka Samhita Sū 1.48.* They are the five *pañcamahābhūtas*, *kāla* (time), *dik* (direction), *manas* (mind) and *ātma* (soul).

Svādu (sweet) is the taste that is the most strengthening. The strengthening effect of the other tastes on the body decrease in the order given.

> *svādu > amla > lavaṇa > tikta > kaṭu > kaṣāyaḥ*
> sweet > sour > salty > bitter > pungent > astringent

The word *yathā pūrvam* indicates that the first half of the list is strengthening. This means that the second half of the list is weakening. Sweet, sour, and salty are strengthening, while pungent, bitter, and astringent are weakening.

How is bitter more strengthening than astringent though it is lighter and the most drying taste? Bitter causes only *dhātu śoṣa* (depletion of *dhātus*), but astringent causes *śoṣa* as well as *stambhana* of the *srotas* (arresting movement in the channels). Astringent is the taste that causes the maximum *bala kṣaya* (loss of bodily strength).

How is *tikta* (bitter) more strengthening than *kaṭu* / *uṣṇa* (pungent) taste?
Bitter causes only *dhātu kṣaya* (depletion of *dhātu*) but pungent causes *dhātu kṣaya* as well as *dhātu pāka* (burning and digestion of *dhātu*).

The details about the six tastes—their properties, actions, examples, combinations—are all described in chapter 10 of *Sūtra sthāna*.
A basic question that one may ask is as follows: "Why are there six tastes? Why not less or more?" The simplest answer to this question is that the human tongue has the ability to perceive only six tastes. There is also another answer to this question in verse 18 of this chapter where the twenty basic qualities are enumerated.

> Every concept in *Āyurveda* stems from the understanding that the entire universe is made up of a matrix of the *guṇas* (qualities).

Moreover there is a cyclical movement of the *guṇas* from origin to destruction and back through the creation-destruction cycle. This can be observed in nature in the cyclic movement of the seasons.The six tastes follow this logic. The healthy condition of life is said to be cool and unctuous. From this stage it progresses to reach a dead state, which is cold and dry. So the six tastes are as follows.

Svādu/madhura (Sweet)	Cold + Unctuous (Oily)	Origin
Amla (Sour)	Unctuous (Oily) + Hot	↓ ↑
Lavaṇa/patu (Salty)	Hot + Unctuous	↓ ↑
Kaṭu/uṣṇa (Pungent)	Hot + Dry	↓ ↑
Tikta (Bitter)	Dry + Cold	↓ ↑
Kaṣāyah (Astringent)	Cold + Dry	Destruction

(In each taste, the first *guṇa* is more predominant and second one is less)

From this we can understand that there is no sharp boundary between the six tastes, and it is in reality a continuum.

Sarvāṅgasundara: That which is perceived by the *rasanendriyas* (sense organs that perceive taste) is called *rasa.* All the *rasas* and *dravyas* are dependent on the *pañcabhūtas* (the five great elements). To understand what the tastes are, one can use these substances. Sweet: ghee, jaggery; sour: tamarind, pomegranate; salty: salt; bitter: *bhūnimba* (Kariyat); pungent: black pepper; astringent: *harītakī*.

Āyurvedarasāyana: Using the example of *kṣāra* (alkali), *Hemādri* explains that the phenomenon of tastelessness is the seventh taste. This is called *dravya viśeṣa* and *rasa viśeṣa* (exceptions to the general rule).

How does *rasa* cause increase or decrease of the *doṣa*?

AH Sū. 1.15–16

How the six tastes affect the *doṣās*

तत्राद्या मारुतं घ्नन्ति त्रयस्तिक्तादयः कफम् ॥१५॥
कषायतिक्तमधुराः पित्तमन्ये तु कुर्वते ॥१६॥

tatrādyā mārutaṁ ghnanti trayas tiktādayaḥ kaphaṁ //15//
kaṣāya-tikta madhurāḥ pitta-manye tu kurvate

tatrādyā – the first three; *mārutaṁ* – *vāta*; *ghnanti* – destroys, pacifies; *trayas* – of the three; *tiktādayaḥ* – bitter and so on (bitter, pungent, astringent); *kaphaṁ* – *kapha*; *kaṣāya* – astringent; *tikta* – bitter; *madhurāḥ* – sweet; *pitta-manye* – curbs *pitta*; *tu* – but; *kurvate* – does

Translation

The first three tastes *(svādu, amla*, and *lavaṇa)* alleviate *vāta*; the last three beginning with bitter *(tikta, uṣaṇa*, and *kaṣāya)* alleviate *kapha*; *pitta* is alleviated by astringent, bitter, and sweet tastes (*kaṣāya, tikta*, and *madhurā*).

Commentary

The same order as given in the last verse is being followed. So when it says, "first three," we should understand that they are

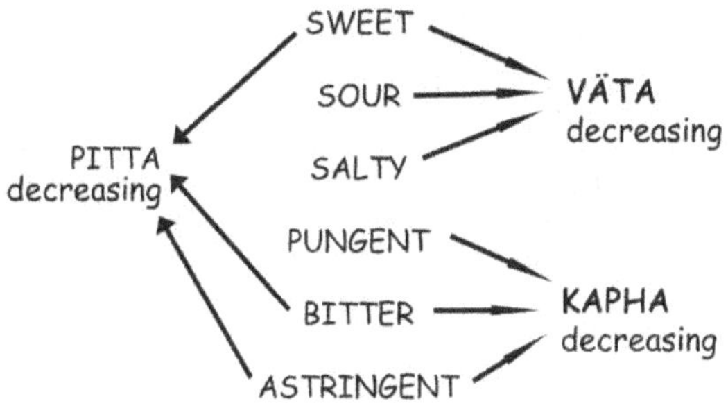

referring to the first three tastes mentioned in the previous verse.

When it says that the first three tastes alleviate *vāta*, it also means that the last three tastes aggravate vāta. (AH Ni 1.14). Similarly with pitta, sour, salty and pungent aggravate it (AH Ni 1.16) and with kapha, sweet, sour and salty tastes aggravate it (AH Ni 1.17)

Vāta is a destructive energy, and *Kapha* is a constructive energy. So when it says, "alleviates *vāta*," it means that those tastes also nourish the body. When it says, "alleviates *kapha*," it also means that it deteriorates the body. Thus sweet, sour, and salty are tastes that nourish the body, while pungent, bitter, and astringent are tastes that disintegrate the body.

Note: Many people think that nourishing is accompanied by weight loss. This is not true with regard to the word used here. Here, nourish means to strengthen the *dhātus*, and deteriorate means to weaken the *dhātus*.

Dravya has been introduced with *rasās* in the last verse. Now we need to understand the behaviour of *dravyas*…

AH Sū. 1.16

Three kinds of substances *(dravya)*

शमनं कोपनं स्वस्थहितं द्रव्यमिति त्रिधा ॥१६॥

śamanaṁ kopanaṁ svastha hitaṁ dravyamiti tridhā //16//

śamanaṁ – palliating, pacifying; *kopanaṁ* – aggravating; *svastha hitaṁ* – beneficial for health; *dravyam* – substances; *iti tridhā* – these three types

Translation

There are three kinds of substances. They are those that are palliating, aggravating, and beneficial for health (strengthening).

Commentary

This is a compact classification of all substances in general from the treatment point of view since *Aṣṭāṅga Hṛdayam* is a practical textbook. There are *dravyas* (substances) that pacify the *doṣas*, those that aggravate the *doṣas*, and those that are for strengthening the *dhātus*. A single substance can also have some *doṣa*-aggravating properties, some *doṣa*-alleviating properties, and some strengthening properties (neither increasing nor decreasing the *doṣas*) as well. For example, *śatāvari* pacifies *vāta* and *pitta* while increasing *kapha* and is especially strengthening for the reproductive system as well.

These three actions are as follows:

1. *Śamanaṁ* (pacifying)
2. *Kopanaṁ* (aggravating)
3. *Svastha hitaṁ* (strengthening) also known as *rasāyana*

There are several ways to understand these three terminologies: *Śamana* (pacifying) substances are medicines used for treating diseases and are known as *pathya*; *kopana* (aggravating) substances are the cause of diseases and known as *apathya*; *svastha hitaṁ* substances are health-promoting foods. Those which are neither too aggravating nor too pacifying are called *svastha hitam*. They are in the middle of the spectrum.

Śamanam is defined as an action that decreases an increased state. *Kopanam* is defined as an action that increases a decreased state. *Svastha hitam* is defined as an action that neither increases nor decreases but maintains the staus quo.

We have introduced the three types of *dravyas* earlier – medicine, poison and food. Medicine causes *śamanam*, poison causes *kopanam* and food causes *svastha hitam*.

***Sarvāṅgasundara*:** Three substances are primarily recommended for the *śamana* of *vāta*, *pitta*, and *kapha*: *tailam* (sesame oil) for *vāta*, *ghṛtam* (ghee) for *pitta*, and *mākṣikam* (honey) for *kapha*. *Tailam* is unctuous, hot, and heavy, which are opposite to the qualities of *vāta*. *Ghee* is sweet, cold, and *manda* (blunt), opposite to the qualities of *pitta*. Honey is dry, sharp, and astringent, which are opposite to the qualities of *kapha*.

The three *doṣas—vāta, pitta*, and *kapha*—aggravate the *dhātus* and *malas*, and this is called *kopanaṁ*.

> These are described in chapter 6 of *Aṣṭāṅga Hṛdayam*: *yava* (barley), *pāṭala (*Stereospermum*), māṣa* (black gram), *matsya* (fish), *mūlaka* (radish), *sārṣapa* (mustard), *manḍaka, dadhi* (yogurt), *kilāṭa* (a preparation made from yogurt), *viruddha matsya payaḥ prabhṛti* (combination of fish and yogurt)—these are examples of substances that cause *kopanaṁ* of the *doṣas, dhātus*, and *malas*.

Those substances that bring the *doṣas, dhātus*, and *malas* into balance are called *svastha hitaṁ*.

> These are described in the chapter on *ṛtucaryā* and in the chapter on *mātrāśitīyam, rakta śāli* (red rice), *ṣāṣṭika śāli* (a type of rice that matures in six months, which is very strengthening), *yava* (barley), *godhūma* (wheat), *jāṅgala māmsa* (meat of animals living in dry regions), *jīvantī, śāka* (leafy vegetables), *divyodaka* (rain water) and *kṣīra* (milk) are some of the examples enumerated. This also includes all the substances that are *ojaskara* (increasing

ojas), *rasāyana* (rejuvenating), and *vājīkaraṇa* (aphrodisiacs).

***Āyurvedarasāyana*:** It is the opinion of *Hemādri* that the effect of *śamanaṁ*, *kopanaṁ* and *svastha hitaṁ* are factually due to the *prabhāva* of the *dravyas* rather than the *rasa*, *guṇa*, *vīrya*, or *vipāka*. Now let us see some examples. The *dravyas* that are of similar *rasa* (taste) or those that sometimes behave as similar but in other situations behave as opposite and pacify the *doṣas* are called *śamanaṁ* by *prabhāva*.

For example, *jīvanti* (*Leptadenia reticulata*), which is *madhura* (sweet) and *śīta* (cold) reduces *kapha*. Note that sweet and cold are properties that would normally be expected to increase *kapha*, but here it does the opposite.

Another example is *rasona* (Garlic), which is *kaṭu rasa* (pungent), *kaṭu vipāka* (effect after digestion), *guru* (heavy), *snigdha* (unctuous/oily) and it reduces *kapha* and *vāta*. Here we see that the *kaṭu rasa* (pungent) of garlic only has an effect on reducing *kapha* but does not increase *vāta*. Similarly, the *guru* (heavy) and *snigdha* (unctuous) of garlic only has an effect on pacifying *vāta* but does not increase *kapha*. This is called *prabhāva* (unique and special action that cannot be explained using conventional logic).

On the other hand, there are *dravyas* that are of opposite *rasa* or *guṇa* but still aggravate the *doṣas—kopanaṁ* by *prabhāva*. For example, *phāṇita* (a kind of sweet drink) is *guru, snigdha*, and *madhura* but aggravates *vāta*. *Māṣa* (black gram) is *guru* but aggravates *pitta*.

The substances that cause increase or decrease of *vāta*, *pitta*, and *kapha* are not *svastha hitaṁ*. Barley, which is *guru, madhura, rūkṣa*, and *śīta* does not disturb healthy *pitta*. Milk, which is *guru, madhura, snigdha*, and *śīta* will not disturb healthy *kapha*. These are all examples for *prabhāva. Prabhāva* is defined in AH Sū. 9.24 (*rasadi samye…*).

A substance can either act as *kopanaṁ, śamanaṁ*, or *svastha hitaṁ* according to how it is used in different situations. So we should not take this is as a rigid classification.

Tip: There can be many ways of classifying the same thing. Here is one classification that is clinically relevant. When you read the rest of the book or other books, you will also find other classifications. In the following verses, there are some more classifications mentioned.

Now some scientific and technical concepts required to study *dravya* are being introduced. One of the ways how *doṣas* are influenced (according to the concept of *rasa*) was described earlier. Now another aspect of *dravya* which influences the *doṣas* is being described - *vīrya*. The student may wonder why two different methods?" The concept of *rasa* is more applicable to *āhāra* (food). There is another way of assessing the action of a *dravya* on an *auṣadha* (medicine). This is called *vīrya*. Both food and medicine are both necessary for health. But food is primary and medicine is secondary. Hence they are mentioned in that order.

AH Sū. 1.17

Two types of potencies *(vīrya)*

उष्णशीतगुणोत्कर्षात्तत्र वीर्यं द्विधा स्मृतम् ॥१७॥

uṣṇa śīta guṇotkarṣāt tatra vīryaṁ dvidhā smṛtaṁ

uṣṇa – hot; *śīta* – cold; *guṇa* – quality; *utkarṣāt* – eminent, prominent; *tatra* – there; *vīryaṁ* – potency; *dvidhā* – two types; *smṛtaṁ* – known as

Translation

Substances are known to possess heating or cooling potencies depending on which one is prominent in them.

Commentary

What is the significance of the word *utkarṣāt* here? This is because there are other opinions about the number of *vīryas* in other textbooks. This is discussed by *ācārya Vāgbhaṭa* in AH. Sū 9.13[3]. But *ācārya Vāgbhaṭa* concludes that hot and cold potencies are the most eminent and significant in terms of practical or clinical understanding and relevance.

---

[3] *vīryaṁ punar-vadanty-eke guru snigdhaṁ himaṁ mṛdu //12//*

laghu-rūkṣoṣṇa-tīkṣṇaṁ ca tad-evaṁ matam-aṣṭadhā

carakastvāha vīryaṁ tat kriyate-yenayā kriyā //13//

nāvīryaṁ kurute kiñcit-sarvā vīryakṛtā hi sā

Vīrya (potency) is nothing but a concentrated manifestation of *guṇa*. Among the twenty *guṇas*, which will be described in AH. Sū 1.18, the most important are *uṣṇa* (hot) and *śīta* (cold). These are denominated as *vīrya.*

Heat and cold are qualities that are perceived by touch in a general sense. When they are perceived in this way, they are called *guṇas*. They can also be present in a substance and at the same time, not be perceivable by touch. In this case they are called *vīrya* (e.g., *māṣa* (black gram) used for heating and *vṛkṣāmla* used for cooling).

Vīrya may or may not be perceived by touch. It refers to the internal effect that a *dravya* creates in the body. So it should not be confused that there is a relation between the two. In most cases it may be similar, but it is not mandatory.

Also refer AH Sū. 9.18–19 to understand the meaning of *uṣṇa* and *śīta vīrya*.

tatroṣṇaṁ bhrama-tṛṅglāni-sveda-dāhāśu-pākitāḥ //18//
śamaṁ ca vāta-kaphayoḥ karoti śiśiraṁ punaḥ
hlādanaṁ jīvanaṁ sthambhaṁ prasādaṁ rakta-pittayoḥ //19//

Sarvāṅgasundara: Central to the twenty *guṇas* are heating and cooling. These two are the most prominent. It is these two *guṇas* that are the cause of all actions (*kāraṇa hetu*). *Vīrya* is the real *śakti* (power to accomplish a result). Basically in this universe there are only two *vīryas* (potencies): heating and cooling, and they possess the character of *agni* and *soma*. Based on the predominance of *uṣṇa* or *śīta*, substances are known for heating or cooling.

Āyurvedarasāyana: It is from the action of *kāyāgni* (*agni* of the body) that all the other *guṇas* manifest. *Vīrya* is dependent on *dravya*.

After the *dravya* is consumed, what is the transformation it undergoes in the body? This is the mechanism by which the *śamanam, kopanam* and *svastha hitam* occur.

AH Sū. 1.17 (contd.)

Three kinds of postdigestive effects *(vipākaḥ)*

त्रिधा विपाको द्रव्यस्य स्वाद्वम्लकटुकात्मकः॥ १७॥

tridhā vipāko dravyasya svādvamla katukātmakaḥ //17//

tridhā - three types; *vipāko* - of post digestive effect; *dravyasya* - of substances; *svādu* - sweet; *amla* - sour; *katuka* - pungent; *ātmakaḥ* - consisting or composed of

Translation

The three types of postdigestive effects (tastes) consist of sweet, sour, and pungent.

Commentary

The question may arise, "Why are there only three postdigestive tastes when there are six *rasas* present?" The clue of the answer for this question is in the next verse which enumerates the *guṇas*.

There are twenty *guṇas* of which four are primary. The progress of life from birth to death can be explained using these four *guṇas*.

- *Śīta snigdha* (sweet): life
- *Snigdha uṣṇa* (sour): youth
- *Uṣṇa snigdha* (salty): middle age
- *Uṣṇa rūkṣa* (pungent): elderly
- *Rūkṣa śīta* (bitter): old age
- *Śīta rūkṣa* (astringent): death

It is said that the healthy *guṇa* combination for life is *śīta* and *snigdha*. The others are all relative levels of deterioration. The last two are too degenerative to be sustained in the body. They are only used in small amounts for temporary periods to break down certain substances. But if the last two combinations stay in the body for longer periods, they will cause rapid deterioration and death. Hence, any substance that is bitter or astringent has to be at least converted to pungent (as a *vipāka*), which is less destructive.[12]

Lavaṇa rasa (salty taste) is formed when the *uṣṇa guṇa* of the sour taste increases more than the *snigdha guṇa*. In one sense, it is actually an inverted *amla rasa* (sour taste)!

Sarvāṅgasundara: The definition of *vipāka* is given in AH Sū. 9.20, "*jāṭhareṇāgninā yogād-yad-udeti rasāntaram, rasānām pariṇāmānte sa vipāka iti smṛtaḥ.*" *Vipāka* is also explained in CS.Sū. 26.68, "*raso nipate….*"

Guṇas have been described earlier while explaining the *doṣas*. All the *guṇas* are enlisted here.

AH Sū. 1.18

Twenty basic qualities (*guṇāḥ*)

गुरुमन्दहिमस्निग्धश्लक्ष्णसान्द्रमृदुस्थिराः॥ १८॥
गुणाः ससूक्ष्मविशदा विंशतिः सविपर्ययाः॥ १८॥

guru-manda-hima-snigdha-ślakṣṇa-sāndra-mṛdu-sthirāḥ
guṇāḥ sa-sūkṣma-viśadā viṁśatiḥ sa-viparyayāḥ //18//

guru – heavy; *manda* – slow; *hima* – cold; *snigdha* – unctuous; *ślakṣṇa* – smooth; *sāndra* – solid; *mṛdu* – soft; *sthirāḥ* – stable; *guṇāḥ* – qualities; *sa-sūkṣma* – subtle; *viśadā* – clear; *viṁśatiḥ* – twenty; *sa viparyayāḥ* – along with their opposite (qualities)

Translation

The twenty qualities are heavy, slow, cold, unctuous, smooth, solid, soft, stable, subtle, and clear along with their opposite counterparts.

Commentary

The twenty qualities are the *"cornerstone of the study"* of *Āyurveda*. All other concepts originate from these. This is the most fundamental aspect of *Āyurveda*. Every concept in *Āyurveda* should be understood in the light of the *guṇas*. This is the huge matrix on which the entire universe is suspended. All diseases, recommendations, and treatments are based on the understanding of *guṇas*.

The first four pairs of *guṇas* are the predominant ones and the rest of them are formed as a result of the combinations of the first four pairs of *guṇas*. Even among those four, hot and cold are the most important and fundamental. The basic qualities from which all others manifest come from *agni* and *soma* or the sun and the moon. Second come dry and wet. The third *guṇa* pair in importance is light and heavy followed by dull and sharp. The rest of the *guṇa* pairs in the list are all derivatives of the four *guṇa* pairs already described.

In the verse above, among the ten *guṇas* enumerated, *sūkṣma* and *viśadā* are catabolic in result, and other eight are anabolic in result.

Anabolic	**Catabolic**
guru (heavy)	*laghu* (light)
manda (dull/slow)	*tīkṣṇa* (sharp)
hima/śīta (cold)	*uṣṇa* (hot)
snigdha (unctuous)	*rūkṣa* (dry)
ślakṣṇa (smooth)	*khara* (rough)
sāndra (solidity)	*drava* (liquidity)
mṛdu (soft)	*kaṭhina* (hard)
sthiraḥ (stable)	*sara* (mobile)
sthūla (gross)	*sūkṣma* (subtle)
picchila (slimy/cloudy/sticky)	*viśadā* (clear)

According to principles of traditional Chinese medicine, these twenty qualities can also be understood as yin and yang.

Why only twenty? Why not more or less? It is only due to convention. *Guṇas* can be unlimited just like the *rasas* (tastes). This grouping has been done for the sake of making it easier to study. As explained earlier, there were many opinions existing that were causing confusion. *Vāgbhaṭa* collated all of them and made a conclusive opinion.

The whole qualitative part of *Āyurvedic* balancing is dependent on this fundamental understanding, that is, to determine the quality of a substance, disease, climate, person, food, and so on and balance it with a substance or practice of the opposite quality. *Āyurveda* studies all foods and medicinal *dravya* (substances) based on five properties (pentad) known as *rasa pañcakam*. These include *rasa* (taste), *guṇa* (attributes), *vīrya* (potency), *vipāka* (postdigestive effect), and *prabhāva* (unique property). This is the best and most comprehensive method to study any substance, and is a special contribution of *Āyurveda* to natural and holistic medicine.

Bhāvaprakāśa: With respect to food, the *guru* quality can be understood as "taking a long time to get digested" and *laghu* quality as "taking less time to get digested." *Manda* quality is understood as "taking a long time to show effect" and *tīkṣṇa* as "quick acting." *Uṣṇa-śīta* (Hot-cold), *mṛdu-kaṭhina* (soft-hard), and *ślakṣṇa-khara* (smooth-rough) are qualities that are understood by touch. *Snigdha-rūkṣa* (oily-dry) is understood by visual observation. *Sandra-drava* (solid-liquid) is known by visual and tactile sensations. *Sthira-sara* (immobile-mobile) can be known by *the quality of spreading*. *Sūkṣma* and *sthūla* (gross and subtle) qualities can be known by their ability to enter or how they enter the *srotas*.

Āyurvedarasāyana by *Hemādri* explains the *karmas* (actions) of each *guṇa*. Note that these are only the primary functions and they can also overlap with the functions of other *guṇas* in a secondary manner.

1. *Guru – bṛmhaṇa* (strengthening, building)
2. *Laghu – laṅghana* (weakening, reducing)
3. *Manda – śamana* (pacifying, palliating)
4. *Tīkṣṇa – śodhana* (cleansing)
5. *Hima – stambhana* (arresting, stopping)
6. *Uṣṇa – svedana* (sweating)
7. *Snigdha – kledana* (moistening, wetting)
8. *Rūkṣa – śoṣaṇa* (drying, parching, withering)
9. *Ślakṣṇa – ropaṇa* (healing, act of growing)
10. *Khara – lekhana* (scraping, scratching, lacerating)
11. *Sāndra – prasādana* (gratifying, calming, sedating)
12. *Drava – viloḍana* (agitating, disturbing, rolling, wallowing, stirring up, churning, splashing)—to cause other substances to dissolve in it
13. *Mṛdu – ślathana* (making loose, laxity, flaccid, relaxed)
14. *Kaṭhina – dṛḍhana* (making hard, fixed, firm, tight)
15. *Sthira – dhāraṇa* (supporting)
16. *Cala – preraṇa* (to set in motion, urging, inciting, impelling)
17. *Sūkṣma – vivaraṇa* (act of uncovering, spreading out, opening up, explaining, interpreting)—hence, the *cūrṇas*

are ground to fine powder to increase ease of absorption through intestinal mucosa

18. *Sthūla – samvaraṇa* (act of covering completely)
19. *Viśada – kṣālana* (washing, cleansing)
20. *Picchila – lepana* (making a layer over something, enveloping, anointing, smearing)

Some other guṇas described in other texts are *vyavāyi* (pervading), *vikāśi* (expanding), *āśukāri* (quick acting), *prasanna* (pleasing), *sugandha* (fragrant), and so on and their opposites. *Vikāśi* (expanding) and *viśada* are properties of alcohol that are opposite to *ojas*. The ten qualities of milk are sweet, cold, soft, unctuous, dense (*bahala*), smooth, slimy, heavy, slow, and pleasing. These are all qualities similar to *ojas* and increase *ojas*. *Vikāśi* has *khara guṇa* (rough); *āśukāri* (quick acting); has *cala guṇa*; and *prasanna* has *sthūla guṇa*.

The term *viśada* includes *śuci* and *vimala*. *Śuci* means to rid of waste that is invisible. *Vimala* means to rid of waste that is visible. *Mṛṣṭam* means that which is palatable (good to taste). *Śivam* means that which has a favorable outcome.

Vyāvāyi means that which is quickly absorbed, circulates all over the body, and then undergoes digestion. *Vikāśi* (expanding) produces laxity of the *dhātus*. *Āśukāri* means quick-acting nature and spreading fast. *Sugandha* (fragrant) is pleasing, subtle, relishing, and mild. *Durgandha (having a foul odor)* is opposite to *sugandha* and causes nausea and anorexia (Sū. S. 46.520–521). The functions of the twenty *guṇas* should be thoroughly understood.

Here ends the description of *pañcamahābhūta dravya* (substances) in chapter 1.

When the *doṣas* were introduced earlier in AH Sū 1.6, it was said that they maintain as well as destroy the body. Now that will be elaborated upon. What are the factors that cause the vitiation of *doṣas*? Now *ācārya* will discuss the broad categories of the causes of *doṣa* vitiation.

AH Sū. 1.19

Three causes of disease and health

कालार्थकर्मणां योगो हीनमिथ्याऽतिमात्रकः॥१९॥

सम्यग्योगश्च विज्ञेयो रोगारोग्यैककारणम्॥१९।

kālārtha-karmaṇāṁ yogo hīna-mithyāti-mātrakaḥ
samyag-yogaś-ca vijñeyo rogārogyaika-kāraṇaṁ //19//

kāla – season or time; *artha* – sense object; *karmaṇāṁ* – activities; *yoga* – method, union; *hīna* – poor, insufficient; *mithyā* – inappropriate, perverted; *ati* – excessive; *mātrakaḥ* – quantity; *samyak* – balanced; *yoga* – interaction; *ca* – and; *vijñeyo* – knowledge of; *roga* – disease; *ārogya* – absence of disease (health); *eka* – only, exclusive; *kāraṇam* – reason, cause

Translation

The deficient, perverted, and excessive interactions of time (*kāla*), sense objects (*artha*), or actions (*karma*) are the only causes of disease. Their balanced interactions are the only causes of health.

Commentary

The three factors that determine disease and health are

1. time (day, season, age, etc.);
2. sense objects (interaction between the sense organs and objects); and
3. activity (occupation, *dinacaryā, ṛtucaryā*, etc.).

Note: According to *Sankhya* philosophy, which explains how the creation took place, there are five sense organs and five sense objects. Sense organs are eyes, ears, nose, tongue, and skin. The sense objects are sight, sound, smell, taste, and touch.

The three factors are also known as *pariṇāma (changes occurring due to the influence of time), asātmya indriyārtha samyoga (unfavorable interaction between the senses and sense objects)*, and *prajñāparādha* (disrespect of one's own intellect). To know more, please see AH Sū. 12.34–43.

The word *eka kāraṇam* is significant. What it means in this context is that although there may appear to be many other apparent reasons for disease, they can be placed under one of these three categories. In this context, the meaning of *eka karaṇa* can also be "primary cause."

In AH Sū 1. 16, by dividing substances into *śamanaṁ, kopanaṁ*, and *svastha hitaṁ*, we explained that substances are the cause for disease or health. In this verse, we are trying to see how exactly these substances interact with the body to cause disease or health.

Three factors causing disease can present in three different ways, which makes a total of nine causes. This is described in the commentaries *Sarvāṅgasundara* and *Āyurvedarasāyana*. Let us take a look at them in detail. These three factors are also described ahead in chapter 12 of *Sūtra sthāna*.

The three factors are

- *hīnayoga*: less than normal;
- *atiyoga*: more than normal; and
- *mithyāyoga*: something different from normal (opposite, unusual, improper, perverted, undesirable).

Kāla* (season or time*)

1. *Hīnayoga* of *kāla*: decreased expression of normal climate (weather) pattern
2. *Atiyoga* of *kāla*: excessive expression of normal climate pattern
3. *Mithyāyoga* of *kāla*: altered expression from normal climate pattern

Kāla are of three types: *varṣa, śīta*, and *uṣṇa*.

Every season has got its own *svarūpa* (normal pattern) of the quantum of cold, heat, and rain.

***Artha* (sense objects)**

1. *Hīnayoga* of *artha*: inadequate contact between the senses and sense objects
2. *Atiyoga* of *artha*: excessive contact between senses and sense objects
3. *Mithyāyoga* of *artha*: improper or unusual contact between senses and sense objects

Artha (sense objects) are of five types: *śabda* (sound), *sparśa* (touch, *rasa* (taste), *rūpa* (form), and *gandha* (smell).

***Karma* (action)**

1. *Hīnayoga* of karma: lack of adequate effort
2. *Atiyoga* of karma: excessive effort
3. *Mithyāyoga* of karma: improper or unusual effort

Karma are of three types: *kāyika* (physically), *vācika* (verbally), and *mānasika* (mentally).

How much is *hīna* and *ati* and what is *mithyā* will have to be determined individually by each person by observing themselves very closely.

Reemphasizing the importance of *doṣas* and a second classification of causative factors of disease is being given in the next verse

AH Sū. 1.20

Definition of disease and health

Two types of diseases—based on origin

रोगास्तु दोषवैषम्यं, दोषसाम्यमरोगता॥२०॥
निजागन्तुविभागेन तत्र रोगा द्विधा स्मृताः॥२०॥

rogastu doṣa vaiṣamyaṁ doṣa-sāmyam-arogatā
nijāgantu vibhāgena tatra rogā dvidhā smṛtāḥ //20//

rogastu – of disease; *doṣa vaiṣamyaṁ* – disturbance or irregularity of *doṣa*; *doṣa-sāmyam* – equilibrium of *doṣa*; *arogatā* – of health; *nija* – internal, endogenous; *āgantu* – external, exogenous; *vibhāgena* – divisions; *tatra* – of that; *rogā* – disease; *dvidhā* – two types; *smṛtāḥ* – it is known

Translation

Disease is the irregularity of *doṣas*; health is the equilibrium of *doṣas*. It is known that there are two categories of diseases: endogenous and exogenous.

Commentary

The concept of *roga* (disease) is being introduced here. Earlier, the term *vṛddhi* was introduced. The word *roga* is derived from the root word '*ruk*' which means to break. *Vaiṣamya* indicates a disturbance from the state of equilibrium.

The state of optimal health is described using the word "*sama*" which indicates a state of balance of the *doṣas, dhātus, agn*i and *mala*. The equilibrium is misunderstood by some, to be a quantitative equality i.e. 33.33% of each of the three doṣas. This is not true. The equilibrium described in *āyurveda* with respect to a healthy state is in fact a dynamic equilibrium. This means that the body adjusts itself constantly in relation to the external environment in order to facilitate optimal functioning of the system. The *sama* (balance) mentioned is a functional equilibrium. This means that each of the *doṣas*, *dhātus*, *agni* and mala are performing their functions in a balanced way – each of them are optimally performing their own functions. It is not the "quantity" of *doṣa.*

One may ask, if *doṣa* disturbance is disease, what about the three *guṇas* which is the index of mental health. The answer is that, *rajas* and *tamas* are also called *mano-doṣa*. So the term *doṣa* also includes the disturbance in the *guṇas of the mind*.

1. Endogenous *(nija)*—internal (arising from within the body)
2. Exogenous *(āgantu)*—external (arising from external sources)

There are seven *āgantu* (extrinsic) causes of diseases described in *Caraka Samhita* Sū. 19.7.

1. Infection/infestation (*kṛmi*)
2. Epidemics (*janapadodhvamsa*)
3. Envirnomental (*kāla*kṛta)
4. Regional (*daiśika*)
5. Occupational (*vyavasāyagat*)

6. Iatrogenic (*vaidyakṛta*)
7. Possession by subtle entities (*grahabādha*)

Nija (intrinsic) causes are eleven in number.

1. Genetic (*bīja bhāga vāyava duṣṭi*)
2. Constitutional (*prakṛti*)
3. Vitiation of *srotas* (*sroto duṣṭi*)
4. Digestive fire abnormalities (*agni duṣṭi*)
5. Corrupted lumen of the channels (*koṣṭha duṣṭi*)
6. Suppression of natural urges (*vega avarodha*)
7. Dietary (*āhāraja*)
8. *Āma (undigested substrates of digestion accumulating in the body)*
9. Age (*vayaḥ*)
10. Gender (*liṅgabheda*)
11. Past life actions (*pūrva janma kṛta*)

Āgantu roga (exogenous) causes are also described in AH Sū. 4.31. These are the nine external causes mentioned in the *Aṣṭāṅga Hṛdayam*. The earlier classification discussed in this commentary was from *Caraka Samhita*.

Note: The broadest definition of *āma* is "a wrong substance, in the wrong place at the wrong time." This definition can then be narrowed down according to the context. If you look at the definition of health from *Suśruta Samhita* (*sama doṣa samāgniśca*...), you will find that *āma* is the exact antithesis of this definition.

The body and mind are explained to be functioning as one complex. We can also see them as different in terms of origin of disease.

AH Sū. 1.21

Foundation of disease *(rogāḍhiṣṭhānam)*

तेषां कायमनोभेदादधिष्ठानमपि द्विधा॥२१

teṣām kāya-mano-bhedād-adhiṣthānam-api dvidhā

teṣām – of that (the two types of diseases mentioned); *kāya* – body; *mano* – of the mind; *bhedād* – is distinctly divided; *adhiṣthānam* – basis or foundation; *api* – also; *dvidhā* – two types

Translation

Of the two types of diseases mentioned, there are two foundations. They are the body and the mind.

Commentary

***Vākyapradīpika*:** The *nija* and *āgantu* diseases mentioned in the last verse can manifest having their foundations on either the mind or the body. *Nija* diseases having their foundation on the body are *jvara, rakta pitta*, and so on. *Āgantu* diseases having their foundation on the body are *jvara* due to traumatic injury, *vidradhī*, and so on. *Nija* diseases having their foundation on the mind are *jvara, unmāda* (stress, madness, etc.), *madātyaya*, and so on. *Āgantu* diseases that have their foundation on the mind are *graha, āveśa*, and so on.

This means that a disease can have its foundation in the body and affect the mind. It can also be vice versa wherein the disease has its foundation in the mind and affects the body. It is very important to differentiate these types in order to give proper treatment and also to avoid relapse. This verse indicates the involvement of body and mind together in any illness, which is now widely accepted by modern science as a psychosomatic connection. This has also been expressed clearly in the invocation verse of this chapter *(rāgādi rogān satatānuṣaktān…)*.

It is of course true that all *āgantu* causes will eventually become *nija* because no disease can result unless the *doṣas* inside are involved.

So far *ācārya* has been explaining about the *doṣas* of the body. What about the mind? Are there any *doṣas* governing it?

AH Sū. 1.21 (contd.)

Two kinds of *doṣas* of the mind *(mānasika doṣa)*

रजस्तमश्च मनसो द्वौ च दोषावुदाहृतौ॥२१॥

rajas-tamas-ca manaso dvau ca doṣāvudāhṛtau //21//

rajas – passion; *tamas* – ignorance, darkness; *ca* – and; *manaso* – of the mind; *dvau* – two in number; *ca* – and; *doṣā* – faults, inadequacies, pathological energies ; *udāhṛtau* – it is said

Translation

It is said that passion (*rajas*) and ignorance (*tamas*) are the two pathological energies of the mind.

Commentary

Vāgbhaṭa has already described the foundation of the physical diseases as *tridoṣa*s earlier. Now he is describing the *manaḥ adhiṣṭhāna*—diseases that arise from the mind. *Rajas* and *tamas* are known in *Āyurveda* as *mano doṣas* since they are the cause of all mental imbalances. Thus, to avoid imbalances of mind, it is important to adopt practices that increase *sattva* and live a *sāttvik* life.

A concise definition of *rajas* and *tamas* is explained by Lord *Kṛṣṇa* in the *Bhagavad Gīta* 14. 7-8.

rajo rāgātmakam viddhi tṛṣṇa-saṅga-samudbhavam
tan nibadhnāti kaunteya karma-saṅgena dehinam

rajas is born of unlimited desires and longings, son of Kunti, and it binds the embodied living entity to the association with fruitive actions.

tamas tv ajñānajam viddhi mohanam sarva dehinām
pramādālasya nidrābhis tan nibadhnāti bhārata

tamas is born out of ignorance, deludes all the living beings and binds using madness, laziness and sleep.

***Sarvāṅgasundara*:** Vitiated *rajas* and *tamas* are the causes of calamities of the mind. The word *ca* indicates the three *doṣas*—*vāta*, *pitta* and *kapha*—can also vitiate the mind. This means that the three *doṣas* are not excluded from the pathogenesis of mental illness. But the *guṇas* are predominantly used to describe mental changes and *doṣas*, to describe physical changes. Of course we should bear in mind that *doṣas* can influence the mind and *guṇas* can influence the body as well. Each of these terminologies has broad as well as narrow connotations. This has to be understood according to context as well. Of the two *guṇas* affecting the mind, *rajas* is more prominent and hence mentioned in the beginning.

This can be illustrated in the six types of *unmāda (mental affliction)* (AH Ut. Ch. 6). The six types of *unmāda* are one each due to the three *doṣas*, one due to the combination of all three *doṣas*, one due to poisoning, and one due to mental stress (*citta ghataja*). The first four are endogenous, and the last two are exogenous according to classification.

***Vākyapradīpika*:** From this verse one can understand that *sattva guṇa* is never harmful. *Rajas* and *tamas* are *doṣas* when out of balance and *guṇas* when in balance. The pure *sattva* is enveloped by *rajas* and *tamas* in this world.

How to understand a disease developing in the body and mind? There are two aspects to it. One is to examine the patient and the other is to examine the disease. Both are important. First let us see how to examine the patient. It is important to note that between *roga* and *rogi*, *ācārya Vāgbhaṭa* is indirectly indicating us to examine the *rogi* before examining the *roga*.

AH Sū. 1.22

Examination of patient (*rogi parīkṣā*)

दर्शनस्पर्शनप्रश्नैः परीक्षेत च रोगिणम्॥२२॥

darśana-sparśana-praśnaiḥ parīkṣeta ca rogiṇaṁ

darśana – inspection; *sparśana* – touch (palpation, percussion); *praśnaiḥ* – interrogation, history taking; *parīkṣeta* – is examined by; *ca* – and; *rogiṇaṁ* – the patient

Translation

The patient is examined using visual, tactile, and interrogatory techniques.

Commentary

After having described the causes of diseases, *Vāgbhaṭa* is now describing how to recognize the symptoms of those causes in the patient.

This is known in *Āyurveda* as *trividha parīkṣa*—examination using three methods, which is a broad classification. It is further expanded into *daśavidha parīkṣa* (ten examination methods).

The clinical examinations within the *daśavidha parīkṣa* also constitute *aṣṭasthāna parīkṣa* (eight examination methods). We will study all these in detail later in the chapters dealing with diagnosis in *Nidāna sthāna.*

In *Āyurveda*, the client who has an imbalance (*rogī*) and the imbalance itself are studied separately and correlated. First the *rogi* (patient) is examined to see whether there is any disease. Next, how they acquired the imbalance is explained (*nidāna* or etiology). Then the disease is examined to find out the stage and nature of its progress. The disease is studied according to five aspects called *nidāna pañcakam*, which will be explained in the next verse.

Sarvāṅgasundara

- *Darśana* is used in *kāsa* (cough), *meha* (polyuria), and so on to examine yellow or white sputum. Stool, urine, and vomit are also examined using this method. This is a *pratyakṣa* (direct perception) type of information.
- *Sparśana* (touch) is used to examine *jvara*, *gulma* (a mass), *vidradhī* (suppurative growth), and so on. This is also *pratyakṣa.*
- *Praśna* (interrogation) is used in finding out about pain, loss of appetite, palpitations, nausea, and so on. This is more of an *anumāna* type of information. Based on the history given by the client, the *Vaidya* will deduce a logical conclusion.

Note: Some of the names of diseases mentioned here may not be understood fully. They will be understood as we progress in the study of *Aṣṭāṅga Hṛdayam*. For now just read them and get familiar with the names.

Āyurvedarasāyana

- By *darśana* (inspection), color, lumps, growths, ulcers, and so on can be assessed.
- By *sparśana* (palpation, touch) cold, heat, rough, smooth, and so on can be assessed.
- By *praśna* (interrogation) pain, fatigue, nausea, and so on can be assessed.

After having examined the *rogi* (patient, let us now examine the *roga* (disease)

AH Sū. 1.22 (contd.)

Examination of disease (*roga parīkṣā*)—*nidāna pañcakam*

रोगं निदानप्राग्रूपलक्षणोपशयाप्तिभिः॥२२॥

rogaṁ nidāna-prāgrūpa-lakṣaṇopaśayāptibhiḥ //22//

nidāna – cause or etiology; *prāgrūpa* or *pūrvarūpa* – prodromal symptoms; *lakṣaṇa* – clinical symptoms; *upaśaya* – diagnostic tests / trial & error; *āpti* or *samprāpti* – pathogenesis

Translation

Etiology, initial nonspecific prodromal symptoms, expressed specific clinical symptoms, diagnostic tests (trial and error), and pathogenesis are the ways to evaluate a disease.

Commentary

This is known in *Āyurvedic* diagnosis as *nidāna pañcakam*, that is, the five steps of etiopathogenesis and symptoms of a disease. They are: cause, nonspecific prodromal symptoms, specific clinical symptoms, diagnostic tests, and pathogenesis. It is important to know the *nidāna pañcakam* of any disease before attempting to chart the treatment plan. The pathogenesis of the disease is explained in six different stages called *ṣaṭ kriyā kāla*. This is explained in the *Suśruta Samhita*, *Sūtra sthāna* (chapter 21).

In the section of the *Aṣṭāṅga Hṛdayam* called *Nidāna sthāna*, several possibilities of pathologies will be discussed and their progression in the human body as well. The *samprāpti* tells us about the entire network of activities going on inside the body and the resultant pathological manifestations. It is very important to understand the pathology from the *Āyurvedic* perspective in terms of *doṣa*, *dhātu*, *mala, srotas*, *agni*, and so on in order to plan an *Āyurvedic* protocol to deal with the illness.

> When he discussed about examining the rogi, ācārya *Vāgbhaṭa* told us about the three fold examination. One of the items in the examination of *rogi* is to ask about the habitat. The significance of this information is described next.

AH Sū. 1.23–24

Three kinds of lands or countries *(deśa)*

भूमिदेहप्रभेदेन देशमाहुरिह द्विधा॥२३॥

जाङ्गलं वातभूयिष्ठमानूपं तु कफोल्बणम्॥२३॥

साधारणं सममलं त्रिधा भूदेशमादिशेत्॥२४॥

bhūmi-deha-prabhedena deśamāhur iha dvidhā

jāṇgalaṁ vāta-bhūyiṣṭhaṁ-ānūpaṁ tu kapholbaṇaṁ //23//

sādhāraṇaṁ sama-malaṁ tridhā bhūdeśam-ādiśet

bhūmi – land; *deha* – body; *prabhedena* – types; *deśamāhur* – all the regions; *iha* – in this world; *dvidhā* – two types; *jāṇgalaṁ* – dry, arid; *vāta bhūyiṣthaṁ* – *vāta* predominant; *ānūpaṁ* – situated near water, watery; *tu* – but; *kapha ulbaṇaṁ* – excessively or predominantly *kapha*; *sādhāraṇaṁ* – moderate type; *sama* – uniformly distributed; *malaṁ* – *doṣa*s; *tridhā* – three types; *bhūdeśam* – land; *ādiśet* – has been said

Translation

Lands and bodies are of three types. One which is dry is *vāta* predominant. The one which is watery is *kapha* predominant. The third is a moderate type where there is equal distribution of the *doṣas.*

Commentary

This is one of the components of the *daśavidha parīkṣa* (ten methods of diagnosis). It is important to know the residential climate and environment of the patient as this is one of the major contributory factors to the disease.

There are two aspects to *deśa*: *bhūmi deśa* and *deha deśa*. *Bhūmi* deśa refers to the regions on the earth. *Deha* deśa refers to different parts of the body or the whole body. We will learn more about *deha deśa* in *śārīra sthāna*. The latter has already been described so now *ācārya* is describing the *bhūmi deśa*. Just like the regions of the earth, the body can be either dry or wet (unctuous).

- *Jāṇgalaṁ*: *vāta*-dominated place (dry, arid)
- *Anūpaṁ*: *kapha*-dominated place (wet, marshy, water logged)
- *Sādhāraṇaṁ*: all three *doṣās* equally present (greenery, good water supply, not too hot or cold)

Why isn't a *pitta*-dominated place described here?
Because *vāta* and *kapha* are two extremes and *pitta* is in the middle. *Pitta* can associate with both *vāta* and *kapha*. Dry and wet cannot associate with each other because they are on opposite ends of the spectrum. *Pitta* is in the middle.
Some experts also explain that a *pitta* habitat is not classified because life cannot exist in a *kevala pitta* atmosphere. Some explain that a *pitta* habitat is not *bheṣaja yogakṛt* (not suitable for administering treatments).
Another reason is given in *Aruṇodaya*: Apart from the three types of lands described there are others which are salty (*ūṣarasa*) and sandy. For example, the desert. These types of

lands which are excessively *pitta* predominant have not been described because these are not usually inhabited by human beings. The lands which are usually inhabited by human beings are classified and described.

Why is it said that it is first divided into two types (*dvidhā*) and then in the end it speaks of three types (*tridhā*)?
First there is a division into two types based on the moisture content. Then comes the third division, which is a description of a place where the moisture is optimal—neither too much nor too little.

It is important to remember that *Āyurveda* considers the human body to be a miniature version of the whole world (or universe). So a certain part of the world or universe can correlate with a certain part of the human body as well according to the principle of microsystems. So in the body also one can identify the three types of regions—*jāṅgalam*, *ānūpam*, and *sādhāraṇam*—just as they are present on the earth.

Āyurvedarasāyana: From this point onward, *auṣadha* (medicine) is going to be described.

After having examined the *rogi* and *roga*, now *ācārya* begins description of the treatments...

AH Sū. 1.24 (contd.)

Determining the right timing for therapies and medicines

क्षणादिर्व्याध्यवस्था च कालो भेषजयोगकृत्॥२४॥

kṣaṇādir-vyādhy-avasthā ca kālo bheṣaja-yoga-kṛt //24//

kṣaṇādi – according to units of time on the clock; *vyādhyāvasthā* – according to stage of the disease; *ca* – and; *kālo* – time for; *bheṣaja* – treatment; *yoga kṛt* – is appropriately administered

Translation

Āyurvedic treatment is administered after considering two aspects of time: as per the units of real time and as per the stage of disease.

Commentary

By using the term *bheṣaja yogakṛt Vāgbhaṭa* is making it clear that the classification and analysis of the intricacies and influences of time and space is meant for the sole purpose of formulating an effective management protocol.

The importance of time in *Āyurvedic* diagnosis and treatment is emphasized here. The calculation of time in *Āyurveda* begins with *kṣaṇa*, which is the smallest unit of time. Transformation is a manifestation of time. Hence the transformation of disease is also a study of time. Preparation and administration of the therapies as well as medications also have to be done taking into consideration the influence of time. We had discussed earlier about the temporal classification of *doṣas* in AH Sū. 1.7, "*te vyāpino'pi...*" with respect to age, time of the day, and stage of digestion. The *doṣa avastha* has to be analyzed according to this understanding.

Kṣaṇādi is external time and *vyādhi avastha* is internal time. *Kṣaṇādi* is measurable time, *vyādhi avastha* is the condition of the *rogi*.

The concept of *kāla* is also utilized in the diagnosis of diseases where the *samprāpti* (pathogenesis) of a disease is analyzed in terms of the the temporal variations like diurnal, seasonal and digestion of food. (Ref. AH Ni 1. 11)

Sarvāṅgasundara: *Kāla is of two types. One is kṣaṇādi kāla (clock and seasonal time) and another is vyādhyāvastha (stage of disease) kāla. Kṣaṇādi kāla* includes *kṣaṇa, lava, truṭi, muhūrta, yāma, ahorātra, pakṣa, māsa*, *ṛtu*, *ayana, samvatsara* (different units of *Vedic* time described further below).

Vedic astronomy divides time based on several different parameters like breathing, blinking of eyelids, movement of the planets, and so on. It gives a very detailed division of time up to the lowest subdivision level of *prāṇa* (respiration), a time lapse of three to four seconds. The astronomical divisions of sidereal time are given in the following table.

1 *paramanu*	=		60,750th of a second
1 *truṭi*	=		29.6296 microseconds
1 *tatpara*	=		2.96296 milliseconds
1 nimesha	=		88.889 milliseconds
45 *nimesha*	=	1 *prāṇa*	4 seconds
6 *prāṇa*	=	1 vinādī	24 seconds
60 *vinādīs*	=	1 *nadī*	24 minutes
60 *nādīs*	=	1 ahorātra	

According to modern standards, twenty-four hours make one day and night; one finds that one *nādi* or *daṇda* is equal to 24 minutes, one *vinādī* is equal to 24 seconds, one *asu* or *prāṇa* is equal to 4 seconds, one *nimesa* is equal to 88.889 milliseconds, one *tatpara* is equal to 2.96296 milliseconds, and finally one *truṭi* is equal to 29.6296 microseconds or 33,750th part of second.

It is really amazing that the Indian astronomers, a long time ago, could conceive and obviously could measure such a small interval of time like *truṭi*. One unit of *prāṇa* is the time an average healthy man needs to complete one respiration or to pronounce ten, long syllables called *guravakṣara* (a group of *Sanskṛt* letters).

The *Purāṇic* division of the day is somewhat different. According to this, *kāla* (time) is born out of sun. The counting starts from *nimesha* (twinkling of an eye).

100 *truṭi* (atoms)	= 1 *tatpara* (speck)
30 *tatpara* (specks)	= 1 nimeṣa (twinkling of eye)
18 *nimeṣa* (twinklings)	= 1 *kāṣṭha* (bit)
30 *kāṣṭha* (bits)	= 1 *kāla* (~minute)
30 *kāla* (minutes)	= 1 *ghaṭika* (~half-hour)
2 *ghaṭika* (half hour)	= 1 *kṣaṇa/muhūrta* (~hour)
30 *kṣaṇa/muhūrta* (hour)	= 1 *ahorātra* (~day).

Source: *Sūrya Siddhānta.*

Truṭi is referred to as a quarter of the time of the falling of an eyelid. One *muhūrta* is equal to 48 minutes; one *ghaṭi* is equal to 24 minutes. One *kāla* is equal to 48 seconds; one *kāṣṭhā* is equal to 1.6 seconds; and one *nimeṣa* is equal to 88.889 milliseconds as obtained above. In its daily motion, the earth rotates around its axis at a speed of nearly 1,660 kilometers per hour and its illuminated half is called *ahaḥ* (day) and the dark half is called *rātri* (night). From the system of units of time given above, one finds that sixty *ghaṭis* or *nādīs* make one day and night. (Refer http://veda.wikidot.com/vedic-time-system.)

These are all different quantitative measurements of time. *Lava* is one-twelfth of a second and *samvatsara* is a year. The duration of symptoms, time of appearance of symptoms, and so on will all be included in *kṣaṇādi. Vyādhi avastha* will include *sāma-pacyamāna-nirāma (with āma, in the process of āma being digested, without āma), mṛdu-madhya-tīkṣṇa (mild, moderate, severe), doṣāvastha (status of doṣa), pakva-nava-purāṇa (ripened, acute, chronic), tīkṣṇa-mrdutva*, and so on.

AS Sū. 13.8–22: This is the last part of the chapter. In these verses the season, the time of the day, and the time of digestion for administering different therapies are given.
For example, *vamana* is given in the morning, *virecana* at midday, and *vasti* also can be given at midday. There is also specificity in the time of administration of medicines. See AH Sū. 13.37 to know more about time of administration of medicines.

There are different calculations of time in *Āyurveda.*
1. Cosmological or chronological time—according to movements of the earth producing the changing seasons
2. Biological time—related to *doṣa*s, organs, digestion, nutrition, aging, and so on.

- *doṣa kāla (doṣa* predominant time)
- *avasthā pāka kāla* (time required for digestion)
- *dhātu poṣaṇa kāla* (tissue nutrition)—mentioned by *Cakrapāṇi*
- *vaya (*aging), stages of life and life-span

- *nidrā jāgaraṇa anna kāla (*sleeping, waking, and eating time*)*

This understanding is used in determining *cikitsa* and is called *cikitsā kāla.*

- *auṣadha kāla*
- *pañcakarma kāla*
- *rasāyana kāla*
- *ṛtucaryā*
- *dinacaryā*

Jyotish or *Vedic* astrology is also study of time. More details about the divisions of time (*kāla*) is given in chapter 2.

The stage of the disease (*vyādhyavastha*) can be described as six in number (*ṣaṭ kriyā kāla*) from *Suśruta's* point of view. They are

1. *caya* (accumulation);
2. *prakopa* (aggravation);
3. *prasara* (spread);
4. *sthāna samśraya* (localization);
5. *vyakti* (manifestation); and
6. *bheda* (differentiation).

Other ways of classifying *avasthās* of disease are *doṣa-avastha* (status of *doṣa* involvement), *āma-avastha* (status of *āma* involvement), *vayasaḥ-avastha* (age-related status), and so on, which have to be taken into consideration before planning the treatment and prognosis. Giving the medicine at the right time, in the right *avastha* of the disease, can increase the effectivity several fold.

Note: Most of the *Āyurvedic* medicines and treatments are time specific and disease-*avastha* specific.

Sarvāṅgasundara: CS Ci. 3.140/AH Ci. 1.21—different treatments to be given in different stages (*avastha*) of fever are mentioned here. CS Ci. 30.287/AH Ci. 1.44—this is the treatment for the *avastha* of mild fever of recent onset.
Vamana is done in the early morning; *virecana* is given in the middle of the day; in the afternoon *vasti* is given (*purvahne vamanam deyam*...).

Āyurvedarasāyana: *Hemādri* explains the different units of time. Two types of *kāla* are *kṣaṇadi rūpa* and *vyādhi avastha rūpa*. *Kṣaṇādi* includes all the units of time as per the real-time calculation. The *kṣaṇādi kāla* system for determining treatment is applicable only if the lengths of day and night are equal. The units of time from *kṣaṇa* to *varṣa* are enumerated below.

1 *mātra* = 1 *nimeṣa* (time required to blink eyelid once)
15 *mātras* = 1 *kāṣṭha*
15 *kāṣṭhas* = 1 *laghu*
15 *laghus* = 1 *daṇḍa* (*nāḍika*)
8 *yāma* = 1 *ahorātra* (30 *muhūrtas*) (day and night)

15 *ahorātra* = 1 *pakṣa* (fortnight)

2 *pakṣa* = 1 *māsa* (month)

2 *māsa* = 1 *ṛtu* (season)

3 *ṛtu* = 1 *ayana* (half year)

2 *ayanas* = 1 *varṣa* (year)

Aruṇodaya: *kṣaṇādis* have already been described above. The life span of a human being has been divided into three stages – *bālya* (childhood), *yauvana* (youth), *vārdhakya* (old age). Ref. *Bhagavad Gīta* 2.13 *dehinosmin yathā dehe kaumāram yauvanam jarā*. In the same way the life span of a disease also has these three stages. It is these three stages of disease that are called *vyādhi avastha*. Another way of saying it is *āma avastha*, *pacyamāna avastha* and *pakva avastha*. *Vaidyas* need to know this to understand the nature of disease and also if the time is favorable, the prognosis is better. Eg. In *jvara*, *kaṣāya* is to be given only in the *pakva avastha* of disease. *Kaṣāya vasti* is given in the afternoon only.

Thus the section describing diseases is over. Now begins the description of treatments.

AH Sū. 1.25

Two kinds of treatments

शोधनं शमनं चेति समासादौषधं द्विधा॥२५॥

śodhanaṁ śamanaṁ ceti samāsād-auṣadhaṁ dvidhā

śodhanaṁ – cleansing; *śamanaṁ* – pacifying, palliating; *ca* – and; *iti* – this; *samāsād* – succinctly grouped; *auṣadhaṁ* – treatments; *dvidhā* – two groups

Treatment

Treatments are succinctly divided into two groups, namely, palliating the *doṣas* and cleansing the *doṣas*.

Commentary

We have been examining the *roga*, *rogi* and understanding their relationship in terms of *deśa* and *kāla* for the purpose of deciding the *cikitsa* (treatment). What those treatments are, is being explained here.

All diseases are due to the vitiation of *doṣas* as explained before. Treatments are described here as two types: the first is that which expels the vitiated *doṣas* out of the body and the second is that which pacifies the vitiated *doṣas* while they remain within the body itself.

The treatments have been classified into *śamana* and *śodhana* on the basis of the quantity of the aggravated doṣas in the body to be dealt with. If the quantity is not much, then *śamana* is preferred over *śodhana*.

Although there are many types of treatments, this is the broadest way of classifying them.

Why is there no mention of *brmhaṇa* (nourishing) therapy? Because it is a type of *śamana* treatment in the case of *vāta* and *pitta* aggravation, also used in *pūrva karma* (initial preparation phase) of *śodhana* therapies. Thus it is inclusive in *śamana* and *śodhana*.

When there is an imbalance due to the aggravation of the *doṣa*s, and the quantitative increase of the *doṣa*s is minimal, it is advised to pacify them by the method of *śamana* (palliation) within the body itself. But when there is a situation called *bahu doṣa* (excessive quantity of vitiated *doṣa* in the body), and palliation is not possible effectively due to the excessive quantitative increase, it is advised to expel them from the body by the process called *śodhana* (cleansing).

Sarvāṅgasundara: The word *samāsad* means concisely. Whatever treatments are available in any kind of medicine or treatment in any healing system in the world can be grouped into two: *śamana* and *śodhana*.

Āyurvedarasāyana: In the case of *vāta* and *pitta*, *bṛmhaṇa cikitsa* (nourishment therapy) causes *śamana* (palliation).

Aruṇodaya: After having said that the correct timing of *cikitsa* will improve the effectiveness of the treatment, now the treatment is being described. Since *roga* has been described as *doṣa vaiṣamya* in 1.20, treatment of the *doṣās* is the same as treatment of the *roga*.

AH Sū. 1.25–26

Three kinds of therapies for *doṣās* in the body

शरीरजानां दोषाणां क्रमेण परमौषधम्॥२५॥

वस्तिर्विरेको वमनं तथा तैलं घृतं मधु॥२६॥

śarīrajānāṁ doṣāṇāṁ krameṇa param-auṣadhaṁ

vastir-vireko vamanaṁ tathā tailaṁ ghṛtaṁ madhu

śarīrajānāṁ – originating from body; *doṣāṇāṁ* – (diseases of the) *doṣas*; *krameṇa* – in the order, by regimen; *param* – ultimate, best; *auṣadhaṁ* – medicine; *vastir* – enema; *vireko* – purgation; *vamanaṁ* – emesis; *tathā* – respectively; *tailaṁ* – oil; *ghṛtaṁ* – ghee; *madhu* – honey

Translation

The best treatments for the (vitiated) *doṣas* in the body are medicated enema (*vasti*), therapeutic purgation (*virecana*), and therapeutic emesis (*vamana*) in that order using oils, ghee, and honey, respectively.

Commentary

It was previously described that diseases can originate with the body or the mind as the foundation. Here the treatment for the diseases *śarīrajānām* (originating from the body) is described. In the next verse, the treatment for diseases originating in the mind will be described. *Tailam* in general means oil and specifically means sesame oil. It should be understood according to context.

The same order of the three *doṣas* as that are mentioned in the previous verses is being followed (i.e., *vāta, pitta, and kapha*).

***Sarvāṅgasundara*:** *Vasti, virecana*, and *vamana* are best for *śodhana* (cleansing); *tailam* (sesame oil), *ghṛtam* (ghee), and *madhu* (honey) are used for *śamana* (palliative) treatment of *vāta, pitta* and *kapha* respectively. For the purification of *kapha*, medicine is given through the mouth and expelled through the mouth. For the purification of *pitta*, medicine is given through the mouth and expelled through the anus. For the purification of *vāta*, the medicine is given through the anus and expelled through the anus.

Āyurvedarasāyana: The word *śarīrajānām* refers to two types of treatment: *śodhana* and *śamana*. For the *śamana* of *vāta, pitta*, and *kapha*, it is recommended to use *tailam, ghṛtam*, and *madhu*, respectively. For the *śodhana* of *vāta, pitta*, and *kapha*, it is recommended to use *vasti, virecana*, and *vamana*, respectively.

AH Sū. 1.26

Three therapies for the *doṣas* of the mind

धीधैर्यात्मादिविज्ञानं मनोदोषौषधं परम्॥२६॥

dhī-dhairyātmādi-vijñānaṁ mano-doṣauṣadhaṁ paraṁ

dhī – intelligence (discrimination); *dhairya* – courage, will power, patience; *ātmādi vijñānam* – knowledge of soul and allied subjects; *mano* – of the mind; *doṣa* – diseases; *auṣadhaṁ* – medicine, therapy; *paraṁ* – best

Translation

The best therapies for the mind are nourishing the intelligence, developing will power, and cultivating spiritual knowledge.

Commentary

After having treated the body in the last verse, it is now time to treat the mind. They are done using three methods. Strengthen the intelligence; cultivate patience; and become enlightened by spiritual realization. In the present day, civilization is suffering more from mental illnesses than physical. People are confused and unable to decide what to do in life like a person who is lost in the darkness. As explained earlier, all the endogenous diseases begin in the subtle body. The subtle body consists of the mind, intellect, and false ego. Three methods are mentioned here to deal with each of them. Patience is for the mind, discrimination is for the intellect, and realization of the self is for the false ego. When the body and mind are perfectly aligned within themselves and with each other, it is the state of perfect health.

1. Intelligence (function of discrimination)
2. Patience or will power (function of determination)
3. Knowledge of self or self-realization (function of direction)

This is the basic principle of *Āyurvedic* counseling therapy. Here it is obvious that *ātma* does not refer to the body. According to the understanding in the *Taittriya Upaniṣad*, there are five layers of existence. They are called *kośas—annamaya, prāṇamaya, manomaya, vijñānamaya*, and *ānandamaya.* They are physical level, interphase between physical and mental, mental (emotional) level, intellectual level, and spiritual level, respectively. The last three levels are mentioned in this verse. *Dhī* is the intellectual platform where discrimination takes place. *Dhairya* is the mental platform as it is the mind that is always restless. The third level is obviously the spiritual platform, because the other two have already been mentioned.

The different levels of the material body are also mentioned in the *Bhagavad Gīta* 3.40

indriyāṇi mano buddhir asyādhiṣṭhānam ucyate

etair vimohayaty eṣa jñānam āvṛtya dehinam

Indriyāṇi is the senses, *mano* is the mind, and *buddhi* is the intelligence. In the *Kaṭha Upaniṣad* 1.3.3–4, the analogy of a chariot driven by five horses is mentioned to describe the different sheaths (*kośas*).

The secret of harnessing the power of the mind is revealed by Lord *Kṛṣṇa* in the *Bhagavad Gīta*. First *Arjuna* divulges the nature of the uncontrolled mind in BG 6.34 by saying, "For the mind is restless, turbulent, obstinate and very strong, O Kṛṣṇa, and to subdue it is, it seems to me, more difficult than controlling the wind." Lord Kṛṣṇa replies to this by saying, "O mighty-armed son of Kuntī, it is undoubtedly very difficult to curb the restless mind, but it is possible by constant practice and by detachment."

More details of how to purify and strengthen the mind, intelligence, and soul are described in the *yoga śāstras*. If one is intelligent, they will patiently cultivate spiritual knowledge. If one has spiritual knowledge, they will patiently discriminate between what is beneficial and not beneficial in every context. Patience is a sign of intelligence and spiritual realization.

If you observe carefully in the last two verses, you will find that *Vāgbhaṭa* is describing the methods to deal with *śarīra-doṣa* and *mano-doṣa*. It is *doṣa* he is talking about and not *roga*. There is a difference between both. These methods are recommended to bring back the balance in the case of mild variations in *doṣa* and prevent aggravation into *roga*. They are more preventive and prophylactic in nature. But when the *doṣa prakopa* progresses to a level of *roga*, we need to employ more than just these techniques. The fundamental difference is that *roga* involves the understanding of *samprāpti* which is influenced by multiple factors beginning from *sthāna samśraya* onwards with *doṣa*-dūṣya *sammūrcchana* (combination of *doṣa* and *dhātu*). For example in the case of a pathological *manoroga* (mental disease), the three methods - *dhī, dhairya, ātmādi vijñānam* - are not sufficient to manage the condition. In the case of *roga* of the mind, the situation has aggravated to the point where the effects have spilled over into physical manifestations. In such cases physical treatments are necessary. But when the condition has not progressed as much and is still in the mind, one can use *dhi*, *dhairya* and *ātmādi vijñānam* to prevent the mind from getting imbalanced. Similarly the *śodhana* and *śamana* mentioned with respect to the *śarīra doṣa* are also explained here in a preventive way to keep the *doṣas* in balance through the days, seasons and so on. *Roga* has to be dealt with using *cikitsa* and this will be explained in the next verse.

ācārya is now explaining how to deal with diseases when they manifest and the factors required to execute a successful treatment.

AH Sū. 1.27

Four limbs of treatment

भिषक् द्रव्याण्युपस्थाता रोगी पादचतुष्टयम्॥२७॥
चिकित्सितस्य निर्दिष्टं, प्रत्येकं तच्चतुर्गुणम्॥२७॥

bhiṣak dravyāṇyupasthātā rogī pāda-catuṣṭayam
cikitsitasya nirdiṣṭaṁ pratyekaṁ taccatur-guṇam //27//

bhiṣak – physician; *dravyāṇi* – medicines; *upasthātā* – paramedical staff, attendant, nurse; *rogī* – patient; *pāda* – legs; *catuṣṭayam* – four types; *cikitsitasya* – to be treated; *nirdiṣṭaṁ* – indicated, declared; *pratyekaṁ* – distinct; *tat* – of each of these; *catur guṇam* – four qualities

Translation

Physician, medicines, nurse, and patient are the four legs of a treatment process. For obtaining indicated results, the four legs should possess four distinct qualities each.

Commentary

After having described the treatments for the body and mind, *Vāgbhaṭa* is now describing the four components required to carry out these treatments.

Each of the four limbs of a treatment possesses four distinct qualities, which are enumerated further. The four limbs of treatment are

1. physician *(bhiṣak/vaidya)*;
2. medicines *(dravyāṇi)*;
3. nurse or care giver *(upasthātā)*; and
4. patient *(rogī)*.

Thus the result of a treatment is determined by a healthy combination of these four limbs or components. If any one of them is improper, it can adversely affect the results.

Āyurvedic treatment process (*cikitsitam*) has four limbs. Each of the four limbs are described as having four features. This is explained in the verses 28–29.

Here we can understand the difference between *auṣadha* and *cikitsa*. *Cikitsa* is a broader term that involves the entire gamut of the management of a diseased condition while *auṣadha* is only one aspect of the treatment. *Vāgbhaṭā* is clearly illustrating that one should never make the mistake of thinking that treatment is all just about giving some medicines.

AH Sū. 1.28

Qualities of physician and other limbs of treatment

दक्षस्तीर्थात्तशास्त्रार्थो दृष्टकर्मा शुचिर्भिषक्॥२८॥
बहुकल्पं बहुगुणं सम्पन्नं योग्यमौषधम्॥२८॥

dakṣas-tīrthātta-śāstrārthe dṛṣṭa-karmā śucir-bhiṣak
bahukalpaṁ bahuguṇaṁ sampannaṁ yogyam-auṣadhaṁ //28//

dakṣas – expert, skilful, efficient by practice; *tīrthātta* – learned from the *gurus (tīrtha – holy abode* i.e. in the presence of the *guru; ātta* – obtained*)*; *śāstrārthe* – all the meanings and interpretations of the texts; *dṛṣṭa-karmā* – observed and experienced (performed) directly; *śucir* – hygienic, pure hearted, having good intentions; *bhiṣak* – healer (*bhiṣaj* – to heal*)*; *bahukalpaṁ* – capable of being used in many pharmaceutical modes and *doṣa*ges; *bahuguṇaṁ* – having many qualities; *sampannam* – easily obtainable, palatable; *yogyam* – suitable for use (according to the situation); *auṣadham* – medicine

Translation

The physician should be an expert who has learned from masters, who knows all the meanings and interpretations of the *Āyurvedic* texts, has observed and practically performed the treatments oneself and pure (in mind and body). The medicinal substance should have the capability to be used in different types of formulations, possess many healing qualities, be easily obtainable and appropriate for use in the particular given situation.

Commentary

Four qualities of a good *vaidya* (physician) are as follows:

1. *dakṣas*—expert, skilful, quick in action, able to do many things in a short time expertly; it also refers to one who is constantly striving to improve the quality of the treatments and trying to make it better and better with each passing day. In other words, a *vaidya* is a perfectionist. If one is

not trying to do that, he or she will simply stagnate and anything that stagnates eventually becomes infected. The word *dakṣa* indicates that the physician is expert in all the different types of medicines, not only *Āyurveda* but other types of medicines and healing systems as well.

2. *tīrthātta-śāstrārthe*—means that he or she has understood the deeper meanings of the science from the *gurus*; it should be noted that the *guru* is not someone who gives us information. That can be understood from books as well. *Guru* is one who teaches us how to see the principle behind what is given in the books. One should approach such a *guru* who gives that vision or ability to see beyond what is written in the books – sometimes called as "reading between the lines". So it is not about learning *śāstra* but about understanding the *artha* behind the *śāstra*. This is what will help in application of the science.
3. *dṛṣṭa-karmā*—directly observed the *gurus* and performed the treatments under their supervision; this appears to be almost the same as *dakṣa*, but it is not. It is not just to mechanically become proficient. That can be done by the therapists as well. It means someone who has seen the principles in action and become fuly convinced of the truths by seeing them coming true in real life. This complete conviction is the essence of *dṛṣṭa karma*.
4. *śuciḥ*—clean in body, words, and mind; clean and honest in dealings and exchanges. There are many types of *śuddhi* (cleanliness) – *dravya śuddhi* (cleanliness in

substances used or acquired), *jñāna śuddhi* (to learn the subject with clarity, to avoid mixing it with other sciences), *karma śuddhi* (activites of body, mind and words should be pure)

Four qualities of a medicine are

1. *bahukalpaṁ*—can be turned into multiple formulations (called *kalpanas*);
2. *bahuguṇaṁ*—possessing multiple qualities (the twenty *guṇas*);
3. *sampannam*—easily obtained (availability), palatable; and
4. *yogyam*—suitable for use, that is, eligible or applicable.

At times the compliance of the treatment becomes dependent on the duration of treatment or the palatability of the formulations. In such a situation, the *vaidya* should be able to change the formulation or treatment to suit the comfort of the patient to ensure continued compliance. This is possible only if the *dravya* has the above mentioned properties.

Sarvāṅgasundara

About the medicine

- *Bahukalpam*—one should be able to administer the medicine in different formulations such as *svarasa, kvātha, cūrṇa*, and so on (called *kalpam*), and they must have the potency to cure diseases.

- *Bahuguṇam*—the medicine should possess as many as possible of the twenty *guṇas*; another meaning is that it should be able to cure many diseases (broad spectrum).
- *Sampannam*—the medicine should be collected properly according to its natural habitat, type of soil, climate, variety, and qualities. It should also be from a clean place (e.g., organic cultivation).
- *Yogyam*—should be given exactly in the right context or *avastha* as described earlier.

There are certain places from where one should and should not collect the medicines. Medicine should be collected from *dhanva* (growing on dry soil), *sādhāraṇa deśa* (place of moderate climate), a clean place, and so on. During ancient times, the concept of growing herbs for business was not practiced. Medicinal herbs were collected from the forest or were found growing freely on the ground, which were freshly collected by clients to make their medicines.

From Caraka Samhita CS Sū. 9.5 (definition of *cikitsa* [treatment])

caturṇāṁ bhiṣagādīnām śastānām dhātu-vaikṛte
pravṛttir-dhātu-sāmyārthā cikitsety-abhidhīyate

Correcting the vitiations in tissues and normalizing their equilibrium using the four items—physician, drug, attendant, and patient—is called treatment.

In regards to *dakṣa, Suśruta* explains in SS Sū. 4.7

ekaṁ śāstram-adhīyāno na vidyāt-śāstra-niścayam
tasmād-bahuśruto śāstraṁ vijānīyāt cikitsakaḥ

One whose assessment is based only on one science cannot understand the conclusion. Therefore a physician should know and hear many different sciences (e.g., *jyotiṣa*, *Vedic* astrology; *vāstu*, *Vedic* architecture; yoga, etc.).

From *Aṣṭāṅga Saṅgraha* Sū. 2.12

śastraṁ śāstrāṇi salilaṁ guṇa doṣa pravṛttaye
pātrāpekṣīṇyataḥ prajñāṁ bāhuśrutyena bṛṁhayet

The good or bad of the weapon, science, and water depend on the user. Hence, one should enhance their knowledge by the study of many sciences.

Just as in modern medicine, a drug can be used in the form of syrup, pill, aerosol, or intravenous form; in *Āyurveda*, a herb can be used as decoction, fermented alcohol, fresh juice, medicated ghee, and so on. If a certain herb or substance is capable of being used in all these forms, it is considered superior.

***Āyurvedarasāyana*:** *Hemādri* has quoted from *Aṣṭāṅga Saṅgraha* (chapter 2, verses 7–17, 20, 24, 33–37) to explain this verse. One who deserves to be called a physician has the following qualities:

1. Invincible in debate
2. Unopposed
3. Steadfast
4. Friendly
5. Polite to all
6. Pleasing in appearance

7. Learned in many different sciences (astrology, *yoga*, etc.)
8. Knows the appropriate time for every activity
9. Knows the deeper meanings of the ancient *Āyurvedic* texts
10. Looks after the sick and destitute as his or her own children
11. Has received permission from his or her *guru* to practice medicine
12. Possesses four kinds of knowledge—causes, symptoms, treatment, and prevention of diseases
13. Does not expect to receive gifts from patients
14. Does not start the treatment without a clear diagnosis of the disease

Next is the description of an incompetent physician:

1. Conversant with the science but unskilled in work
2. Gets disillusioned when approaching patient
3. Audacious
4. Not respected by the wise elders

Science alone is insufficient. *Suśruta* compares the person who has a lot of information but does not know their practical application to a donkey that carries heavy loads without knowing what it is carrying. The physician must learn to use his or her intelligence coupled with training under wise gurus to interpret the knowledge appropriately.

AH Sū. 1.29

Four qualities of a nurse

अनुरक्तः शुचिर्दक्षो बुद्धिमान् परिचारकः॥२९।

anuraktaḥ śucir-dakṣo buddhimān paricārakaḥ

anuraktaḥ – loving; *śuciḥ* – hygienic, having pure intentions; *dakṣa* – skilled; *buddhimān* – intelligent (able to understand quickly the instructions of the physician); *paricārakaḥ* – nurse, caretaker, assistant

Treatment

The nurse or caretaker should be loving, pure, clean, skilled, and intelligent.

Commentary

The role of the nurse or caregiver cannot be underestimated. This includes all the people who are involved in the care of the patient including family members. The behavior of a nurse should be caring and loving. This means to have a positive frame of mind, using loving words, encouraging, and giving mental strength to the patient. Sometimes the patient may become unwilling to take the treatment. At such a time, the nurse should be able to convince the patient cleverly and continue the treatment uninterrupted. A nurse should also have pure intentions and maintain hygiene of body and environment. It need not be emphasized that good intention alone is not sufficient, but the nurse should also be skilled in his or her work. Intelligence means to understand and carry out the instructions of the physician with diligence, precision, and speed. At times it is also important to be able to understand what has not been told by the physician and do accordingly. A nurse should have a good presence of mind.

AH Sū. 1.29 (contd.)

Four qualities of a patient

आढ्यो रोगी भिषग्वश्यो ज्ञापकः सत्त्ववानपि॥२९॥

āḍhyo rogī bhiṣag-vaśyo jñāpakaḥ sattvavān-api //29//

āḍhyo – wealthy enough to afford treatment, possessing what is required; *rogī* – patient; *bhiṣak-vaśyo* – willing to be controlled by the physician (obedient); *jñāpakaḥ* – communicative; *sattvavān* – mentally strong, stable and peaceful (having sattvic qualities); *api* – also

Translation

The patient should be affording, obedient, communicative as well as mentally pure and strong.

Commentary

Here it is mentioned that ideally a patient should be *sattvavān* meaning one who is *sattvic* in thoughts and actions. The patient should also be able to afford the treatment. This should be clarified before starting the treatment to avoid misunderstanding and frustration midway. It is important that the patient is compliant with the instructions of the physician without which no treatment will be effective. Treatment is a team work. The communication should be open and frank. One should not hide any information from the physician as it may influence the treatment decisions. Regular updates are also important.

The word *āḍhyo* has often been translated as wealth in terms of money. There is a deeper meaning to this. Poor means a person who always feels that whatever she or he has is enough and desires more and more. Wealthy means a person who is satisfied with what she or he has and is peaceful. It means poverty in mind. It means increased attachment to objects of the senses.

AH Sū. (supplemental verse)

Prognosis of diseases

साध्योऽसाध्य इति व्याधिर्द्विधा, तौ तु पुनर्द्विधा॥
सुसाध्यः कृच्छ्रसाध्यश्च, याप्यो यश्चानुपक्रमः॥

sādhyo'sādhya iti vyādhir-dvidhā tau tu punar-dvidhā
susādhyaḥ kṛcchra-sādhyaśca yāpyo-yaścānupakramaḥ //??//

sādhyo – curable; *asādhya* – incurable; *iti* – thus; *vyādhir* – diseases; *dvidhā* – classified into two types; *tau* – those; *tu* – but; *punar-dvidhā* – again two types; *susādhyaḥ* – easily curable; *kṛcchra-sādhyaś* – cured with difficulty; *ca* – and; *yāpyo* – not curable but kept under control with medicines, diet and lifestyle changes; *yaśca* – and those; *anupakramaḥ* – incurable or fatal (those in which nothing can be done)

Translation

Diseases are classified into two types: curable and incurable. The two types are again classified into two each. Curable is divided into easily curable and cured with difficulty. Incurable diseases are divided into those can be kept under control and fatal.

Commentary

Rarely do people who even know about *Āyurveda* turn to it at the very early signs of disease. Most of the clients who turn to *Āyurveda* in the present times, have eventually reached the advanced incurable stage. Due to this reason, long-term, continuous treatments along with diet and lifestyle changes are inevitable to keep their diseases under control. In my humble opinion, almost all chronic diseases should initially be treated with *Āyurvedic* methods and turned over to modern medicine only when *Āyurveda* does not give desired results. This is because almost all chronic diseases are *yāpya* even in their early stages from the perspective of modern medicine, but they can be cured using *Āyurveda* if detected at an early stage.

It is very important for a practitioner to recognize the four categories and give a realistic expectation to the client. This is why *dṛṣṭa karma* or practical experience on the part of the *vaidya* as explained earlier is important. This will improve the credibility of the practitioner and avoid disappointment for the client.

The definition of *yāpya* is given in SS Sū. 23.10–11,

yāpanīyaṁ vijānīyāt kriyā dhārayate tu yaṁ

kriyāyāṁ tu nivṛttāyāṁ sadya eva vinaśyati

prāptā kriyā dhārayati yāpya-vyādhi-tam-āturaṁ

prapatiṣyad-ivāgāraṁ viṣkambhaḥ sadhu-yojitaḥ

"The *yāpya* diseases are those which can be kept under control with the help of treatment but will become fatal as soon as the treatment is withdrawn just as the house is supported as long as the pillars are properly placed but will collapse as soon as the pillars are removed."

Even if all the four limbs (*catuṣpada*) of treatment are perfect, there are some more factors which determine the prognosis of the disease and success of treatment.

AH Sū. 1.30

Features of curability and incurability

Factors suggesting good prognosis

सर्वौषधक्षमे देहे यूनः पुंसो जितात्मनः॥ ३०॥

अमर्मगोऽल्पहेत्वग्ररूपरूपोऽनुपद्रवः॥ ३०॥

sarvauṣadha-kṣame dehe-yūnaḥ puṁso jitātmanaḥ

amarmago'lpa-hetvagra-rūpa-rūpo'nupadravaḥ //30//

sarva – complete; *auṣadha* – medicine; *kṣame* – effectiveness, ability to tolerate the potency; *dehe* – by the body; *yūnaḥ* – along with; *puṁso* – person (the patient); *jitātmanaḥ* – self controlled;

amarmago – not on any vital body parts; *alpa* – trivial; *hetu* – cause; *agra-rūpa* – (pūrva rūpa) prodromal symptoms; *rūpa* – signs and symptoms; *anupadravaḥ* – not having complications

Translation

The body of the person should have the ability to tolerate the potency of the medicine and treatments. The person should be self - controlled; the vital body parts, uninjured; have very few causative factors; and, though having prodromal and visible signs of disease, not having any complications. (This suggests good prognosis.)

Commentary

Many times it is not possible to perform *śodhana* treatments (pañcakarma) due to the fact that the person is too weak and will be unable to digest the medicines or withstand the severity of the treatments, which further weakens the body. This is called *balaḥ* (strength) and is one of the items of the patient examination. This is also why the second point mentioned is *yūnaḥ* (youthful), as small children, pregnant women, the elderly, and those who are excessively weakened due to the disease are usually contraindicated from strong cleansing therapies due to a lack of strength.

The word *pumsaḥ* indicates a male body. There is a scientific reason why a male body has greater resilience and ability to recover from illness. This could appear as a male chauvinistic statement. But it is not. *Āurveda* recognizes the physiological and psychological differences between both the sexes which is confirmed by modern research as well. The reasons are detailed in *śārīra sthāna* of the *Aṣṭāṅga Hṛdayam.*

It is mentioned that a person receiving *Āyurvedic* treatment should be self-controlled (*pumso jitātmanaḥ*). Self-control is an important aspect of the treatment. When one is ill, the mind is also affected and tends to be fickle. One should be realistic and have faith in the physician and treatment. Some people are often quick to criticize *Āyurvedic* treatment with incomplete understanding, saying, "I tried it, but I did not get well, and *Āyurveda* is not effective." This can discourage patients who are trying to receive treatment and genuine *vaidyas* who are offering authentic treatment. It is unhealthy and offensive to hear such negative comments about *Āyurveda* and Lord *Dhanvantari.* One should keep a respectful distance from such people whose faith is disturbed.

Self-control also implies the willingness to accept the difficulties involved in carrying out the treatment. One must be willing to undergo discipline and do whatever is required in order to get cured from the illness. It may not be easy to follow the rules and regulations prescribed, but they have to be done without any doubt or consideration.

Who is *jitātmana*? "*Jitātmana praśātasya paramātmā samāhita...*" (BG 6.7). So in order to become *jitātmana*, one must cultivate some spiritual understanding.

There are several vital energy points and organs in the body that if affected can make the situation worse. A physician should be able to check and confirm whether there has been any injury to the *marmas*. There are specific treatments prescribed for conditions involving injury or trauma to the *marmas*.

The causative factors can be divided into modifiable and nonmodifiable. For example, age is a factor that cannot be modified. Diet is a factor that can be modified. And the severity of the factors should also be assessed.

The earlier one approaches the *vaidya*, the better it is in terms of prognosis as described earlier. The early symptoms of disease are called *agrarūpa* or *pūrvarūpa*. If one can identify the disease at this stage, there is an almost guaranteed curative response.

Sarvāṅgasundara: *sarva auṣadha kṣamate* includes the ability to tolerate (*kṣamate*) *tīkṣṇa*, *madhya* and *mṛdu* medicines. Medicines grown in different places. *Śamana* and *śodhana* medicines. The word *pumsaḥ* means that men will have better prognosis than women. (this could be because women's bodies are generally softer – *mṛdu*).

AH Sū. 1.31

Factors suggesting good prognosis (contd.)

अतुल्यदूष्यदेशर्तुप्रकृतिः पादसम्पदि॥ ३१॥

ग्रहेष्वनुगुणेष्वेकदोषमार्गो नवः सुखः॥ ३१॥

atulya-dūṣya-deśa-ṛtu-prakṛtiḥ pāda-sampadi

graheṣv-anuguṇeṣv-eka-doṣa-mārgo navaḥ sukhaḥ //31//

atulya – dissimilar; *dūṣya* – vitiated body tissues; *deśa* – habitat or place of residence; *ṛtu* – season; *prakṛti* – constitution; *pāda* – limbs (the four limbs of treatment); *sampadi* – in excellent condition, beneficial, in abundance; *gṛheṣv-anuguṇeṣu* – favorable planetary astrological influence; *eka doṣa* – arising from only a single *doṣa*; (*eka*) *mārgo* – manifesting in one disease pathway (of the *doṣa*); *navaḥ* – newly manifested (early stage of disease); *sukhaḥ* – is easy (to cure)

Translation

The factors for good prognosis of a disease are dissimilarity (incongruence) between the vitiated tissues, habitat, season and constitution. Having the four limbs of treatment in excellent condition, favourable planetary influences, imbalance of only a single *doṣa*, the disease manifesting in only one pathway and being of recent onset are also factors for good prognosis.

Commentary

Twelve factors are mentioned here for good prognosis. The more number of factors that are present, the better is the prognosis. The *pāda-sampadi* (four limbs of treatment) are physician, medicine, paramedical staff, and patient (ref AH Sū.1.27). Here the importance of medical astrology is also clearly indicated by saying that it is also important for the planets to be favorably disposed to have good results with the treatment. That is called *daiva vyapāśraya cikitsa*. Sometimes, the treatment given is correct and yet the disease is not cured. Then one should understand that it may not be favorable astrologically.

The three *doṣa mārgas* (pathways of disease)—*abhyantara* (internal), *bāhya* (external), *and madhyama* (middle)—are described in AH Sū. 12.44–48, and the prognosis depends on the pathway/s which the *doṣa/s* has/have traversed in the body. The word *mārga* can also refer to *srotas* or channels.

Astrology can indicate the diseases that have formed due to sinful activities of past life. The astrological chart can also indicate the parts of the body which are weak, the types of imbalances that can occur, and the times during life when they could manifest. If the astrological combinations are not favorable, even the best treatments will be futile. In such cases, there are certain *pūjas* (rituals) that need to be done before the treatment to try to correct the astrological inconsistencies. These are described in books such as *Hārita Samhita, Vīrasimhāvalokanam, Sāyaṇīyam*, and so on.

It is also mentioned that when similar properties of tissues, location, season, and constitution converge to produce a disease, it becomes difficult to cure as all the factors contribute to exacerbate the condition. In such a case the prognosis is bad (e.g., a disease affecting a *vāta* tissue, in a *vāta* location, in a *vāta* season, in a person with *vāta* constitution *(prakṛti)*). And when there is dissimilarity, it indicates good prognosis, because one factor will not support the other to exacerbate disease. This is also described using the terminologies *prākṛta* or *vaikṛta*. *Prākṛta* means having the same qualities as and *vaikṛta* means the opposite. Eg. The prognosis of *vāta* predominant *jvara* varies with respect to *kāla* (time or season). *Āyurvedadīpikā* explains that all *vāta* predominant *jvaras* are *kṛcchrasādhyaḥ* (difficult to cure) in the rainy season and so it is called *vaikṛta* (You will learn the qualities of the different seasons in Chapter 3) where as in spring and autumn it is *sukhasādhya* (easy to cure) and hence called *prākṛta*.

AH Sū. 1.32

Difficult prognosis

Curable with difficulty (*kṛcchra sādhya*) and incurable (*yāpya*) but manageable diseases

शस्त्रादिसाधनः कृच्छ्रः सङ्करे च ततो गदः॥ ३ २॥
शेषत्वादायुषो याप्यः पथ्याभ्यासाद्विपर्यये॥ ३ २॥

śastrādi-sādhanaḥ kṛcchraḥ saṅkare ca tato gadaḥ
śeṣatvād-āyuṣo-yāpyaḥ pathyābhyāsād-viparyaye //32//

śastrādi sādhana – requiring surgical instruments; *kṛcchraḥ* – difficult to cure; *saṅkare* – mixed together (more than one *dūṣya*, *mārga* etc); *ca* – and; *tato* – that which; *gadaḥ* – disease; *śeṣatvād* – what is left or remaining; *āyuṣo* – of the life-span; *yāpyaḥ* – to remain cured; *pathyābhyāsād* – following the suitable rules of diet and lifestyle; *viparyaye* – reversed, altered, to turn around.

Translation

Diseases requiring surgery, with multiple involvement of *doṣas*, *dhātus*, and pathways (*rogamārga*) are difficult to cure. They can be kept under control for the remaining life-span by following a strict regimen, which is opposite to the disease.

Commentary

Here again the role of medical astrology or destiny is indicated by the word *āyuṣo*. In spite of all the factors being unfavorable, if the person is *destined to live*, they can be managed on rules of diet and lifestyle. This is the most powerful factor—time. Destiny is also called *karma*, which can be understood by studying the astrological chart of the patient to calculate their life-span. If they are destined to live, there is a good chance of cure.

The strength of this single most important factor is to be specially noted with respect to all the others. That also means that if all the other factors are favorable but this one factor is not, then there is little chance of recovery. A *vaidya* cannot change the destiny of a person. He or she can only act as an instrument of destiny for the patient. This is a humbling truth.

In the traditional system, when a patient comes to the *vaidya*, the first thing he or she often looks at is the astrological chart to determine whether there is a *yoga* (astrological combination of planets) indicating long life. If the chart indicates that the life-span of the body is completed, then it is not advisable to attempt intensive treatments. The patient only needs to be made comfortable and prepared to die.

Life is like a journey and the astrological chart is like the map. The body is like a car. The car is required only until the destination is reached. Each car has its own expiry date and the driver has to change the vehicle to continue the journey. This is understood from astrology.

Why is *vyādhi saṅkara* (combination of one or more diseases in the same person) considered *kṛcchra sādhya (difficult to cure)?* This is because the treatment for one will contradict the other disease (*viruddha upakramatva)*

In such disease, the most important factor as mentioned here is the *pathyābhyāsa* of the lifestyle and regimen to avoid any factor that can aggravate the condition. Without following a strict regimen, any medicine will be of little use. First of all one should find a *vaidya* who is able to prescribe such a regimen specific for the condition (*ātura vṛtti*). This is not easily found these days where more emphasis is on medicines and less on the lifestyle and diet regimen. By following the correct regimen, one cuts out all the causative factors that aggravate the disease, and thus, the disease is arrested where it is unable to progress further.

The words *śeṣatvād āyuṣo* indicate that the person is only alive because the life span is not complete. In such cases, practising *pathya* opposite to that of the *roga* is recommended. The death of a person is said to occur when the *āyus* and *puṇya* is exhausted. If there is a severe affliction on the body, death is possible even if there is *āyus* remaining due to the impact of the affliction. *Cikitsā* can only help in such cases where *āyus* is still remaining. This is why it is also advised to check the *āyuḥ* of the person before beginning the treatment, especially in the case of serious illnesses. If there is no *āyuḥ* remaining, *cikitsā* cannot help.

There are some disease conditions where surgery is warranted. A good *vaidya* should be able to differentiate these conditions and refer the *rogī* to a surgeon to avoid wastage of time. The details about *doṣas*, *dhātus*, and disease pathways are described in chapters 11 and 12.

AH Sū. 1.33

Incurable and fatal diseases (*anupakrama*)

अनुपक्रम एव स्यात्स्थितोऽत्यन्तविपर्यये॥ ३ ३॥
औत्सुक्यमोहारतिकृद् दृष्टरिष्टोऽक्षनाशनः॥ ३ ३॥

anupakrama eva syāt-sthito'tyanta-viparyaye
autsukya-mohārati-kṛd dṛṣṭariṣṭo'kṣa-nāśanaḥ //33//

anupakrama – incurable, unmanageable, not to be entertained; *eva* – certainly; *syāt* – of these; *sthito* – situated; *atyanta* – severely; *viparyaye* – opposite, perverse, contrary to; *autsukya* – anxiety; *moha* – delusion; *ārati* – restlessness; *kṛt* – showing; *dṛṣṭa* – able to see; *ariṣṭa* – visible signs and symptoms of end of life; *akṣa nāśanaḥ* – when the sense organs stop functioning

Translation

When the situation is severely opposite (gravely contrary), the disease is said to be incurable. One will be able to perceive the visible signs of the end of life such as anxiety, delusion, and restlessness.

Commentary

The word used in AH Sū 1.32 is *viparyaye* (opposite) and those used in AH Sū 1.33 are *atyanta viparyaye* (severely opposite).

Here you can see the use of the three words that were used in the invocation verse, which are the initial causes of all diseases. These three symptoms are observed in both the beginning of a disease as well as the end of life. They are also called *ariṣṭa lakṣaṇā* (omens of death). Patients who are at the end of their lives are seen to exhibit delusions, restlessness, anxiety, and so on.

Āyurvedic physicians supposedly had the ability to predict death in advance using the science of *ariṣṭa lakṣaṇa*. This is why treatment is stopped to avoid further inconvenience to the patient. Many details of the science of predicting the end of life are given in *Aṣṭāṅga Hṛdayam*, *Śārīra sthāna* (chapters 5 and 6); *Caraka Samhita*, *Vimāna sthāna*; and *Suśruta Samhita*, *Sūtra sthāna.*

The indriyas (sense-organs) function properly only in the presence of adequate ojas. During the end of life, there is severe depletion of ojas and hence the sense organs begin to shut down. This is called akṣa nāśanaḥ.

> Chapter 1 is the essence of the entire content of *Aṣṭāṅga Hṛdayam* and the *ācārya* closes the description by making the point that one should exercise careful discrimination in accepting patients for various reasons.

AH Sū. 1.34

Situations when patients may be avoided

त्यजेदार्तं भिषग्भूपैर्द्विष्टं तेषां द्विषं द्विषम्॥ ३४॥

हीनोपकरणं व्यग्रमविधेयं गतायुषम्॥ ३४॥

चण्डं शोकातुरं भीरुं कृतघ्नं वैद्यमानिनम्॥ ३५॥

tyajedārta bhiṣag-bhūpair-dviṣṭaṁ teṣāṁ dviṣaṁ dviṣaṁ

hīnopakaraṇaṁ vyagram-avidheyaṁ gatāyuṣaṁ //34//

caṇḍaṁ śokāturaṁ bhīruṁ kṛtaghnaṁ vaidyamāninaṁ

Translation

These are the situations in which a physician may decide to reject a patient

tyajet: – must be rejected; *ārta* – one who is distressed (patient)

1. *bhiṣag (physician) bhūpair (king) dviṣṭaṁ* - one who is hated by physician & king (public enemy, criminal, etc.). Here the word *king* represents the *state*. This is related to the social situation of the day, so it should be interpreted as present-day laws and government structures.
2. *Teṣāṁ dviṣaṁ dviṣam*—patient who has feelings of animosity toward the physician or vice versa (ideally both should have positive feeling toward each other) or patient who has some other hidden agenda apart from healing
3. *Hīna upakaraṇaṁ*—if the *vaidya* is deprived of equipments, prerequisites, and facilities for treatment

4. *Vyagraṁ*—restless, busy with other activities (not having time for treatment), distracted, unwilling to make treatment a priority, not sticking to the instructions of the *vaidya*
5. *Avidheyaṁ*—unregulated patient (doesn't follow the *vidhi*, *pathya*, *apathya*, etc.) due to lack of faith or other reasons, This is the opposite of *bhiṣak vaśya* explained in AH Sū 1.29
6. *Gatāyuṣaṁ*—whose life-span has run out (one who is at the end of life), for example, showing end-of-life symptoms (*ariṣṭa lakṣaṇa*)
7. *caṇdaṁ*—angry, wrathful, impetuous, evil minded, violent, destructive, cruel
8. *śokāturaṁ*—afflicted with grief (always negatively thinking, pessimistic, and complaining)
9. *bhīruṁ*—fearful. This indicates a person who lacks *sattva bala* explained in AH Sū 1.29

10. *kṛtaghnaṁ*—ungrateful (for the hard work of the physician and assistants)

11. *vaidya-māninaṁ*—thinks himself to be a physician *or vaidya-amāninam* (does not respect the physician)

Commentary

In today's world we find several patients in this category. There are few who have genuine faith in *Āyurveda*. Most of the patients turn to *Āyurveda* as a final resort (a last-ditch stand) when they run out of options in modern medicine. This could also probably be due to a lack of awareness among modern physicians about other healing systems, thus being unable to refer the patient to receive *Āyurvedic* treatment for suitable ailments.

Another reason for this is that *Āyurveda* has not been properly practiced. Untrained and/or unqualified people claiming to be *vaidyas* have inflicted great harm upon the science by disturbing the faith of the general populace and the medical doctors. It is the responsibility of the custodians of *Āyurveda* to make sure that the authenticity of the science is preserved and education is conducted along those lines. In spite of that, there are still many, who have implicit faith in *Āyurveda* and the number is growing.

Note: Qualification does not only mean having a university degree, but it more importantly means having the qualities of a *vaidya* as enumerated in the textbooks.

There is an apparent contradiction between what is being said here and what is said in AH. 2.24, "*vimukhān-nārthīnaḥ kuryāt,*" meaning one should never reject a patient and it is also said elsewhere that a patient should be treated as your own child. The mention in AH 2.24 is not only related specifically to a physician-patient relationship. It is a general principle of *sadvṛtta* (good behavior).

Those who are ungrateful are befitting to be rejected because, in spite of the hard work of the physician and others, they may not hesitate to malign the physician and the science of *Āyurveda*. If they are not cured, they may be spiteful not considering that the physician has tried his or her best. If they are cured, they may discredit the physician by proclaiming it as being due to their destiny or saying it is a placebo effect. The physician's work can sometimes be a thankless job. Due to this reason, an ungrateful person can be rejected.

Now *ācārya* gives a narration of the sequential arrangement of the chapters in the book.

Index of the 120 chapters of the *Aṣṭāṅga Hṛdayam (35 to 48)*

AH Sū. 1.35

तन्त्रस्यास्य परं चातो वक्ष्यतेऽध्यायसङ्ग्रहः॥ ३५॥

tantrasyāsya param cāto vakṣyate'dhyāya-sangrahaḥ //35//

tantrasya – of the science; *asya* – of that; *param* – superior; *ca* – and; *ataḥ* – thus; *vakṣyate* – is described; *adhyāya* – chapters; *sangrahaḥ* – compilation

Translation

Thus this supreme science (of *Āyurveda*) has been explained in the following compilation of chapters.

Commentary

The book called *Aṣṭāṅga Hṛdayam* is divided into six sections. They are

1. *Sūtra sthāna*—section of aphorisms;
2. *Śārīra sthāna*—section of the descriptions of the body,
3. *Nidāna sthāna*—section of etiologies of diseases,

4. *Cikitsā sthāna*—section of treatments,
5. *Kalpa siddhi sthāna*—section on preparation of medicines,
6. *Uttara sthāna*—the final section.

AH Sū. 1.36

Section 1: Sūtra sthānam: 36 to 39

आयुष्कामदिनर्त्वीहारोगानुत्पादनद्रवाः॥ ३६॥
अन्नज्ञानान्नसंरक्षामात्राद्रव्यरसाश्रयाः॥ ३६॥

āyuṣkāma-dina-rtvīhā rogānutpādana-dravāḥ
annajñānānnarasaṁ-rakṣā mātrā-dravya-rasāśrayāḥ //36//

āyuṣkāma – quest for longevity; *dina* – *dinacaryā* (daily regimen); *ṛtu* – *ṛtucaryā* (seasonal regimen); *ihā* – these; *rogānutpādana* – *roga anutpādana* – prevention of diseases; *dravāḥ* – *dravadravya vijñānīya* – knowledge of liquids; *annajñāna* – knowledge of nature of food materials); *annarasaṁ rakṣā* – protection of food; *mātrā* – *mātrāśitīyam* – quantity of food; *dravya* – *dravyādi vijñānīyam* (principles of pharmacology); *rasāśrayāḥ* – *rasabhedīyam* (taste and its varieties)

AH Sū. 1.37

दोषादिज्ञानतद्भेदतच्चिकित्साद्युपक्रमाः॥ ३७॥

शुद्ध्यादिस्नेहनस्वेदरेकास्थापननावनम्॥ ३७॥

doṣādi-jñāna-tad-bheda-tac-chikitsā-dvyupakramāḥ
śudhyādi-snehana-sveda-rekāsthāpana-nāvanaṁ //37//

doṣādi-jñāna – *doṣādi vijñānīyam* (knowledge of *doṣa,* etc.); *tad-bheda* – *doṣa bhedīyam* (subclassification of *doṣas*); *tac-chikitsād* – their treatment; *doṣa upakramaṇīyam* (treatment of *doṣas*); *dvi* – *upakramāḥ* – (two types of treatment); *śudhyādi* – *śodhana sangrahaṇīyam* (drugs for therapies); *snehana* – *sneha vidhi* (norms for unction); *sveda* – *sveda vidhi* (norms for sudation); *reka* (*vireka*) and *vamana* (norms for emesis and purgation); *āsthāpana* – *vasti* (enema); *nāvanam* – *nasyam* (nasal medication)

AH Sū. 1.38

धूमगण्डूषदृक्सेकतृप्तियन्त्रकशस्त्रकम्॥ ३८॥
सिराविधिः शल्यविधिः शस्त्रक्षाराग्निकर्मिकौ॥ ३८॥

dhūma-gaṇḍūṣa-dṛk-seka tṛpti-yantraka-śastrakaṁ
sirā-vidhi-śalya-vidhi śastra-kṣārāgni-karmikau //38//

dhūma – *dhūmapāna* (inhaling herbal smoke); *gaṇḍūṣa* – buccal retention; *dṛkseka* – *aścottanāñjana vidhi* (eye drops and collyriums); *tṛpti* – *tarpaṇa puṭapāka* (norms for retention therapies on eye); *yantraka* – blunt surgical instruments; *śastrakam* – sharp surgical instruments; *sirā-vidhi* – venesection; *śalya-vidhi* – foreign body removal; *śastra* – surgical practice; *kṣārāgni-karmikau* – using alkalis and heat

AH Sū. 1.39

सूत्रस्थानमिमेऽध्यायास् त्रिम्शत्...

sūtrasthānam-ime'dhyāyās-trimśat...

sūtrasthānamime – in the *Sūtra sthānam*; *adhyāyās* – chapters; *trimśat* – thirty

Translation

These are the thirty chapters in the section called S*ūtra sthāna.*

Commentary

The thirty chapters in the first section of *Aṣṭāṅga Hṛdayam* called *Sūtra sthāna* are enumerated here. They are

No.	Word in the *Sanskṛt* verse	Name of the chapter	English translation
1.	*Āyuṣkāma*	*Āyuṣkāmīyaṁ*	Quest for longevity
2.	*Dina*	*Dinacaryā*	Daily regimen
3.	*Ṛtu*	*Ṛtucaryā*	Seasonal regimen
4.	*Rogānutpādana*	*Rogānutpādanīya*	Prevention of diseases

5.	*Dravāḥ*	*Drava dravya vijñānīyam*	Knowledge of liquids
6.	*Annajñāna*	*Annasvarūpa vijñānīyam*	Knowledge of nature of food materials
7.	*Annarasaṁ rakṣā*	*Anna rakṣā*	Protection of foods
8.	*Mātrā*	*Mātrāśitīyaṁ*	Quantity of food
9.	*Dravya*	*Dravyādi vijñānīyaṁ*	Knowledge of substances, etc.
10.	*Rasāśrayāḥ*	*Rasabhedīyaṁ*	Classification of tastes
11.	*Doṣādi-jñāna*	*Doṣādi vijñānīyaṁ*	Knowledge of *doṣās*, etc.
12.	*Tad-bheda*	*Doṣa bhedīyaṁ*	Divisions of *doṣas*
13.	*Tad cikitsā*	*Doṣopakramaṇīy aṁ*	Treatment of *doṣas*
14.	*Dvyupakramāḥ*	*Dvividhopakrama ṇīyaṁ*	Two types of treatments

15.	*Śudhyādi*	*Śodhanādisaṅgra haṇīyaṁ*	Groups of drugs for purificatory therapies
16.	*Snehana*	*Sneha vidhi*	Norms for oleation therapy
17.	*Sveda*	*Sveda vidhi*	Norms of sudation therapy
18.	*Reka*	*Vamana virecana vidhi*	Norms of therapeutic emesis and purgation
19.	*Āsthāpana*	*Vasti vidhi*	Norms of therapeutic enema
20.	*Nāvana*	*Nasya vidhi*	Norms of nasal medications
21.	*Dhūma*	*Dhūmapāna vidhi*	Norms of herbal smoke therapy
22.	*Gaṇḍūṣa*	*Gaṇḍūṣādi vidhi*	Norms for mouth gargles, etc.
23.	*Dṛk-seka*	*Āścottana añjana vidhi*	Norms for eyedrops and collyriums

24.	*Tṛpti*	*Tarpaṇa puṭapāka vidhi*	Norms for nourishing therapies of eye
25.	*Yantraka*	*Yantra vidhi*	Norms of blunt surgical instruments
26.	*Śastrakam*	*Śastra vidhi*	Norms of sharp surgical instruments
27.	*Sirā-vidhi*	*Sirāvyadha vidhi*	Norms of venesection
28.	*Śalya-vidhi*	*Śalyāharaṇa vidhi*	Norms of foreign-body removal
29.	*Śastra*	*Śastra karma vidhi*	Norms of surgical practice
30.	*Kṣārāgni-karmikau*	*Kṣārāgni karma vidhi*	Norms of using alkalis and thermal cautery

AH Sū. 1.39 (contd.)

Section 2: Śārīra sthānam

............................शारीरमुच्यते॥ ३९॥
गर्भावक्रान्तितद्व्यापदङ्गमर्मविभागिकम्॥ ३९
विक्रितर् दूतजम् षष्टम्.........................

....*śārīram-ucyate*

garbhāvakrānti-tad-vyāpad-aṅga-marma-vibhāgikaṁ //39//
vikṛtir-dūtajaṁ ṣaṣṭham..

śārīram – of the development of body; *ucyate* – called; *garbhāvakrānti* – embryology; *garbha-vyāpat* – complications of pregnancy; *tad* – that; *aṅga-vibhāga* – anatomy; *marma* – science of vital points; *vibhāgikam* – sections; *vikṛtir* – section on imbalances; *dūtajaṁ* – omens and natural signs, signs of death; *ṣaṣṭham* – six chapters

No.	Word in the *Sanskṛt* verse	Name of the chapter	English translation
31.	*Garbhāvakrānti*	*Garbhāvakrānti śārīra*	Embryology
32.	*Tad-vyāpad*	*Garbha vyāpad śārīra*	Disorders of pregnancy
33.	*Aṅga vibhāga*	*Aṅga vibhāga śārīra*	Classification of body parts
34.	*Marma vibhāga*	*Marma vibhāga śārīra*	Classification of vital points
35.	*Vikṛtir-*	*Vikṛti vijñānīya śārīra*	Knowledge of bad prognosis
36.	*Dūtajaṁ*	*Dūtādi vijñānīyaṁ śārīra*	Knowledge of messengers, etc. (Omens)

AH Sū. 1.40–41

Section 3: Nidāna sthānam

..............................निदानं सार्वरोगिकम्॥४०॥
ज्वरासृक्श्वासयक्ष्मादिमदाद्यर्शोतिसारिणाम्॥४०॥
मूत्राघातप्रमेहाणां विद्रध्याद्युदरस्य च॥४१॥
पाण्डुकुष्ठानिलार्तानां वातास्रस्य च षोडश ॥४१॥

.. nidānaṁ sārvarogikaṁ
jvarā-sṛk-śvāsa-yakṣmādi-madādy-arśo-'tisāriṇāṁ //40//
mūtrāghāta-pramehāṇāṁ vidradhyādy-udarasya ca
pāṇḍu-kuṣṭhānilārtānāṁ vātāsrasya ca ṣoḍaśa //41//

nidānaṁ – *nidāna sthānam*; *sārvarogikam* – all the diseases; *jvarā* – fever; *asṛk* – bleeding; *śvāsa* – breathlessness; *yakṣmādi* – wasting; *madādy* – intoxication; *arśo* – hemorrhoids; *atisāriṇām* – diarrhea; *mūtrāghāta* – urinary disorders; *pramehāṇāṁ* – diabetic and other polyuria disorders; *vidradhyādy* – suppurative infection; *udarasya* – abdominal disorders; *ca* – and; *pāṇḍu* – diseases causing pallor and others; *kuṣṭha* – skin disorders; *anilārtānāṁ* – *vāta* disorders; *vātāsrasya* - of *vāta rakta* disorders; *ca* - and; *ṣoḍaśa* – sixteen (chapters)

No.	Word in the *Sanskṛt* verse	Name of the chapter	English translation
37.	*Sārvarogikam*	*Sarvaroga nidānaṁ*	Diagnosis of diseases in general
38.	*Jvarā*	*Jvara nidānaṁ*	Diagnosis of *jvara (inflammatory pathologies)*
39.	*Asṛk*	*Rakta pitta kāsa nidānaṁ*	Diagnosis of bleeding disease and cough
40.	*Śvāsa*	*śvāsa hidhmā nidānaṁ*	Diagnosis of dyspnea and hiccup
41.	*Yakṣmādi*	*Rājayakṣma, svarabheda, arocka, chardi, hṛdroga, tṛṣṇa nidānaṁ*	Diagnosis of wasting diseases, etc.
42.	*Madādy*	*Madātyaya nidānaṁ*	Diagnosis of alcoholic intoxication
43.	*Arśo*	*Arśas nidānaṁ*	Diagnosis of hemorrhoids

44.	*Atisāriṇām*	*Atisāra grahaṇi nidānaṁ*	Diagnosis of diarrheal diseases and *grahaṇi* (inability to hold the food in the intestines)
45.	*Mūtrāghāta*	*Mūtrāghāta nidānaṁ*	Diagnosis of obstruction/retention of urine
46.	*Pramehāṇāṁ*	*Prameha nidānaṁ*	Diagnosis of turbid polyuria
47.	*Vidradhyādy*	*Vidradhi, vṛddhi, gulma nidānaṁ*	Diagnosis of abscess, hernia, hydrocele, tumors etc.
48.	*Udarasya*	*Udara nidānaṁ*	Diagnosis of abdominal enlargement
49.	*Pāṇḍu*	*Pāṇḍu roga, śopha, visarpa nidānaṁ*	Diagnosis of pallor diseases, edema, rapidly spreading skin lesions
50.	*Kuṣṭha*	*Kuṣṭha, śvitra, kṛmi nidānaṁ*	Diagnosis of skin disease, whitish skin lesions, microbial infections

51.	*Anilārtānāṁ*	*Vāta vyādhi nidānaṁ*	Diagnosis of *vāta* diseases
52.	*Vātāsrasya*	*Vāta śoṇita nidānaṁ*	Diagnosis of *vāta rakta* syndrome

- Chapter on *madātyaya* includes *madaṁ* (intoxication), *mūrccha* (fainting), and *sannyāsa* (coma).
- Chapter on *rājayakṣma* includes *svara bhedam* (speech abnormality), *arocakaṁ* (indigestion), *chardi* (vomiting), *hṛd rogaṁ* (heart disease), *tṛṣṇa* (thirst).
- Chapter on *vidradhi* includes *vṛddhi* (scrotal enlargement), *gulma* (mass in abdomen).
- Chapter on *vāta vyādhi* includes diseases such as *ākṣepaka, apatantraka, āntrāyāma, bahirāyāma, vraṇāyaṁa, hanusramsa, jihvāsthamba, ardita, sirāgraha, pakṣavadha, daṇḍaka, apabāhuka, viśvacī, khañjā-paṅgu, kalāva-khañja, ūrusthambha, kroṣṭuka śīrṣaka, vāta kaṇṭaka, gṛdhrasī, khalli, pādaharṣa, pādadāha* (these are all different diseases occurring due to *vāta vitiation*. They will be discussed later).

Section 4: Cikitsā sthānam: 42 and 43

चिकित्सितं ज्वरे रक्ते कासे श्वासे च यक्ष्मणि॥४२॥
वमौ मदात्ययेऽर्शःसु विशि द्वौ द्वौ च मूत्रिते॥४२॥
विद्रधौ गुल्मजठरपाण्डुशोफविसर्पिषु॥४३॥
कुष्ठश्वित्रानिलव्याधिवातास्रेषु चिकित्सितम्॥४३॥

द्वाविंशतिरिमेऽध्यायाः... ....

cikitsitaṁ jvare rakte kāse śvāse ca yakṣmaṇi
vamau madātyaye-'rśaḥsu viśi dvau dvau ca mūtrite //42//
vidradhau gulma-jaṭhara-pāṇḍu-śopha-visarpiṣu
kuṣṭha-śvitrānila-vyādhi- vātāsreṣu-cikitsitaṁ //43//
dvāvimśatir-ime-'dhyāyāḥ ....

cikitsitaṁ – in the section on management; *jvare* – on inflammation; *rakte* – on blood; *kāse* – on cough; *śvāse* – on breathlessness; *ca* – and; *yakṣmaṇi* – on emaciation, and so on; *vamau* – vomiting; *madātyaye* – intoxication; *arśaḥsu* – hemorrhoids, and so on; *viśi dvau* – two types of intestinal disorders (*atisāra* and *grahaṇi*); *dvau ca mūtrite* – two types of urinary disorders (*mūtṛaghāta* and *prameha*)
vidradhau – deep rooted painful swellings in skin, and so on; *gulma* – round motile or immobile swelling in abdomen changing in size; *jaṭhara* – (*udara*) – abdominal diseases; *pāṇḍu* – vitiated disease of blood accompanied by anemia; *śopha* – edema; *visarpiṣu* – quickly spreading inflammatory painful skin lesions (eg erysipelas);
kuṣṭha – skin diseases; *śvitra* – *tridoṣic* non exudative skin disease resembling leucoderma; *ānila-vyādhi* – *vāta* diseases; *vāta-asreṣu* – a syndrome called *vāta rakta*; *cikitsitam* – treatment (is described); *dvāvimśatir* – twenty two; *ime* – in these; *adhyāyāḥ* – chapters

No.	Word in the *Sanskṛt* verse	Name of the chapter	English translation
53.	*Jvare*	*Jvara cikitsā*	Treatment of *jvara* (inflammatory pathologies)
54.	*Rakte*	*Rakta pitta cikitsā*	Treatment of bleeding diseases
55.	*Kāse*	*Kāsa cikitsā*	Treatment of cough
56.	*śvāse*	*śvāsa hidhma cikitsā*	Treatment of dyspnea and hiccup
57.	*Yakṣmaṇi*	*Rājayakṣmādi cikitsā*	Treatment of wasting diseases, etc.
58.	*Vamau*	*Chardi hṛdroga tṛṣṇa cikitsā*	Treatment of vomiting, heart disease, and intense thirst
59.	*Madātyaye*	*Madātyaya cikitsā*	Treatment of alcoholic intoxication
60.	*Arśaḥsu*	*Arśas cikitsā*	Treatment of hemorrhoids
61.	*Viśi dvau*	*Atisāra cikitsā*	Treatment of diarrheal diseases

62.		*Grahaṇi cikitsā*	Treatment of *grahaṇi* (inability to sustain food in the intestines)
63.	*Dvau ca mūtrite*	*Mūtrāghāta cikitsā*	Treatment of urinary obstruction
64.		*Prameha cikitsā*	Treatment of turbid polyuria disorders
65.	*Vidradhau*	*Vidradhi vṛddhi cikitsā*	Treatment of abscess and *vṛddhi* (the term means enlargement, which is used to indicate inguinal hernia, scrotal hernia, hydrocele, femoral hernia, etc.)
66.	*Gulma*	*Gulma cikitsā*	Treatment of abdominal swellings
67.	*Jaṭhara*	*Udara cikitsā*	Treatment of enlargement of abdomen
68.	*Pāṇḍu*	*Pāṇḍu roga cikitsā*	Treatment of diseases causing pallor
69.	*śopha*	*śvayathu (śopha) cikitsā*	Treatment of edema

70.	*Visarpiṣu*	*Visarpa cikitsā*	Treatment of fast-spreading skin lesions
71.	*Kuṣṭha*	*Kuṣṭha cikitsā*	Treatment of localized skin diseases
72.	*śvitra*	*śvitra kṛmi cikitsā*	Treatment of systemic skin disease causing whitish discoloration and parasites
73.	*Ānila-vyādhi*	*Vāta vyādhi cikitsā*	Treatment of *vāta* diseases
74.	*Vāta-asreṣu*	*Vāta śoṇita cikitsā*	Treatment of *vāta* rakta

In this verse *atisāra* and *grahaṇi* are jointly called *viśi*. This is because both the conditions are imbalances of the digestive system.

In this verse we find that *vidradhi* and *vṛddhi* are jointly called *vidradhau*. This is because both conditions are together in the same chapter, and *vṛddhi*, if not treated, can progress into the condition called *vidradhi*.

AH Sū. 1.44

Section 5: Kalpa siddhi sthāna

.... कल्पसिद्धिरतः परम् ॥४४॥

कल्पो वमेर्विरेकस्य तत्सिद्धिर्वस्तिकल्पना॥४४॥
सिद्धिर्वस्त्यापदां षष्ठो द्रव्यकल्पोऽत उत्तरम्॥४५॥

.... kalpasiddhir-ataḥ paraṁ
kalpo vamor-virekasya tat-siddhir-vasti-kalpanā //44//
siddhir-vastyāpadāṁ ṣaṣṭho dravya-kalpo'ta uttaraṁ

kalpasiddhir – manufacturing and use of medicines; *ataḥ* – thus; *paraṁ* – next; kalpo – making of; vamo – (*vamana*) medicines for therapeutic emesis; *virekasya* – for therapeutic purgation; *tat siddhir* – their accomplishment; *vasti* – therapeutic enemas; *kalpanā* – preparation of formulations; *siddhir* – how to manage; *vastyāpadāṁ* – complications arising from *vasti* procedure; *ṣaṣṭho* – six types; *dravya-kalpo* – making of medicines; *ata uttaram* – now is *Uttara sthāna*

No.	Word in the *Sanskṛt* verse	Name of the chapter	English translation
75.	*Vamor*	*Vamana kalpana*	Emetic recipes
76.	*Virekasya*	*Virecana kalpana*	Purgative recipes
77.	*Tat-siddhir*	*Vamana virecana*	Management of complications of

		vyāpat siddhi	purgation and emesis therapies
78.	*Vasti kalpana*	*Vasti kalpana*	Enema recipes
79.	*Vastyāpadāṁ*	*Vasti vyāpat siddhi*	Management of complication of enema therapy
80.	*Dravya-kalpo*	*Dravya kalpana*	Pharmaceutics

AH Sū. 1.45–46

Section 6: Uttara sthāna: 45 to 48

बालोपचारे तद्व्याधौ तद्ग्रहे, द्वौ च भूतगे॥४५॥
उन्मादेऽथ स्मृतिभ्रंशे द्वौ द्वौ वर्त्मसु सन्धिषु॥४६॥
दृक्तमोलिङ्गनाशेषु त्रयो द्वौ द्वौ च सर्वगे॥४६॥

bālopacāre tad-vyādhau tad-grahe dvau ca bhūtage //45//

unmāde'tha smṛti-bhramśe dvau dvau vartmasu sandhiṣu

dṛk-tamo-liṅganāśeṣu trayo… ....

bālopacāre - care of the new born baby; *tad* - of that; *vyādhau* - diseases; *tad* - of that; *grahe* - planets, evil spirits; *dvau* - two (chapters); *ca* - and; *bhūtage* - two chapters on *bhūtas* (ghosts etc);

unmāde - of depression; *atha* - thus; *smṛti-bhramśe* - loss or aberration of memory; *dvau* - two (chapters); *dvau* - two (chapters); *vartmasu* - eye lids; *sandhiṣu* - of the junctions (i.e. sclera, cornea etc);

dṛk - vision; *tamo* - darkness (eg. cataract); *liṅganāśeṣu* - and of blindness; *trayo dvau dvau* - two chapters each; *ca* - and; *sarvage* - of the whole (eye)

dvau ca bhūtage - two chapters of bhūta vijñānīya and bhūta pratiṣedha

unmāde'tha smṛti-bhraṁśe dvau - two chapters, namely, *unmāda* and *apasmāra*

uvau vartmasu sandhiṣu - two chapters of *vartma and sandhi*

dṛk-tamo-liṅganāśeṣu trayo - three chapters of *dṛṣṭi roga vijñānīya, timira pratiṣedha and linganāśa pratiṣedha*

AH Sū. 1.47

कर्णनासामुखशिरोव्रणे भङ्गे भगन्दरे॥४७॥
ग्रन्थ्यादौ क्षुद्ररोगेषु गुह्यरोगे पृथग्द्वयम्॥४७॥

....*dvau dvau ca sarvage //46//*
karṇa-nāsā-mukha-śiro-vraṇe bhaṅge-bhagandare
granthyādau kṣudra-rogeṣu guhyaroge pṛthak-dvayaṁ //47//

karṇa - ear; *nāsā* - nose; *mukha* - mouth; *śiro* - of head; *vraṇe* - on wound care; *bhaṅga* - bone fracture; *bhagandare* - fistulas; *granthyādau* - cystic swellings, tumors, and so on; *kṣudra* - minor diseases; *rogeṣu* - diseases of; *ca* - and; *guhyaroge* - diseases of genital organs; *pṛthak* - separately; *dvayam* - two (chapters)

- *dvau dvau ca sarvage karṇa nāsa mukha śiro - two chapters each of eye, ear, nose, face and head*

AH Sū. 1.48

विषे भुजङ्गे कीटेषु मूषकेषु रसायने॥४८॥
चत्वारिंशोऽनपत्यानामध्यायो बीजपोषणः॥४८॥

viṣe bhujaṅge kīṭeṣu mūṣakeṣu rasāyane
catvāriṁśo'napatyānām-adhyāyo bīja-poṣaṇaḥ //48//

viṣe - poison of; *bhujaṅge* - of snakes; *kīṭeṣu* - insects, spiders, and so on; *ca* - and; *mūṣakeṣu* - and rodents; *rasāyane* - rejuvenation; *catvāriṁśo* - forty chapters; *anapatyānām* - for those who are devoid of offspring; *adhyāyo* - a chapter; *bīja-poṣaṇaḥ* - on nourishing the seed, that is, semen and ovum (increasing fertility and virility)

No.	Word in the *Sanskṛt* verse	Name of the chapter	English translation
81.	*Bālopacāre*	*Bālopacaraṇīya*	Care of newborn baby
82.	*Tad-vyādhau*	*Bālāmaya*	Treatment of children's diseases
83.	*Tad-grahe*	*Bālagraha pratiṣedha*	Treatment of children afflicted by negative forces

84.	*Dvau ca bhūtage*	*Bhūta vijñānīya*	Knowledge of evil spirits
85.		*Bhūta pratiṣedha*	Treatment of possession by evil spirits
86.	*Unmāde*	*Unmāda pratiṣedha*	Treatment of insanity
87.	*Smṛti-bhramśe*	*Apasmāra pratiṣedha*	Treatment of apasmāra
88.	*Dvau vartmasu*	*Vartma roga vijñānīya*	Knowledge of diseases of eyelids
89.		*Vartma roga pratiṣedha*	Treatment of diseases of eyelids
90.	*Sandhiṣu*	*Sandhi-sitāsita roga vijñānīya*	Knowledge of diseases of fornices, sclera, cornea
91.		*Sandhisitāsita roga pratiṣedha*	Treatment of diseases of fornices, sclera, cornea

92.	*Dṛk*	*Dṛṣṭi roga vijñānīya*	Knowledge of diseases of vision
93.	*Tamo*	*Timira pratiṣedha*	Treatment of *timira*
94.	*Liṅganāśeṣu*	*Liṅganāśa pratiṣedha*	Treatment of blindness
95.	*Sarvage*	*Sarvākṣi roga vijñānīya*	Knowledge of diseases of whole eye
96.		*Sarvākṣi roga pratiṣedha*	Treatment of diseases of whole eye
97.	*Karṇa*	*Karṇa roga vijñānīya*	Knowledge of diseases of ear
98.		*Karṇa roga pratiṣedha*	Treatment of diseases of ear
99.	*Nāsa*	*Nāsa roga vijñānīya*	Knowledge of diseases of nose
100.		*Nāsa roga pratiṣedha*	Treatment of diseases of nose
101.	*Mukha*	*Mukha roga vijñānīya*	Knowledge of diseases of mouth

102.		*Mukha roga pratiṣedha*	Treatment of diseases of mouth
103.	*śiro*	*śiro roga vijñānīya*	Knowledge of diseases of head
104.		*śiro roga pratiṣedha*	Treatment of diseases of head
105.	*Vraṇe*	*Vraṇa pratiṣedha*	Treatment of wounds
106.		*Sadyo vraṇa pratiṣedha*	Treatment of wounds due to external trauma
107.	*Bhaṅga*	*Bhaṅga pratiṣedha*	Treatment of fractures
108.	*Bhagandare*	*Bhagandara pratiṣedha*	Treatment of fistula
109.	*Granthyādau*	*Granthi, arbuda, ślīpada, apaci, nāḍi vraṇa vijñānīya*	Knowledge (diagnosis) of mass lesion, huge *granthis*, swelling in the feet, small swellings in the neck region, sinus/fistula

110.		*Granthyādi pratiṣedha*	Treatments of mass lesion, huge *granthis*, swelling in the feet, small swellings in the neck region, sinus/fistula
111.	*Kṣudra rogeṣu dvayaṁ*	*Kṣudra roga vijñānīya*	Knowledge (diagnosis) of minor diseases (this is huge group of diseases that do not fall under any other category)
112.		*Kṣudra roga pratiṣedha*	Treatment of minor diseases
113.	*Guhyaroge dvayaṁ*	*Guhya roga vijñānīya*	Knowledge (diagnosis) of diseases of genital organs
114.		*Guhya roga pratiṣedha*	Treatment of diseases of genital organs
115.	*Viṣe*	*Viṣa pratiṣedha*	Treatment of poisoning

116.	*Bhujaṅge*	*Sarpa viṣa pratiṣedha*	Treatment of snake poisoning
117.	*Kīṭeṣu*	*Kīṭa lūtādi viṣa pratiṣedha*	Treatment of poison of insects, spiders, etc.
118.	*Mūṣakeṣu*	*Mūṣika alarka viṣa pratiṣedha*	Treatment of poison of rats, rabid dogs, etc.
119.	*Rasāyane*	*Rasāyana vidhi*	Rejuvenation therapy
120.	*Bīja-poṣaṇaḥ*	*Vājīkaraṇa vidhi*	Virilification therapy

Commentary

The *Uttara sthāna* is the last part of the *Aṣṭāṅga Hṛdayam* and deals with seven branches of *Āyurveda across* forty chapters. The seven branches are

1. *Bāla* (pediatrics)—includes pregnancy and women's health as well;
2. *Graha* (about evil spirits);
3. *Ūrdhvāṅga* (diseases of the upper part of body—above the shoulder);
    a. Ophthalmology (eye);
    b. Rhinology (nose);
    c. Otology (ear);
    d. Lips, gums, teeth, tongue, palate, throat;

e. Head;

4. *Śalya* (surgery)—part of it is dealt within the last part of *Sūtra sthāna;*
5. *Viṣa* (toxicology and neutralizing of poisons);
6. *Jara* (rejuvenation and overcoming senility); and
7. *Vṛṣa* (aphrodisiacs and enhancing sexual prowess/virilification).

Here it is clearly mentioned that the chapter on *vājīkaraṇa* or increasing virility is especially meant for procreation of strong and healthy children. This means that *Aṣṭāṅga Hṛdayam* does not advocate the use of the techniques mentioned in the chapter on *vājīkaraṇa,* for the purpose of indiscriminate sex. The descriptions given in the text about superior sexual prowess is only to illustrate the strengthening effects of the treatments.

AH Sū. 1.48½

इत्यध्यायशतं विंशं षड्भिः स्थानैरुदीरितम् ॥४८ १/२॥

ityadhyāya-śataṁ viṁśaṁ ṣadbhiḥ sthānair-udīritam //48½ //

itydhyāya - in these chapters; *śataṁ viṁśaṁ* - one hundred and twenty; *ṣadbhiḥ sthānair* - in six sections; *udīritam* - (all these topics) have been described

Translation

Thus, 120 chapters in six sections have been described.

Names of *Vāgbhaṭa* and chapter

इति श्रीवैद्यपतिसिंहगुप्तसूनु मद्वाग्भटविरचितायामष्टाङ्गहृदय
संहितायां सूत्रस्थाने आयुष्कामीयो नाम प्रथमोध्यायः ॥१॥

iti śrī vaidyapati simhagupta sūnu śrī Vāgbhaṭa viracitāyām-aṣṭāṅga-hṛdaya saṁhitāyāṁ sutra-sthāne āyuṣkāmīyaṁ nāma prathamodhyāyaḥ

iti: - *this; śrī vaidyapati simhagupta sūnu* - *the son of Śrī vaidyapati Simhagupta; śrī Vāgbhaṭa viracitāyām* - *composed by Śrī Vāgbhaṭa; aṣṭāṅga-hṛdaya saṁhitāyāṁ* - *of the aṣṭāṅga hṛdayam samhita; sūtra-sthāne* - *of the Sūtra sthāna; āyuṣkāmīyaṁ nāma* - *named ayuskamiya; prathamodhyāyaḥ* - *the first chapter*

Translation

Thus ends the first chapter of the *Sūtra sthāna* of the *Aṣṭāṅga Hṛdayam* samhita, composed by *Śrī Vāgbhaṭa*, the son of *Śrī vaidyapati Simhagupta.*

Topics in the Chapter

- *Maṅgalācaraṇaṁ* (Invocation)
- Name of chapter and blessings of the sages—1
- Purpose of *Āyurveda*—2
- Advent of *Āyurveda*—3, 4a
- Why was the *Aṣṭāṅga Hṛdayam* written?—4b, 5a
- Eight branches of *Āyurveda*—5b, 6a
- Three *doṣas* maintain and destroy the body—6b, 7a

- The locations of three *doṣās* in body – 7a
- *Doṣa* periods related to age, day, night, and digestion—7b, 8a
- Four types of fires (*agni*)—8b
- Three types of channels: *koṣthas*—9a
- *Prakṛtiḥ* (Individual body constitution)—9b, 10
- Qualities of three *doṣās*—11, 12a
- Types of imbalances—12b
- Seven *dhātūs* (also known as *dūṣyas*)—13a
- Three *malās*—13b
- Increase and decrease of *doṣa* (*deha-paripālanoṣaya*)—14a
- Six tastes enumerated—14b, 15a
- How the six tastes affect the *doṣās*—15b, 16a
- Three kinds of substances (*dravya*)—16b
- Two types of potencies (*vīrya*)—17a
- Three kinds of postdigestive effects (*vipākaḥ*)—17b
- Twenty basic qualities (*guṇāḥ*)—18
- Three causes of disease and health—19
- Definition of disease and health—20
- Two types of diseases, based on origin—20
- Foundation of disease *(rogāḍhiṣṭhānam)*—21a
- Two kinds of *doṣas* of the mind *(mānasika doṣa)*—21b
- Examination of patient *(rogi parīkṣā)*—22a
- Examination of disease *(roga parīkṣā), nidāna pañcakam*—22b
- Three kinds of lands or countries *(deśa)*—23, 24a

- Determining the right time for therapies and medicines—24b
- Two kinds of treatments—25a
- Three kinds of therapies for *doṣās* in the body—25b, 26a
- Three therapies for the *doṣas* of the mind—26b
- Four limbs of treatment—27
- Qualities of physician and other limbs of treatment—28
- Four qualities of a nurse—29a
- Four qualities of a patient—29b
- Prognosis of diseases (supplemental verse)
- Features of curability and incurability
    - Factors suggesting good prognosis—30
    - Factors suggesting good prognosis (contd.)—31
- Difficult prognosis
    - Incurable but manageable diseases (*kṛcchra sādhya* and *yāpya*)—32
    - Incurable and fatal diseases (*anupakrama*)—33
- Situations when patients may be avoided—34, 35a
- Index of the 120 chapters of the *Aṣṭāṅga Hṛdayam*—35b onward

---

1. *"lobh-erṣyā-dveṣa-mātsarya-rāgādināṁ."*
2. *rāga dveṣa vimuktaistu…*
3. *"aśvatthamenam suvirūḍha mūlam asaṅga śastreṇa dṛḍhena chittvā."*
4. In Ā*yurveda* the whole myriad of disease is often addressed using the term *rāgādi.*
5. Imperfect senses, tendency to err, tendency to cheat, become illusioned.
6. Direct perception, inference, comparison, and hearing from authorized persons (*Tarka sangraha).*
7. *Paaram artha* literally means the highest result, that is, spiritual.

8. *Pāṭha, avabodha and anuṣṭhāna*

9. http://www.harekrishna.com/col/books/CLAS/bhag/12_2.html.

10. BG 1.40–43.

11. The three phases of digestion are sweet phase, sour phase, and pungent phase (*madhura avasthāpāka, amla avasthāpāka*, and *kaṭu avasthāpāka*).

12. This is only the inference of *Dr. Sanjay* and not the *ācārya's* explanation.

Chapter 2

दिनचर्या

Dinacaryā

Daily Regimen

Summary of the chapter

The topics described in brief in chapter 1 will be elaborated in the rest of chapters of *Aṣṭāṅga Hṛdayam* of which daily regimen, seasonal regimen and prevention of diseases form chapters 2, 3, and 4. There are external and internal causes of health and disease. The first to be described are the external causes. The external causes have two divisions: diet and lifestyle. Lifestyle has two divisions: for *niyata kāla* (regular or usual) and for *aniyata kāla* (irregular or unusual). Routine or usual activities have two divisions: daily and seasonal. Hence in this chapter the author begins with daily regimen (*dinacaryā*). Since chapter 1 began with the instruction that everything should be done with an aim to attain long life, the daily activities that prolong life are being described.

In short, the daily regimen asks us to wake up before sunrise, empty bowels, brush teeth, apply *nasya* (nasal drops), gargle, massage, exercise, take bath, and apply *añjana* (eye ointment) twice a week. The rest of the chapter details how one should conduct oneself during the day and maintain a positive mental attitude. There are a lot of recommendations on moral, ethical, social, and financial etiquettes of life in this chapter. This is referred to in the *Vedic* fold as *nīti*. There are several books dealing with *nīti* and *Śrī Vāgbhaṭa* has advised us to consult them for elaborate understanding, since it is beyond the scope of this book to go into their details. (Some examples have been included in the commentaries.) Finally the benefits of following this lifestyle are enumerated.

Note: Many of the practices mentioned in the next two chapters were followed hundreds of years ago when the lifestyle, living environments, social structure, and values were much different. The student should study them with the intention of

1. being informed about what was practiced during the ancient times;
2. discovering the unchanging universal principle behind these practices; and
3. innovating ways to adapt and apply these principles in a practical way to modern times

Blindly trying to copy the same practices in the modern scenario may not be always practical or recommended. It is said that, "In matters of principle one should stand like a rock and in matters of style one must flow like the river." In most cases, the conflicts and disagreements occur on the level of application only. Everyone generally agrees with the principle.

Dinacaryā (daily regimen) recommendations involve practices aimed toward achieving a balance of action, speech, and mind. Some of the recommendations are for a healthy body, some for healthy speech, and some for creating a healthy mind-set. All the three have bearing on each other, and they involve personal as well as social aspects.

Sections in the chapter

I. Physical cleansing and nourishment—1 to 20, 32, 33

II. Being virtuous in thought, word, and deed—21 to 26

III. Interpersonal relationships—27 to 29

IV. Synchronizing with the four *puruṣārthās*—30, 31

V. Constant awareness and discrimination of time, place, and person—34 to 45

VI. Conclusion—46 to 49

Key *Sanskṛt* words in this chapter

muhūrta, śauca, ajīrṇa, añjana, nāvana, gaṇḍūṣa, abhyaṅga, vyāyāma, udvartana, snāna, dharma, pāpa, upakāra, karuṇā, trivarga, madhyamam, deha, vāk, cetasā, ceṣṭā, sadvṛtta, āyuḥ, ārogya, aiśvarya

Title Verse

अथातो दिनचर्याध्यायं व्याख्यास्यामः ।
इति ह स्माहुरात्रेयादयो महर्षयः ॥ (गद्य सूत्रं २)

athāto dinacaryādhyāyam vyākhyāsyāmaḥ
iti ha smāhur-ātreyādayo maharṣayaḥ

athāta – therefore; *dinacaryā* – daily regimen; *adhyāyaṁ* – chapter; *vyākhyāsyāmaḥ* – will describe; *iti* – this; *ha sma-āhur* – as spoken by; *ātreyādayo* – *Ātreya ṛṣi* and others; *maharṣayaḥ* – the sages

Translation

Therefore as advised/spoken by the great hermit *Ātreya* and the group of sages, thus is described the chapter on daily regimen.

Commentary

Sarvāṅgasundara: What we do on a daily basis is called *dinacaryā*. The previous chapter was named "quest for longevity" and it was established as the purpose of *Āyurveda*. Longevity is possible only if there is proper lifestyle. Following the daily regimen will be of benefit not only in this world but also the next (i.e., it will also bestow us with spiritual emancipation). One must adopt or adapt to a *dinacaryā* that suits one's body constitution and the environment around.

The discussion of lifestyle in *Āyurveda* is divided into *svastha vṛtta* (regimen for healthy individuals) and *ātura vṛtta* (regimen for diseased individuals). Since prevention of diseases is better than curing, *svastha vṛtta* is given primary importance over *ātura vṛtta*.

The definition of *svastha* is the state when the body, mind, and their various components are in their natural and undistorted state functioning in the optimal manner. The regimen mentioned in chapters 2 and 3 are primarily meant for a *person who is healthy.*

Those who are diseased should follow a modified regimen according to their requirements as advised by their *vaidya* (physician). The only phrase mentioned in the previous chapter about *svastha vṛtta* is "*doṣa sāmyam arogataḥ*" (AH Sū. 1.20)

The subjects in the *Āyurvedic* texts are divided into four: *śarīra* (body), *dravya* (substances), *roga* (diseases), and *cikitsa* (treatment), respectively.

AH Sū. 2.1a

Time of waking up from sleep

ब्राह्मे मुहूर्ते उत्तिष्ठेत्स्वस्थो रक्षार्थमायुषः ॥१॥

brāhme muhūrte uttiṣṭhet svastho rakṣārtham āyuṣaḥ

brāhme muhūrte – a certain time period before sunrise; *uttiṣṭhet* – must wake up; *svastho* – a healthy person; *rakṣārtham* – for the purpose of protecting; *āyuṣaḥ* – longevity

Translation

A healthy person must wake up during the *brahma muhūrta* (last part of the night) for the purpose of protecting health and increasing longevity.

Commentary

According to the *Vedic* calculation of time, there are thirty *muhūrtas* in twenty-four hours. In the case where the days and nights are equal (during equinox) there will be fifteen *muhūrtas* in the day and fifteen in the night. The *Śathapatha Brāhmaṇa* defines muhūrta as one-fifteenth part of the day (Ref. 10.4.2.18 and 12.3.2.5). In *Taittriya Upaniṣad* the fifteen names of the *muhūrtas* are mentioned. *Brahma muhūrta* is the last *muhūrta* of the night.

One *muhūrta* is commonly accepted as forty-eight minutes before sunrise if the duration of day and night are equal. This time of the day is quiet and best for meditation since the *prāṇic* energy flows through the *suṣmna nāḍi* (central energy channel along the spine) readily at this time and your mind will not be distracted easily. Practicing *yoga* and *prāṇāyāma* during *Brahma muhūrta* gives more benefits than during other times of the day. It is a time when the atmospheric energy undergoes transition from predominantly *vāta* to *kapha*.

One can experience lightness and clarity (*vāta*) and have stability (*kapha*) also. It is also not advisable to sleep during the *sandhis* (transition periods—the four transition periods are sunrise, sunset, midnight, and noon) except the one at midnight. In the case of midnight *sandhi*, one should not be staying awake. The word *uttiṣṭhet* indicates that it is a *requirement* for all healthy persons to wake up early and not an option. During *Brahma muhūrta*, there is a predominance of *sattva guṇa* in the atmosphere. This predominance of *sattva guṇa* is the reason why it is advised to get up early and make the most of this time for progressive activities, since *sattva* is an energy of clarity and knowledge.

***Aruṇodaya*:** There are various opinions regarding the duration of *Brahma muhūrta*. One opinion by *Govinda vaidya* is that it is different for different kinds of people. Before sunrise, the final (7½ *nazhika*[1]) 180 minutes are for those who have renounced the world desiring liberation; (5 *nazhikas*) 120 minutes are for those who are great thinkers trying to understand the world and for students; (3¾ *nazhika*) 90 minutes are for ideal *gṛhasthas* (those living with family—householders); (2½ *nazhika*) 60 minutes, for common people; and the last *nazhika* (24 minutes) is for lazy people.

The word *svastho* is significant. Only a *svastha* (healthy person) is advised to wake up early. If you are *asvastha* (unhealthy), you are allowed to take extra rest. It also means that the way you wake up in the morning is an indicator of your health, and spontaneously rising early feeling fresh and energetic is one of the fifteen indicators of good health.

The definition of *svastha* is given in *Suśruta Samhita*:

> *sama doṣa samāgniśca sama dhātu mala kriya*
> *prasannātmendriya manaḥ svasthā ityabhidhīyate*
> —*Suśruta Saṁhita*, *Sūtra sthāna*, Ch. 15, verse 41

"A functional equilibrium of the *doṣa*, *agni*, *dhātu*, and *mala kriya* along with pleasantness of the soul, senses, and mind is known as the state of *svastha*."

The fifteen indicators of health as given by *Kaśyapa* and *Nāgārjuna* are as follows:

annābhilāṣo bhuktasya paripākaḥ sukhena ca
sṛṣṭa-viṇ-mūtra-vātatvaṁ śarīrasya ca lāghavam
su-prasann-indriyatvaṁ ca sukha-svapna-prabodhanam
bala-varṇāyuṣaṁ lābhaḥ saumanasyaṁ samāgnitā
vidyād-ārogya-liṅgāni viparīto viparyayam

—*Kāśyapa Samhita, Khila sthānam*, Ch. 5, verse 6.2–8

Desire for food, easy digestion of ingested food, proper excretion of feces, urine, flatus, lightness of body, clarity of the sense organs, comfortable sleep and waking, strength, complexion and longevity, pleasing mind, and balanced digestion and metabolism are known to be features of good health and the opposite of these features is the opposite of good health.

tal-lakṣaṇaṁ pañcadaśa prakāra
āhāra kāṅkṣa svadanaṁ vipāka
purīṣa mūtrānila sṛṣṭatā ca
tadendriyārtha grahaṇe ca śakti
manaḥ sukhatvam bala varṇa lābha
svapna sukhena pratibodhanam ca
upāyataḥ sādhanam asya vidyā
snehādi yat karma mayā pratiṣṭham

—*Nagārjuna*

"The symptoms of good health are fifteen in number. They are as follows: to have a healthy appetite; to digest the food consumed; expulsion of feces, urine, and flatus; all the senses strong enough to perceive sense objects; pleasant mind; strength; immunity; complexion; and to fall asleep effortlessly at night and wake up feeling rejuvenated in the morning. The technique to achieve this is to follow the daily routines like oleation, and so on."

Kaśyapa and *Nāgārjuna* are both stating the same points about positive health. Often we hear definitions about health where absence of disease is the focus. But here we find a positive definition of health where the factors indicating health are emphasized over absence of disease.

The result of getting up early in the morning is described as *āyuṣa rakṣa* meaning "protection of longevity." It is worth a research study to observe the effects of waking up early in the morning on the quality of life of individuals in comparison to waking up late in the morning.
What should one do in places where the days and nights are very much different in duration and keep changing all through the year? In such cases, it is best to follow a discipline of dividing the twenty-four hours into equal halves and follow that rather than to follow the rising and setting of the sun. For example in a place like Denmark, during the winter the sun sets at about 11:00 p.m. and rises at about 4:30 a.m.

Dealing with daylight saving time

These are artificial adjustments made to make the most of the available day time. The clock time has nothing to do with the way the *doṣas* are changing. That has to be understood by minutely observing the changes taking place in the body in response to changes in the environment. Often people are not in touch with themselves and are unable to recognize these responses. There needs to be development of more sensitivity. That is the only way to deal with it.

As far as waking up is concerned, if the difference is only an hour or so, one can make the adjustments easily.

AH Sū. 2.1b

What to do immediately upon rising?

शरीरचिन्तां निर्वर्त्य कृतशौचविधिस्ततः ॥१॥

śarīra cintāṁ nirvartya kṛta śauca vidhis-tataḥ //1//

śarīra cintāṁ – analyzing one's body; *nirvartya* – after having accomplished or brought about; *kṛta* – perform; *śauca vidhi* – acts of cleansing; *tataḥ* – therefore, from that time

Translation

After waking up one should analyze one's own body carefully and then perform all the procedures for cleansing oneself.

Commentary

When we wake up in the morning, it is advised to take a while to gather our thoughts and situate ourselves properly in our body. While the body is asleep, it is not uncommon for the mind to travel out of the body. But as soon as we wake up, the mind returns to the body and may need some time to settle. If we rush things at this time, it can lead to disorders due to the mind being disconnected from the body.

Śauca vidhi or cleansing schedule indicates that as soon as you wake up, it is a sign of good health to naturally get the urge to pass stool. There are many other types of cleansing to be done that are described ahead. It is very common these days to be constipated and accept it as *normal*. Many people only pass stool once every two to four days. This is the first sign of ill health and its repercussions will be described in chapter 4.

The sitting posture while emptying the bowels is also important. The western toilet (chair position) is not conducive to proper emptying of the bowels compared to the squatting posture. The squatting position relaxes the puborectalis muscle that helps for easier elimination by straightening the canal. This has been proven by research.[2]

Sarvāṅgasundara: By *śarīra cinta*, it is meant that one should analyze whether the food consumed on the previous day has been completely digested or not. If it has not been digested completely, one will feel some heaviness in the body, fullness in the abdomen, lazy, unenergetic, and so on. This is called *rasa ajīrṇa*. In that case one is advised to go back to sleep for some more time till the digestion is completed. (ref. AH Sū 8.29)

AH Sū. 2.2

Herbs used for cleansing oral cavity

अर्कन्यग्रोधखदिरकरञ्जककुभादिजम् ॥२॥

प्रातर्भुक्त्वा च मृद्वग्रं कषायकटुतिक्तकम् ॥२॥

arka-nyagrodha-khadira-karañja-kakubhādijam

prātar-bhuktvā ca mṛdvagraṁ kaṣāya-kaṭu-tiktakam //2//

arka nyagrodha khadira karañja kakubhādijam – names of plants that can be used for brushing the teeth; *prātar* – early in the morning; *bhuktvā* – by chewing; *ca* – and; *mṛdu* – soft; *agram* – tip; *kaṣāya* – astringent; *kaṭu* – pungent; *tiktakam* – bitter

Translation

Herbs like *arka, nyagrodha, khadira, karañja, kakubha*, and so on, which are astringent, pungent, and bitter may be used. Early in the morning, one should chew the tip of the brush to make it soft.

Commentary

Great importance is given to oral care in *Āyurveda*. It is the initial point of entry of the digestive tract, which is the most important channel of the body. A lot of people have problems related to teeth and gums these days. Expensive dental treatments have become common. If these recommendations are followed, one can avoid almost all problems related to teeth, gums, or the oral cavity.

After completing the cleansing in the morning, it is time to brush our teeth. These are the herbs/trees mentioned here:

1. *Arka—Calotropis procera*—Sodom apple
2. *Nyāgrodha—Ficus bengalensis*—Banyan tree
3. *Khadira—Acacia catechu*—Khayir gum
4. *Karañja—Pongamia pinnata* (recently moved to the genus *Milletia*)
5. *Kakubha—Terminalia arjuna*—Kahua bark

The word *ādijam* indicates that these are not the only options and there are many more. The roots of these plants are to be used. The twigs are also used in some places. The roots or twigs can be used as they are or they can be dried and powdered and used with a toothbrush.

All the substances recommended for cleaning the teeth and mouth are *kaṣāya* (astringent), *tikta* (bitter), and *kaṭu* (pungent). These are ideal tastes for cleansing as they have a scraping action and a *kapha* reducing action (as opposed to the sweet toothpastes that are commonly used these days). They cause closure of the tissues by contraction and strengthen the gums to hold the teeth strongly. This is for balancing the *bodhaka kapha* and digesting the *āma* that lodges in the oral cavity. They are also anti-infective. *Neem* (*nimba*) and *babool* (*arimeda*/Sweet Acacia) are also commonly used for brushing. Sweet taste is also recommended by *Suśruta Samhita* in case of children for the sake of palatability.

***Aruṇodaya*:** By the term *ādi*, it should be understood that all the other plants mentioned in the *Aṣṭāṅga Saṅgraha*, namely, *vāta* (banyan tree), *asana* (*myristica*), *arka* (*calotropis*), *khadira* (*acacia*), *karavīra* (*nerurium*), and so on can also be used to brush the teeth. In addition, *koṭṭam*, *triphala*, *trikaṭu*, and *trijāta* can be powdered, mixed with honey, and used for brushing the teeth.

In Kerala, the husk that remains after dehusking and cleaning the paddy is dry roasted till it is charred and is used for cleaning teeth. The midrib of the coconut leaf is used for scraping the tongue as well. This has been a traditional practice for many hundreds of years. Alum is also used for brushing teeth in many areas due to its astringent property.

Bhāvaprakāśa advises to take the root of one of these plants, dip its tip in a mixture of honey and *triphala-kaṭukādi cūrṇa*, and use for cleaning the teeth.

Sarvāṅgasundara: Names of many other herbs are given in *Aṣṭāṅga Ṣaṅgraha* and *Suśruta Samhita.*

AH Sū. 2.3

Size of the brush twig and method of brushing

कनीन्यग्रसमस्थौल्यं प्रगुणं द्वादशाङ्गुलम् ॥ ३॥

भक्षयेद्दन्तपवनं दन्तमांसान्यबाधयन् ॥ ३॥

kanīny-agra-sama sthaūlyaṁ praguṇaṁ dvādaśāṅgulam

bhakṣayed-danta-pavanaṁ danta-māmsāny-abādhayan //3//

kanīnya – the little finger (pinky); *agra* – tip of; *sama* – equal to, similar to; *sthaūlyam* – thickness, width; *praguṇam* – in good condition, straight; *dvādaśa* – twelve; *aṅgulam* – fingers; *bhakṣayet* – after every meal, after chewing; *danta* – teeth; *pavanam* – clean; *danta-māmsāni* – the teeth and gums; *abādhayan* – without hurting or injuring

Translation

The brush should be such that the thickness of the tip is of the size of the little finger, in good condition, straight, and twelve fingers in length. Teeth and gums should also be cleaned after every meal without hurting or injuring them.

Commentary

One should brush carefully without injuring the gums. In some versions the word *sakūrcam* is used instead of *praguṇam*. *Sakūrcam* means "with the brush."

The importance of brushing teeth after every meal is stressed here; *bhakṣa-yet* indicates a *compulsory mood*, which means *must*—an emphasis

AH Sū. 2.4

Contraindications for brushing teeth

नाद्यादजीर्णवमथुश्वासकासज्वरार्दिती ॥४॥

तृष्णास्यपाकहृन्नेत्रशिरःकर्णामयी च तत् ॥४॥

nādyād-ajīrṇa-vamathu śvāsa-kāsa jvarārditī /

tṛṣṇāsya-pāka-hṛn-netra-śiraḥ karṇāmayī ca tat //4//

na – not; *adyād* – by these (*na adyāt* - contraindicated in); *ajīrṇa* – indigestion; *vamathu* – nausea, vomiting; *śvāsa* – dyspnea; *kāsa* – cough; *jvara* – fever; *arditī* – one who has facial palsy; *tṛṣṇā* – thirst; *asya-pāka* – ulcerations and boils in mouth, stomatitis; *hṛd* – heart; *netra* – eyes; *śiraḥ* – head; *karṇa* – ears; *āmayī* – diseases with *āma* toxins; *ca* – and; *tat* – that

Translation

Brushing teeth (according to the procedure mentioned here) is contraindicated in those having indigestion, nausea, vomiting, dyspnea, cough, *jvara*, facial palsy, thirst, mouth ulcers, and diseases of heart, eyes, head, and ears.

Commentary

Āsyapāka: ulcerations in mouth (boils in the mouth) since we are talking about the cleaning of mouth, *āsya* will mean *the mouth*. *Pāka* means cooked or boiled, which means boils or ulcers in this context. *Āmayī*: having a disease

Why are these people not allowed to brush teeth? Possible answers are given below

Brushing teeth is NOT recommended in the following conditions:

- *Ajīrṇa*—indigestion
- *Vamathu*—nausea
- *Śvāsa*—breathlessness
- *Kāsa*—cough
- *Jvara*—an inflammatory reaction

- *Ardita*—facial paralysis
- *Tṛṣṇa*[4]—thirst
- *Āsya pāka*—ulcers in mouth/stomatitis
- *Hṛd netra śiraḥ karṇa āmayī*—diseases of heart, eyes, head, and ears

Ajīrṇa (indigestion)—astringent is heavy and can increase indigestion.

Vamathu (vomiting)—bitter taste increases *vāta* and can aggravate vomiting.

Śvāsa (breathlessness)—all three tastes can cause *vāta* aggravation and so they are especially avoided in *kṣayaja śvāsa.*

Kāsa (cough)—all three tastes cause *vāta* aggravation, which is main cause of *kāsa.*

Jvara (inflammations)—pungent increases *pitta*, astringent is a heavy taste and not good in *agni māndya.*

Ardita (facial palsy)—*vāta* aggravation can increase the problem.

Tṛṣṇa (excessive thirst)—pungent and bitter are drying and hence increase thirst.

Āsya pāka (mouth ulcers)—pungent taste increases *pitta* and can cause ulcers

Hṛd roga (cardiac disorders)—all three can cause increase of *vyāna vāta.*

Netra roga (eye diseases)—*pitta* aggravation can aggravate eye disorders, which are *pitta* predominant.

---

[4] when we say intense thirst for tṛṣṇā in Āyurveda, what is meant is that the entire head region including the tālu and śṛṅghāṭaka marma are drying

Śiro roga (diseases affecting the head)—only if they are *vāta-pitta* type of issues.

Karṇa roga (ear diseases)—ear is a *vāta*-predominant organ, and hence, one should be careful.

The clue to understanding the reason for all the contraindications is in the three tastes that are used for cleansing the mouth—*tikta, kaṭu, kaṣāya* (bitter, pungent, astringent). The excessive use of these tastes cause certain pathologies, and they are mentioned in AH Sū. 10.14–21. Especially see the symptoms of *atiyoga*. That will explain all these conditions. Some of the conditions mentioned will be absolute contraindications, and some will be relative.

Āyurvedarasāyana: Certain types of trees are contraindicated for use in brushing because of their poisonous effects, *madhura, amla, or lavaṇa* (sweet, sour, or salty taste).

AH Sū. 2.5–2.6a

Eye care

सौवीरमञ्जनं नित्यं हितमक्ष्णोस्ततो भजेत् ॥५॥

लोचने तेन भवतः सुस्निग्ध घनपक्ष्मणी ॥५॥

व्यक्त त्रिवर्णे विमले मनोज्ञे सूक्ष्म दर्शने ॥६॥

sauvīram-añjanaṁ nityaṁ hitam-akṣṇos-tato bhajet

locane tena bhavātaḥ susnigdha-ghanapakṣmaṇī //5//

vyakta-trivarṇe vimale manojñe sūkṣma-darśane //6//

sauvīram – made from antimony sulphide; *añjanaṁ* – collyrium; *nityaṁ* – regularly; *hitam* – beneficial; *akṣṇos* – for the eyes; *tataḥ* – then; *bhajet* – put on (repeatedly); *locane* – in the eyes; *tena* – by that; *bhavātaḥ* – occurs, results in; *susnigdha* – unctuous; *ghana* – thick; *pakṣmaṇī* – eye lashes; *vyakta* – well defined; *trivarṇe* – three colors; *vimale* – in cleaning; *manojñe* – making them attractive (to the mind); *sūkṣma-darśane* – bestowing minute or fine vision

Translation

Collyrium made from antimony sulphide should be applied regularly (daily) and is very beneficial for the eyes. By using it, the eye lashes become lubricated and thick, improving the acuity of vision, looking very attractive and pleasing to the mind.

Commentary

Bhajet—also means *to repeat* in an emphatic mood. Some say that *sauvīra* is prepared out of *dehusked yava* (barley), either boiled or unboiled. In some places *sauvīra* is also prepared from *godhūma* (wheat). Another meaning of *sauvīra* is fruit of jujube. Why is the word *trivarṇe* used here?

It means that one will be able to see all the three basic colors—red, blue, yellow—clearly. This indicates that the *ācāryas* knew about the existence of three primary colors and these colors combine to form the entire spectrum of colors.

The eye tends to accumulate *kapha.* These herbs are astringent and help to reduce the *kapha* in the eyes. One to two drops of honey or pomegranate juice can also be used. Pomegranate juice is kapha and pitta pacifying.

Eyes, though pitta predominant organs and fiery in nature, are part of the head region, which is a *kapha*-predominant area (ref. AH Sū 1.7) and hence always at the risk of *kapha* accumulation, thus reducing the fire. *Kapha* will always try to dominate over *pitta* due to the reason that head is the home of *kapha*. Eyes which are fiery organs (*āgneya*) situated on the head are like two fireballs immersed in water and always at risk due to *kapha*, which is watery in nature.

AH Sū. 2.6b–7a

Protecting the eyes from excess *kapha*

चक्षुस्तेजोमयं तस्य विशेषात् श्लेष्मतो भयम् ॥ ६॥

योजयेत्सप्तरात्रेस्मात्स्रावणार्थं रसाञ्जनम्

cakṣus-tejomayaṁ tasya viśeṣāt śleṣmato bhayam //6//

yojayet sapta-rātre 'smāt srāvaṇārtham rasāñjanam //7//

cakṣus – of the eyes; *tejomayam* – (will bestow tejas to the eyes) full of *tejas*; *tasya* – of that; *viśeṣāt* – especially; *śleṣmato* – from *kapha*; *bhayam* – danger, at the risk of; *yaḥ* – that; *jayet* – cures; *sapta rātre* – within seven nights; *asmāt* – thus, due to; *srāvaṇārthe* – for the purpose of draining out (*kapha*); *rasāñjanam* – collyrium

Translation

The eyes are full of *tejas* (fiery energy) and are especially at the risk of *kapha* accumulation. Due to this reason, *rasāñjanam* should be applied once a week for the purpose of draining out the accumulated *kapha*.

Commentary

Viśeṣāt means especially having the risk of accumulation of *śleṣma* (*kapha*). *Tejas* is the refined essence of *pitta*, and the eye is described as *tejomayam* meaning *full of tejas*.

The *kapha* that travels through the *srotas* during daytime stagnates in the night due to sleep and may turn into waste. This waste must be liquefied and expelled using *rasāñjanam* once in seven days.

The upper part of the body has been described to be *kapha* predominant in chapter 1. So here is a special situation where a fiery organ (eyes) is situated in a watery location (*kapha*). So the fire is always under threat of being diminished by the water surrounding it.

What is *rasāñjanam*? The bark of *dārvī* (*chitra*) is made into a *kaṣāya* (decoction) and concentrated into a paste. When *sauvīram* powder (antimony sulphide) is added, it is called *rasāñjanam*.

Many homes in India make their own collyrium out of the black soot formed by the burning of wood fire and processed with medicinal oils. In India we still find men in certain communities applying collyrium in their eyes as a regular practice.

We can also see that the concept of a seven day week was known during the earlier days as well. The number seven is also utilized in many other areas of *Āyurveda* – *dhātus*, oleation, *snehapāna* (treatment involving drinking of *ghee*) and so on.

Aruṇodaya: During daytime, the excess *kapha* is excreted out of the eyes through the concerned *srotas*. But during the night (while sleeping), when the *manovaha* and certain other *srotas*es become nonfunctional, the *kapha* has a tendency to accumulate. This accumulated *kapha* should be removed using *rasāñjanam*.

AH Sū. 2.7b

Nasal irrigation and Gargles and chewing betel leaf

ततो नावनगण्डूषधूमताम्बूलभाग्भवेत् ॥७॥

tato nāvana-gaṇḍūṣa-dhūma-tāmbūla-bhāg-bhavet //7//

tataḥ – after that, then; *nāvana* (*nasya*) – nasal drops; *gaṇḍūṣa* – mouth gargle; *dhūma* – smoke (inhalation); *tāmbūla* – betel nut (chewing); *bhāg* – separately; *bhavet* – should be done

Translation

After that, nasal drops, mouth gargle, inhalation of herbal smoke, and chewing of betel nut should be done separately, one after another.

Commentary

The elaboration of these procedures will come later in *Sūtra sthāna*.

- *Nāvana*—chapter 20

- *Dhūma*—chapter 21
- *Gaṇḍūṣa*—chapter 22

An elegant sequence

The *nasya*, performed after the application of *añjana* in the eyes, will help to expel the *doṣa*s that are brought out from the eyes into the nasopharynx. The *gaṇḍūṣa* done after *nasya* is meant to expel the *doṣa*s brought out by *nasya* from the oropharynx. The *dhūma pāna* (taking in herbal smoke) is meant to pacify the residual *doṣa*s that have remained behind after the previous procedures. Then *betel* leaf is to be chewed along with *pūgādi* (*pūga*, etc—*Areca catechu*) as a final detoxification and to correct the *agni*, which becomes low as a result of the cleansing.

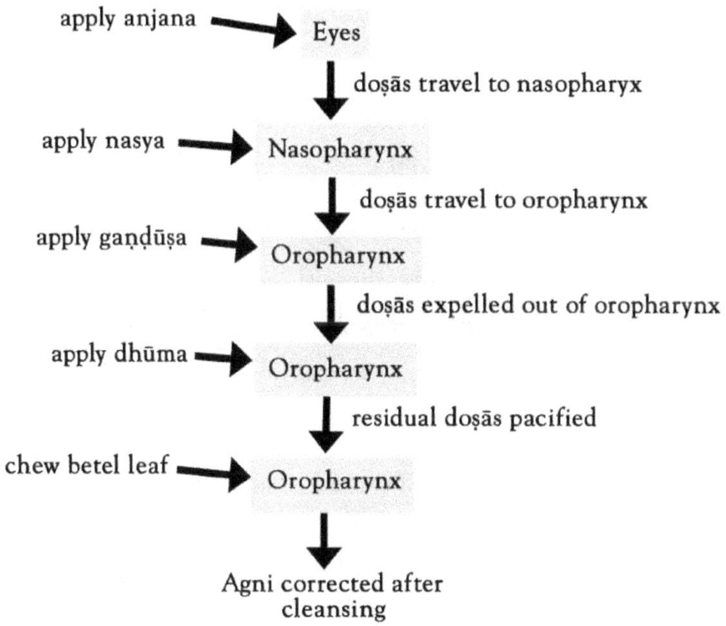

The cleansing goes downwards from the eyes to nose to mouth to pharynx and finally use *betel* leaf which has the special properties to purify and detoxify.

In *yoga* there is a method of cleansing the nasopharynx and associated structures by the method of *jala neti* (flushing the nose with salt water from a *neti* pot). The effect of this practice is different from *nasya*. *Jala neti* causes only local cleansing while *nasya* pulls the *doṣās* from all the surrounding *srotas* into the nasopharynx and pushes it down to the oropharynx.

A common oil used in south India for *nasya* in most households is called *aṇu tailam* (*aṇu*: subtle; *tailam*: oil). It has the ability to balance all the three *doṣa*s. For daily use, two drops in each nostril, after steam inhalation, sixty minutes before bathing is recommended.

For *dhuma*, the simplest method is to smear a piece of cotton cloth with a paste of ghee and turmeric, dry it in shade, roll it into a cigar shape, and use for *dhūma*.

Sarvāṅgasundara: *Betel* leaf is said to have a property called *vaiśadya* (cleansing the *srotas*), *aruci haratva* (improving appetite and taste perception), and *saugandhya* (good odor).

Āyurvedarasāyana: It is explained in *Aṣṭāṅga Saṅgraha* that first *aṇu tailam* should be used for *nasya*. The result is *ghana unnata* (increased compactness), *prasanna tvak* (healthy skin), *skanda* (shoulder), *grīvā* (neck), *āsya* (face), and *vakṣasaḥ* (chest). *Gaṇḍūṣa* is to be done in the order of oil, decoction, and warm water.

Note: Please read the procedure for *nasya* and *dhūma* properly, or consult your practitioner before trying out any of the recommendations.

1. 1 nazhika = approx. 24 minutes.
2. http://www.ncbi.nlm.nih.gov/pmc/articles/PMC4017696/.

AH Sū. 2.8

Contraindications for chewing betel leaf

ताम्बूलं क्षतपित्तास्ररूक्षोत्कुपितचक्षुषाम् ॥८॥

विषमूर्च्छामदार्तानामपथ्यं शोषिणामपि ॥८॥

tāmbūlaṁ kṣata-pittāsra-rūkṣotkupita-cakṣuṣām

viṣa-mūrcchā-madārtānām-apathyaṁ śoṣiṇām-api //8//

tāmbūlam – betel leaf; *kṣata* – wounded, *pittāsṛa* – corruption of *rakta dhātu* due to *pitta* aggravation (a pathological condition called *rakta pitta*); *rūkṣo* – those who have excessive dryness; *utkupita cakṣuṣām* – those with aggravated (inflammatory) eye disorders, *viṣa* – poisoned; *mūrcha* – fainting; *mada* – intoxicated; *ārtānām* – those distressed with; *apathyam* – not allowed to eat; *śoṣiṇām* – those afflicted with wasting type of diseases; *api* – also

Translation

Betel leaf is contraindicated in the wounded and those afflicted by *rakta pitta*, excessive dryness, inflammatory eye disorders, poisoning, fainting, intoxication, and wasting diseases.

Commentary

Ārtānām is a common term for all the conditions mentioned here. These are all *pitta*-aggravated conditions. Betel leaf chewing increases *pitta* and *rūkṣa* (dryness). Hence all the conditions that are *pitta* and *rūkṣa* aggravated are contraindicated. Traditionally betel leaf was chewed after lunch for improving digestion since it increases *pitta*.

Why is it said that one should not eat betel leaf in case of fainting? Fainting is usually due to *pitta* aggravation (ref. AH Sū 12.52). *Betel* leaf aggravates *pitta* due to its *uṣṇa* (hot), and *tīkṣṇa* (sharp) qualities. It also spreads very fast due to *laghu* (light) quality.

In the ***Bhāva prakāśa*** qualities of betel leaf are mentioned as follows:

- *tīkṣṇa*, uṣṇa (sharp/penetrating, heating);
- best among *rocana* (appetizer/digestive) drugs;
- intensifies taste perception;
- *sara* (laxative/mobilizing) property;
- has the taste of *tikta, kṣāra, kaṭu* (bitter, alkaline, and pungent);
- *uṣṇa, madhura, kaṣāya* (hot, sweet, astringent);
- alleviates *vāta*, *kapha*, parasites, and foul smell;
- excites erotic passion, aphrodisiac;
- beautifies and cleanses mouth;
- enhances libido;
- causes bleeding disorders;
- *laghu* (light);

- *vaśyam* (enchanting), used to charm others;
- relieves *kapha*, bad odor, intestinal gas, tiredness;
- clarity of oral cavity;
- fragrance, glow, and grace;
- brightness and charm;
- removes dirt from teeth (tartar) and jaws;
- cleanses tongue; and
- controls regurgitation and throat diseases.

AH Sū. 2.9

Benefits of body massage—with oil

अभ्यङ्गमाचरेन्नित्यं, स जराश्रमवातहा ॥९॥

दृष्टिप्रसादपुष्ट्यायुःस्वप्नसुत्वक्त्वदार्ढ्यकृत् ॥९॥

abhyaṅgam-ācaren-nityaṁ sa jarā-śrama-vātahā

dṛṣti-prasāda-puṣtyāyuḥ-svapna-sutvaktva-dārḍhya-kṛt //9//

abhyañgam – oil massage; *ācaret* – must be performed; *nityaṁ* – regularly; *sa* – that; *jarā* – aging; *śrama* – exertion, exhaustion; *vāta* – (aggravation of) *vāta*; *hā* – destroys; *dṛṣṭi prasāda* – improves vision, *puṣṭi* – nourishment; *āyuḥ* – longevity; *svapna* – (sound) sleep; *sutvaktva* – good skin; *dārḍhya kṛt* – makes strong and sturdy

Translation

Oil massage should be performed regularly. It destroys aging, exhaustion and *vāta*. It improves vision, nourishment, longevity, sleep, health of skin and makes the body strong.

Commentary

After removal of the *sthūla malas* (gross wastes), the *sūkṣma malas* (subtle wastes) are being cleansed now. It is advised to first apply oil on the body and then exercise. Oil will trap the heat inside the body, which allows for sweating when exercising.

The word *kṛt* is common to *puṣṭi* (nourishment), *āyuḥ* (longevity), *svapna* (sleep), *sutvaktva* (healthy skin), and *dārḍhya* (firmness).

How does massage improve vision? There is a *nāḍi* that goes all the way from the feet up to the eyes. When the feet are massaged, these *nāḍi* are stimulated and thus improves the vision.

Whenever the word ends with *-et*, it implies an emphasis or order that *it should be done*. In this verse we can see *ācaret*. -*et* is a potential mood, which is used to express a wish, advice, a request, a possibility, or the near future. It is also used for conditional clauses, for example, "if he would go."

While massaging the body with oil, it is usually done in the direction of the body hairs and this is called *anuloma* in technical language. This helps to move the toxins toward the *koṣṭha* and get eliminated. But in the case of *udvartanam* (AH Sū 2.16), the movement of massage is in the opposite direction of the body hairs and is called *pratiloma* in *Sanskṛt*.

Regular massage is one of the best ways to pacify *vāta* aggravation, which causes degeneration of the body. This is the reason why regular massage is the single most effective antiaging technique. The skin is the largest sense organ of the body, and thus, the application of oil on the skin will help to make a significant impact.

Āyurvedarasāyana: The process of *abhyaṅga* stimulates the appetite. The oil enters into the *srotas* of the body through the pores of the skin and spreads all over the body and is digested by the *agni*. *Aṣṭāṅga Sangraha* states that the effects are good appetite, *vāta* pacification, good body odor and that the skin becomes pleasant to touch. *Abhyaṅga* also prevents wrinkling of skin. *Abhyaṅga* should be done in a way that is soothing and pleasing to the touch (*sparśa sukha*).

The example of leather, wheel, and pot has been given to illustrate the benefits of *abhyaṅga*. All these three are regularly oiled—leather, for increasing the softness; wheel, for smooth functioning; and pot, for increasing its strength.

According to *Suśruta Samhita*, the duration taken for the oil to be absorbed is given as

three hundred *mātras*—stays on skin, not absorbed;

four hundred *mātras*—to travel through skin;

five hundred *mātras*—to reach *rakta*;

six hundred *mātras*—to reach *māmsa*;

seven hundred *mātras*—to reach *medas*;

eight hundred *mātras*—to reach *asthi*; and

nine hundred *mātras*—to reach *majja*.

one *mātra* = three seconds (approximately), or the time taken to blink an eyelid (two different opinions).

Sarvāṅgasundara: The word *nityam* (regularly) can mean that one may practice *abhyaṅga* once in one, two, or three days.

AH Sū. 2.10a

Where to massage?

शिरःश्रवणपादेषु तं विशेषेण शीलयेत् ॥१०॥

śiraḥ-śravaṇa-pādeṣu taṁ viśeṣeṇa śīlayet //10//

śiraḥ – head; *śravaṇa* – ears; *pādeṣu* – legs; *taṁ* – those parts; *viśeṣeṇa* – especially; *śīlayet* – is to be made into a habit

Translation

Especially the head, ears, and feet should be massaged regularly.

Commentary

If there is no time or facility to massage the whole body, then at least one should massage the head, ears, and feet. This will also give very good benefit. Actually according to the correspondence theory and microsystem theory, the whole body is represented in a miniature form on the ear and feet (hands also), and massaging them will stimulate and benefit the whole body.

Hands are not mentioned here, because hands will be used for massaging and hence will automatically come in contact with oil. *Śīlayet* again is indicating a potential mood expressed by the author meaning that one *must* do it.

Pādeṣu can also be referring to foot massage that has evolved from *kalari* (a type of Indian martial art practiced in Kerala).

Benefits of oil massage of the head (CS Sū. 5.81):

One who applies sesame oil regularly on the head will not have headache, baldness, graying, or hair fall. Strength of head and forehead will be enhanced. Deep-rooted hair, sense organs that are working well, bright facial skin, sound sleep, and happiness are other characteristics. It also relieves scalp diseases.

Benefits of massaging feet (*Bhāva prakāśa*)

Removes *khara-tva, sthira-tva, rūkṣa-tva* (roughness, immobility, dryness), fatigue and numbness of feet, rigidity and contractions are removed instantly.

There are different oils that may be chosen for the oil massage. The Kerala tradition of *Āyurveda* has given us a wide variety for oils for each condition and also different oils for the head and body. Some of the common oils are *dhanvantaram tailam, Prabhañjanam tailam, Bala tailam, Daśamūla tailam, Ketakīmūlādi tailam,* and *Triphalādi tailam* for the body and *Nīlibhṛṅgādi tailam, Balādhātryādi tailam, Tenginpuṣpādi tailam, Dhurdhurapatrādi tailam,* and so on for the head. It is an old saying in Kerala that a *Vaidya* is considered an expert only when he or she is confident of prescribing an oil for the head.

Prescribing an oil for the head is a serious matter because it influences the *prāṇa*.

Āyurvedarasāyana: *Ācārya Hemādri* has especially mentioned the head because all the sense organs are situated on the head and application of oil on the head will nourish all the sense organs (*indriya tarpaṇaḥ*). The pain of the jaw, nape of neck, head, and ear are relieved by instilling oil in the ears. The benefits of oil application on the feet are eradication of *pāda supti* (numbness of feet), *śrama* (tiredness), *stambha* (stiffness arresting movement), *sankoca* (contraction, foot drop), and *sphuṭana* (cracking).

AH Sū. 2.10b

Contraindications for massage

वर्ज्योऽभ्यङ्गः कफग्रस्तकृतसंशुद्ध्यजीर्णिभिः ॥१०॥

varjyo'bhyaṅgaḥ kapha-grasta-kṛta-saṁśuddhy-ajīrṇibhiḥ //10//

varjyo – contraindicated for; *abhyaṅga* – massage; *kapha grasta* – those having aggravated *kapha*; *kṛta samśuddhya* – those who have undergone purification treatments or cleansing therapies (*pañcakarma*); *ajīrṇibhiḥ* – those suffering from indigestion

Translation

Oil massage is contraindicated in those who have *kapha* aggravation, after having undergone *pañcakarma* cleansing therapies and those suffering from indigestion.

Commentary

Abhyaṅga is done only after *agni dīpana* (correcting the digestive fire) and *pācana* (digestion of *āma* toxins), or else it can increase the *āmatva* (accumulation of undigested substances) in the body. Those who have *kapha* aggravation and those who have undergone *pañcakarma* or other cleansing procedures have tendency toward *manda agni* (low *agni*), and hence, *abhyaṅga* is contraindicated. Those suffering from fever or any other type of inflammation in the body should never be given an oil massage due to the same reason.

How to recognize a *kapha grastha*?

Sarvāṅgasundara says that this condition can be recognized by the presence of excess sleepiness and laziness. The signs of *kapha* aggravation are explained in AH Sū. 11.7 (*śleṣmāgnisāda*...), which are low digestion, increased salivation, laziness, heaviness, pallor, cold feeling internally or externally to touch, laxity of organs or body, breathlessness, cough (respiratory pathologies), and excessive sleep.

***Āyurvedarasāyana*:** One should avoid oil massage in the case of acute fever and after *vamana* and *virecana* as well. One who performs *abhyaṅga* should exercise after that. Hence, the benefits of exercise are described next.

This is a general rule for daily use, however there are special oils that are used to treat inflammations, *kapha* and other ailments and those may be employed as per the prescription of the expert *Vaidya*.

AH Sū. 2.11

Benefits of exercise

लाघवं कर्मसामर्थ्यं दीप्तोग्निर्मेदसः क्षयः ॥११॥

विभक्तघनगात्रत्वं व्यायामादुपजायते ॥११॥

lāghavaṁ karma-sāmarthyaṁ dīpto 'gnir-medasaḥ kṣayaḥ

vibhakta-ghana-gātratvaṁ vyāyāmād-upajāyate //11//

lāghavam – lightness (of body); *karma sāmarthyaṁ* – ability to work (hard), work efficiency; *dīpto-agnir* – ignites digestive fire; *medasaḥ kṣayaḥ* – depletion of fatty tissue; *vibhakta* – finely chiseled contours (muscles can be seen separately); *ghana gātratvam* – dense (strong) body; *vyāyāmad* – of exercise; *upajāyate* – as a result of

Translation

Lightness of the body, increased capacity to work, kindling of digestive fire, reduction of fat, and a finely sculpted or well-shaped and compact body are the results of exercise.

Commentary

Vibhakta also means separated, ornamented, isolated, symmetrical, distinct, and decorated. Exercising after applying oil is especially practiced in *kalari*, which is the martial-art form of Kerala. This indicates that *Vāgbhaṭa* lived in Kerala.

According to *Aruṇodaya* or *Govinda vaidya*, exercise is especially required for those who are involved in a sedentary job. For those whose regular activities include a lot of walking or physical activity, their daily activity itself is sufficient for exercise. *Yogāsana* and *prāṇāyāma* may be included in the daily regimen as a form of exercise. There are several aspects of yoga, which are included in the daily regimen in the present day, and there is nothing wrong with that. In this book we are only elaborating on the items mentioned in the classical *Āyurvedic* texts.

It is to be noted that if one engages in exercise without oil massage, eventually all the lubricating elements in the body will dry up and induce degenerative changes.

Āyurvedarasāyana says that the oil enters deep into the tissues and promotes density of the *dhātus* and thus provides strength. (Refer chart in AH Sū 2.9)

AH Sū. 2.12a

Contraindications for exercise

वातपित्तामयी बालो वृद्धोजीर्णी च तं त्यजेत् ॥१२॥

vāta-pittāmayī bālo vṛddho'jīrṇī ca taṁ tyajet //12//

vāta pitta āmayi – those suffering from *vāta* and *pitta* diseases, *bālaḥ* – child; *vṛddhaḥ* – elderly person; *ajīrṇī* – person having indigestion; *ca* – and; *tam* – (*vyāyāmam*) here indicates exercise; *tyajet* – contraindicated

Translation

Exercise is contraindicated in those suffering from *vāta-pitta* diseases, in case of indigestion, in children, and in the elderly.

Commentary

All the nouns are used in singular meaning that the discussion here is about specific situations. *Tyajet* is a potential mood, which means that it is not an option. This is a general instruction, and it can be modified if required for special circumstances.

The process of exercise involves aggravation of *vāta* and *pitta* and decrease of *kapha*. One example of a breach of this principle is the hot *yoga* that is practiced around the world. This should not be practiced by those who have an aggravation of *vāta* and *pitta.*It could be beneficial for others.

When one breaks these rules, one may not necessarily experience an immediate adverse reaction. The effects accumulate gradually and manifest eventually in the form of chronic degenerative and inflammatory diseases.

After discussing who should and should not exercise, the next verse describes how much and when to exercise.

AH Sū. 2.12b–13a

Who should exercise, how much, and when?

अर्धशक्त्या निषेव्यस्तु बलिभिः स्निग्धभोजिभिः ॥१२॥

शीतकाले वसन्ते च, मन्दमेव ततोन्यदा ॥१३॥

aṛdha-śaktyā niṣevyastu balibhiḥ snigdha-bhojibhiḥ //12//

śīta-kāle vasante ca, mandam-eva tato'nyadā //13//

ardha-śaktyā – with half of the strength; *niṣevyaḥ* – should be performed; *tu* – indeed; *balibhiḥ* – by strong people; *snigdha bhojibhiḥ* – by those having a fatty or oily diet; *śīta-kāle vasante ca* – during the winter and spring seasons; *mandam-eva* – certainly very slow or light (exercise); *tato-anyadā* – in all other cases apart from the above mentioned.

Translation

Exercise should be performed in the winter and spring seasons, up to half of the strength by those who are strong and those who engage in eating fatty foods. In all other seasons, one should perform only light exercise (less than half the strength).

Commentary

Here the concepts of who, when and how much exercise to be performed are explained. The words *ardha śaktyā* and *mandam eva* emphasize the fact that one should never exercise to the point of complete exhaustion. It should ideally be up to half of the exhaustion limit. Body-building exercises, which push you to the extreme, are *atiyoga* and can result in many illnesses in the long term as mentioned in verse 13.

Exercise is here specifically recommended for *balibhiḥ* and *snigdha bhojibhiḥ*—that is, those who are strong and those who indulge in fatty foods, and that too only in the winter and spring. This means that those who are weak and who do not indulge in rich foods need less exercise.

According to *Āyurveda*, health is neither about having a sculpted or chiseled body nor about being slim, or having bulging muscles or six-pack abdominal muscles. This is misleading. A certain amount of fat is essential for the body and should be maintained.

We will learn in *nidāna sthāna* that many diseases are caused by excessive exercise causing the aggravation of *vāta* and *pitta*. This could be a clue for many of the modern lifestyle diseases.

How can we understand what constitutes half the strength (*ardha śakti*)? *Suśruta*[1] explains that when the *vāyu* situated in the heart starts coming up through the mouth, it indicates expenditure of half the strength. This will be explained in chapter 4 of this book as *śrama śvāsa* (dyspnea on exertion). It means that one feels a pressure on the chest, and there is heaving while breathing. It also means the use of accessory respiratory muscles (muscles of the neck as well as the sides of the chest) during breathing, which indicates that one has gone beyond half strength. This capacity of *ardha śakti* can be increased with regular training but prematurely going beyond this limit is not advisable. What to do after exercise is covered next.

Note: The winter and spring seasons mentioned here correspond to the external and internal changes of the seasons mentioned in Chapter 3. In some regions of the world, though there is a so called summer season, it is not actually summer because it does not manifest all the characteristics of summer mentioned in the *Āyurvedic* texts and thus cannot be technically accepted as summer. In such cases, this rule of exercise may not be applicable.

AH Sū. 2.13b

What to do after exercise

तं कृत्वानुसुखं देहं मर्दयेच्च समन्ततः ॥१३॥

taṁ kṛtvā 'nusukhaṁ dehaṁ mardayecca samantataḥ //13//

tam kṛtvā – after having done that (exercise); *anusukham* – comfortably/ lightly; *deham* – on the body; *mardayet* – strong massage; *ca* – and; *samantataḥ* – from all sides (i.e. whole body)

Translation

After exercise one should have a strong, full-body massage from all sides in a comfortable manner.

Commentary

Anusukham means as comfortable as each individual's preference. *Mardayet* describes not just application but strong rubbing. So according to the order above, first there is soft application of oil, then exercise, and then finally a strong massage again with the oil that is already on the body. The strength of the massage should be comfortably tolerated by the receiver.

Suśruta explains that *mardana* should be done after exercise over the sweating body (*svinna gātrasya*), and diseases will flee away from you just as swift animals escape from a lion.

AH Sū. 2.14

Consequences of too much exercise

तृष्णा क्षयः प्रतमको रक्तपित्तं श्रमः क्लमः ॥१४॥

अतिव्यायामतः कासो ज्वरच्छर्दिश्च जायते ॥१४॥

tṛṣṇā kṣayaḥ pratamako rakta-pittaṁ śramaḥ klamaḥ

ativyāyāmataḥ kāso jvara-cchharddiśca jāyate //14//

tṛṣṇa – thirst; *kṣayaḥ* – emaciation; *pratamaka* – (*pratāmyati*) become exhausted or severely breathless/ faint or lose consciousness; *rakta pittam* – diseases of blood due to increased heat in circulation (increase of *pitta doṣa* in *rakta dhātu*); *śrama* – physical fatigue; *klama* – mental fatigue; *ativyāyāmataḥ* – due to excessive exercise; *kāsa* – cough; *jvaraḥ* – fever; *chardiḥ* – vomiting; *ca* – and; *jāyate* – originates, it causes

Translation

Thirst, emaciation, breathlessness due to exhaustion, *rakta pitta* diseases, tiredness and fatigue, cough, inflammation (fever), and vomiting are the results of excessive exercise.

Commentary

How will you know that you are performing too much exercise? You have to look for the symptoms enumerated here. The right amount of exercise changes according to season. As a rule of thumb, it should be up to half of the physical strength, which is understood by the amount of exercise required to just break sweat on the forehead. This has also been explained in the previous verse.

Sarvāṅgasundara: *Tṛṣṇa* is the first symptom that appears due to excessive exercise. It also depends on the time, place, and quantity of exercise that a person performs.

In many cases a person may be genetically predisposed to a certain disease. But he or she most probably will not suffer from the disease if his or her diet and lifestyle are healthy. This means that the genetic predisposition alone is not enough in most cases; it also takes a vitiated internal environment created by faulty *dinacaryā* and *ṛtucaryā* to manifest the disease. The list given here enumerates the diseases that can result as a result of excessive exercise.

Clinically if you find a client presenting with these symptoms, you should always look for exertion, overexercising, or overwork in his or her lifestyle. If this is not stopped, any amount of medicine given may not be helpful. You can read about these pathologies in the *Nidāna sthāna.* They will be explained in later volumes of this series.

- *Tṛṣṇa* (thirst)—AH Ni. Ch. 5
- *Kṣaya* (emaciation)—AH Ni. Ch. 5
- *Pratamaka* (a type of breathlessness)—AH Ni. Ch. 4
- *Rakta pitta* (vitiation of blood by *pitta*)—AH Ni. Ch. 3
- *Kāsa* (cough)—AH Ni. Ch. 3
- *Jvara* (inflammations)—AH Ni. Ch. 2
- *Chardi* (vomiting)—AH Ni. Ch. 5

Note: these translations are literal but not the *Āyurvedic* equivalents. Though the literal meaning helps to give a proximal idea of the disease, the *Āyurvedic* concept may be slightly different in many cases.

AH Sū. 2.15

Causes of untimely death

व्यायामजागराध्वस्त्रीहास्यभाष्यादि साहसम् ॥१५॥

गजं सिंह इवाकर्षन् भजन्नति विनश्यति ॥१५॥

vyāyāma jāgarādhva-strī hāsya bhāṣyādi sāhasaṁ

gajaṁ siṁha ivākarṣan bhajannati vinaśyati //15//

vyāyāma – (too much) physical exercise; *jāgara* – keeping awake in the night; *adhvaga* – traveling on foot (walking long distances); *strī* – woman (excessive sexual indulgence); *hāsya* – laughing; *bhāṣya* – talking; *ādi* – etc (other strenuous activities); *sāhasam* – taking too much risk; *gajam* – of elephant; *simha* – lion; *iva* – just like; *ākarṣan* – attracting; *bhajan-ati* – participating excessively; *vinaśyati* – destroys completely (death); *vyāyāmam sāhasam* – too much exercise

Translation

Indulging excessively in physical exercise, staying awake at night, traveling long distances, sexual activity, laughing, talking, engaging in other strenuous activities, and taking too much risk attract one's own destruction (death), just as an elephant is attacked by a lion.

Commentary

While prohibiting excessive exercise, the other items which also have the same consequences are enumerated.

A lion attacking an elephant is a very good analogy. Although the elephant is a bigger animal, it can be killed by the lion. But if the lion is not careful, it can get killed by the elephant. No matter how healthy one is, if one participates in the above activities excessively, destruction of life is certain.

How excessive exercise can cause disease has been explained in the previous verse. The effects of staying awake at night (AH Sū. 7.64) and excessive speaking have been described as *vāta* aggravating in AH Ni. Ch. 1.14. The results of *vāta* aggravation are described in AH Sū. 11.6 and 12.49–50.

Here sex is referred to as *stri*. According to some *Vedic* literatures, the female body is capable of enjoying sex without getting as depleted as a male body does. There is also a description of a special benediction given to women by Lord Indra for the same (ref. Srimad Bhāgavatam 6.9.9). *Cāṇakya Pandita*, a famous Indian philosopher and thinker, has written that a woman who has regular sex is able to remain more youthful compared to a man.

> *adhvā jarā manuṣyāṇām vājīnām bandhanam jarā*
> *amaithunam jarāstrīṇām vastrāṇām ātapo jarā*
> (*Chanakya Niti* 4.17)

"Constant travel brings old age upon a man, a horse becomes aged by being constantly tied up, lack of sexual intercourse brings old age upon a woman, and garments become old upon being exposed to the sun."

But in the case of men, it is explained in the *Vedic* writings that abstention from sex helps to keep them more youthful and vibrant. Here we are only discussing the effect of celibacy on health. In this way we can understand the effect of sex on both men and women are different.

Modern interpretation

A modern study revealed that women who had sex at least four times a week scored as looking up to ten years younger than their natural age.[2] This refers to regular intercourse with the same partner and not casual encounters with multiple partners. Dr. Weeks, head of old-age psychology at the Royal Edinburgh

Hospital, says that in women sex produces a human growth hormone, which helps the process of rejuvenation.[3]

It is also observed that after sex, there is a more depleting effect on the male hormonal system in comparison with the female system. So excessive sex could have a more depleting effect on males compared to females. This has been observed as a decrease in prostaglandin E_1, elevated PSA (prostate-specific antigen) levels, and excessive DHT levels (dihydrotestosterone), among other hormones.[4]

These are some suggestions to inspire further study, which is required in this subject to come up with conclusive answers.

All the causes of untimely death enumerated here are degenerative processes controlled by *vāta*. All six activities mentioned here will aggravate *vāta* and initiate premature degenerative processes in the body. As indirectly indicated here, one of the good ways to reduce *vāta* is to undertake *mauna vrata* (vow of silence) for a few days and avoid too much laughter. The word *ādi* indicates that much more can be added to this list. These are only some prominent examples.

In the *Vidura nīti* section of the *udyoga parva* of *Mahābharata*, it is said that six types of people are affected by loss of sleep.

kaccid etair mahādoṣair na-spṛṣṭo'si nirādhipa
kaccinna paravitteṣu gṛdhyan-viparitapyase

"One who is attacked by a strong person, a weak person, one who has failed to achieve one's goal, one who has lost one's wealth, one tormented by lust, and a thief are affected by loss of sleep."

During the olden days, people often traveled long distances by walking. In today's context, where everyone is flying around, the meaning of the word *adva* could also include *vimāna gamanam* (airplane travel) or *vāhana gamanam* (vehicle travel).

One should make a special note that it is only excessive indulgence in these activities that will result in depletion or degeneration. In optimal amount, they will help keep the person healthy and balanced.

Aruṇodaya: The lion kills the elephant in a unique manner, by attacking from behind. But if the lion decides to deliberately test its strength against the elephant and attacks from the front, the elephant will catch the lion using the trunk, trample the lion, and kill it. In the same way, if the *vyāyāmādis* are used in the proper way, they can strengthen the body, but if not used properly, they can cause death.

AH Sū. 2.16

Udvartanam (Dry-powder massage)

उद्वर्तनं कफहरं मेदसः प्रविलायनम् ॥१६॥
स्थिरीकरणमङ्गानां त्वक्प्रसादकरं परम् ॥१६॥

udvartanaṁ kaphaharaṁ medasaḥ pravilāyanaṁ
sthirīkaraṇam-aṅgānāṁ tvak-prasāda-karaṁ param //16//

udvartanam – powder massage; *kapha haram* – destroys *kapha*; *medasaḥ pravilāyanam* – liquefies fat; *sthirīkaraṇam angānām* – makes the body stable and sturdy (compact); *tvak prasāda* – excellence of skin; *karam* – does (bestows/ promotes); *param* – ultimate, best

Translation

Massage with herbal powder removes *kapha*, melts *medas* (fatty and lubricating tissues), gives stability to the body, and bestows excellent texture on the skin.

Commentary

One of the common herbal powders used for this purpose is *triphala*. We will learn in chapter 6 that *triphala* is good for all skin diseases, absorbing excess moisture in the skin and reducing obesity and excess *kapha*. Any herbal powder that has *kaṣāya* (astringent) taste and is good for skin (*tvacya*) can be used for *udvartana*. It is excess moisture and fat that makes the body flabby and loose. When this is taken out, the body again becomes firm and sturdy.

Powder massage is usually done in the opposite direction to that of the hairs on the body (called *pratiloma*). While doing this, one should take special care not to disturb the *prāṇa* flow in the body, which is in the direction of the hair (*anuloma*) direction. So after massaging three to four times in the opposite direction, one should massage once at least in the direction of the hairs.

This treatment is commonly done for quick weight reduction, and one can expect to reduce about three to four kilograms during a ten- to fifteen-day treatment. The effect takes place especially in relation to subcutaneous fat deposits. It also helps to break the cellulite for beauty treatments in women and reduce the size of thighs and arms.

In this context it is done to scrape away the excess oil before bathing.

---

1. Sū. S. Ci. 24.47.
2. http://www.mirror.co.uk/lifestyle/sex-relationships/having-regular-sex-can-keep-157110 5th Jan 2012.
3. http://dazeinfo.com/2010/06/18/can-sex-keep-you-young/.
4. http://www.herballove.com/articles/science-aftermath-sexual-exhaustion-how-excessive-ejaculation-causes-damaging-chemical.

AH Sū. 2.17

Snānaṁ (benefits of bathing)

दीपनं वृष्यमायुष्यं स्नानमूर्जाबलप्रदम् ॥१७॥

कण्डूमलश्रमस्वेदतन्द्रातृड्दाहपाप्मजित् ॥१७॥

dīpanaṁ vṛṣyam-āyuṣyaṁ snānam-ūrjā-balapradam

kaṇḍū-mala-śrama-sveda-tandrā-tṛṅg-dāha pāpmajit //17//

Six items obtained by bathing

dīpanam – ignites digestive fire (improves appetite); *vṛṣyam* – sexual capacity; *āyuṣyam* – life span; *snānam* – bathing; *ūrjā* – energy, mental refreshment, enthusiasm; *bala* – strength, prāṇa; *pradam* – bestows;

Eight items removed by bathing

kaṇḍū – itching; *mala* – dirt; *śrama* – fatigue, exhaustion/weariness; *sveda* – sweat; *tandrā* – lethargy; *tṛṭ* –

thirst; *dāha* – burning sensation; *pāpma* – sins; *jit* – cures, removes

Translation

Ignition of digestive fire, sexual vigor, increased life-span, strength, and refreshment of the mind are obtained by bathing. Itching, dirt, fatigue, sweat, lethargy, thirst, burning sensation of the body, and sins are removed by bathing.

Note: Here it is mentioned that sin is also cleansed by bathing and it brings a sense of holiness in life.

Commentary

After massage it is now time to take the morning bath. All the physical and emotional benefits are mentioned in the beginning. The words *pāpmajit* indicates that bathing is not just a physical activity. Not only are the physical impurities cleansed but one is also emotionally rejuvenated, and even spiritual obstacles are cleared due to the removal of sins.

In India many people visit holy rivers like the Ganges and Yamuna to bathe in their waters and become purified of sins. It is also seen in many other religions that holy water is sprinkled on the body in order to purify and free from sins. This is because water has a special property of being a vehicle to carry the vibrations and energies of what it is associated with. This was proved in the experiments on water conducted by the Japanese scientist Masaru Emoto.

Regular bathing increases the *sattva guṇa*, which prevents the tendency to commit sin. If we do not bathe regularly, we promote the increase of *tama guṇa*, which invites lower and sinful tendencies to take birth and thrive in our hearts and minds. In some areas of the world, bathing is not a regular feature. This may be due to the climatic variations and culture.

The mechanism of *dīpana* (kindling the digestive fire) by bathing is similar to how *agni* is increased during winter. When the external body becomes cool and the skin pores are closed or blocked, the *agni* is drawn inward to the center from the periphery. Also note that this effect is described in the case of a *svastha* (healthy person) and not *ātura* (diseased person) in this context. In *ātura avastha*, bathing is avoided, for example, *Jvara* (AH Ci. 1.17). (Refer *tyajet...snānābhyaṅga-pradeśāmśca pariśeṣam ca laṅghanam.*)

Bathing with special medicated water boiled with herbs like neem, mañjiṣṭa and so on is used during *Āyurvedic* treatments to cure itching.

Sarvāṅgasundara: Bathing is a little sweet (*kiñcit madhuram*), nourishing (*bṛmhaṇam*), unctuous (*snigdham*), strengthening (*bala vardhanam*), and pleasing to the mind (*manaso harṣaṇam*). Hence it is called *vṛṣyam*. Bathing increases *agni* by two mechanisms: (1) closing the skin pores and directing *agni* inward and (2) increasing the *bhrājaka pitta* (the subdivision of *pitta* that is present in the skin). Warm water is advised for bathing to achieve this effect, but it is only temporary. A similar redirection of *agni* and increase of *bhrajaka* *pitta* happens in cold climates, during the winter and rainy seasons, where there is the dampening of *jathara agni* (digestive fire) (CS Sū. 4.36).

Āyurvedarasāyana: *Dīpanam* is the *prabhāva* (special property) of bathing. *Vṛṣyam* means that it is beneficial for associating with women (*strī prasaṅga*), that is, sexual intercourse, and it qualitatively and quantitatively nourishes semen. *Tandrā* means an obstruction to the interaction of the mind and *karmendriyas* (four limbs, anus, and genitals) as the *buddhi (*intellect*)* and *jñāna indriya (*sense organs*)* cease to function. A burning sensation of the body is called *dāha*.

AH Sū. 2.18

Use of hot water for bathing

उष्णाम्बुनाऽधःकायस्य परिषेको बलावहः ॥१८॥

तेनैव तूत्तमाङ्गस्य बलहृत्केशचक्षुषाम् ॥१८॥

uṣṇāmbunā 'dhaḥ kāyasya pariṣeko balāvahaḥ

tenaiva-tūttamāṅgasya bala hṛt-keśa cakṣuṣām //18//

uṣṇa – hot; *ambu* – water; *nā* – with; *adhaḥ* – lower part; *kāyasya* – of the body; *pariseko* – pouring; *balāvahaḥ* – renders strength; *tena* – of that; *iva* – also (*tenaiva*: the same activity); *ūttamāṅgasya* – on the upper part of body; *bala hṛt* – takes away strength; *keśa* – hair; *cakṣuṣām* – and eyes

Translation

Pouring hot water over the lower part of the body (below the neck) gives strength to that part and doing the same on the upper part of the body takes away strength, especially of the hair and eyes.

Commentary

Never pour hot water on the head and eyes. Never pour cold water over the body.

Pair garam aur sar ṭhanḍa, māro vaid ko ḍanḍa (**पैर गरम और सर ठण्डा, मारो वैद को डण्डा**) is an old Indian saying that means, "If you keep your feet warm and your head cool, you can keep the physician away," just as in English, we have the saying "An apple a day keeps the doctor away."

Pouring hot water on the head causes loss of strength to the eyes and to the hair on the head (causing hair fall). The use of pressurized heated water in shower is so common these days. One must make an effort to keep the head out of hot water spray or keep body away from cold spray.

Aruṇodaya: The word *tenaiva* indicates that to whatever extent the warm temperature of water is strengthening to the body, to the same extent, it is harmful to the hair and eyes if used on the head.

AH Sū. 2.19

Contraindications to bathing

स्नानमर्दितनेत्रास्यकर्णरोगातिसारिषु ॥१९॥

आध्मानपीनसाजीर्णभुक्तवत्सु च गर्हितम् ॥१९॥

snānam-ardita netrāsya karṇa rogātisāriṣu
ādhmāna pīnasājīrṇa bhukta-vatsu ca garhitam //19//

snānam – bathing; *ardita* – facial palsy; *netra* – of the eyes; *āsya* – oral cavity; *karṇa* – ears; *roga* – disease; *atisāriṣu* – with diarrhea; *ādhmāna* – abdominal distention; *pīnasa* – rhinitis; *ajīrṇa* – indigestion; *bhukta vatsu* – immediately after food; *ca* – and; *garhitam* – forbidden

Translation

Bathing is contraindicated in those having facial palsy; diseases of the eyes, oral cavity, and ears; diarrhea; abdominal distention; rhinitis; indigestion; and immediately after having had a meal.

Commentary

The reasons for the contraindications mentioned above are

- *ardita*—because it is a *kapha āvṛta* (*vāta* enveloped by *kapha*) disease;
- *netra roga*—*kapha-pitta* pathology;
- *āsya roga*—mouth ulcers are due to *kapha-pitta*;
- *karṇa roga*—*kapha āvṛta*;
- *atisāra*—especially in sticky diarrhea (*āma* and kapha involvement);
- *ādhmāna*—this happens just after food (kapha phase) when bathing is contraindicated;
- *pīnasa*—rhinorrhea is a *kapha-vāta* disease;

- *ajīrṇa*—especially in *ajirna* (indigestion) due to *kapha* aggravation (whenever there is *kapha* aggravation, low digestive fire and *ajirna* are seen); and
- *bhuktavatsu*—immediately after intake of food is the *kapha* stage of digestion.

These are all conditions where there is *kapha vṛddhi* (aggravation of *kapha*) or *kapha āvaraṇa* (enveloped by *kapha*) or *utkliṣṭa kapha* (distressed or distorted *kapha*) and *pitta* being expelled from the body, that is, conditions where *stambhanam* (arresting movement) type of treatment is contraindicated. Here the *utkliṣṭa doṣa*s (the state when the *doṣas* that were in a compounded state with the *dhātus*—in *sammūrcchana*—are separated and ready for expulsion) are being expelled from the body, so one should not arrest their expulsion by bathing, which will contract the *srotas* and cause *stambhana*.

Note that though two verses earlier it was said that bathing causes *dīpanam* (igniting digestive fire), bathing is contraindicated here in case of *ajīrṇa* (indigestion). In case of *ajīrṇa, pācanam* (digestion) is also required. So unless the *āma* is digested, there is no point in increasing appetite by bathing. Moreover the *dīpanam* (igniting digestive fire) effect of bathing is only temporary.

Here is an example, where we can see that there is a distinction between *dīpanam* (igniting digestive fire) and *pācanam* (digestion). They are two separate phenomena and *dīpana* (igniting digestive fire) can occur without *pācana* (digestion) but not vice versa.

One should remember that the contraindications given here are a general list. It is possible that in certain specific variations of the conditions mentioned here, bathing is not contraindicated.

AH Sū. 2.20

Good eating habits and dealing with natural urges

जीर्णो हितं मितं चाद्यान्न वेगानीरयेद्बलात् ॥२०॥

न वेगितोऽन्यकार्यः स्यान्नाजित्वा साध्यमामयम् ॥२०॥

jīrṇe hitaṁ mitaṁ cādyānna vegān-īrayed-balāt

na vegito'nya-kāryaḥ syān-nājitvā sādhyam-āmayam //20//

jīrṇe – after digestion (of previous meal); *hitaṁ* – wholesome, beneficial; *mitaṁ* – adequate, moderate quantity; *ca* – and; *adi* – etc; *anna* – food; *vegān* – the natural urges; *īrayed* – (*īrayati*) to agitate, initiate; *balāt* – by force; *na* – not; *vegito* – one has the urges; *anya-kāryaḥ* – any other activity or involvement; *syāt* – be; *na* – not; *ajitvā* – without curing; *sādhyam* – curable; *āmayam* – disease

Translation

Eat only after the previous meal is digested; food should be beneficial and moderate in quantity. Do not artificially initiate or withhold natural urges by force. Avoid performing any other activity without relieving the urges when they present in a natural manner. Diseases should be cured before doing anything else.

Commentary

Aruṇodaya: After bathing, the next thing is to have food. Before eating one should check if the previous meal has been digested, and if not, do not eat.

Cāṇakya Paṇḍita says in his *nīti*, chapter 4, verse 16:

ṛṇa-śeṣas cāgni-śeṣo vyādhi-śeṣas tathaiva ca
punaśca vardhate yasmāt tasmācccheṣaṁ na rakṣayet

"Debt of money should be completely paid back, fire should be removed completely, and remnants of illness should be removed completely. Otherwise these three will grow up again."

na anya kārya syāt (not doing any other work) is common to both suppressing as well as initiating the urges.

This is one of the most important verses for one who wants to maintain good health. How to go about three vital things for health are mentioned here—first is about eating, second is about natural urges, and third is about disease. The word *hitam* in relation to food is a broad term that includes eating foods according to *kāla* (time), *deśa* (place), *ṛtu* (season), *prakṛti* (body constitution), *agni* (digestive ability), and so on. The sign of previous meal having been digested is that one will feel hungry. So it is recommended not to eat if there is no hunger. One should also be able to differentiate between food cravings, addictions, emotional hunger and physical hunger.

The details about the same will be described in the chapters ahead:

- *Jīrṇe* (after digestion)—AH Sū. 8.25–26
- *Hitam* (beneficial)—AH Sū. Ch.5, 6, 7, 8
- *Mitam* (appropriate quantity)—AH Sū. 8.1–6
- *Vega dhāraṇa* (suppression of urges)—AH Sū. Ch. 4

***Āyurvedarasāyana*:** Food should be digestible. Food should be *kriyā and dravya pradhāna*. What are *kriya* and *dravya pradhāna*, and *āhāra* and *vihāra*? *Vihāra* is *kriyā pradhāna*. *Āhāra* is *kriyā* and *dravya pradhāna*. This is the difference between *vihāra* and *āhāra*. In the *Vedic* culture, there is great importance to who has cooked the food, who is offering it, where it is being consumed, and so on. Here the description is that one should not accept food that is not cooked, offered, and so on without the proper etiquettes. As far as possible, one should try to cook one's own food.

Food that is consumed should be digested. *Hitam* indicates that the food should be appropriate according to the place, season, and so on.

He quotes from AS Sū. 3.46 (*annapānavidhānena*...) that one should take food according to the prescribed rules, without hurrying, after offering prayers, with a pleasant mind, and after feeding the poor and hungry as charity.

One should also avoid food from a person who does not have the ability to think and act using their own intelligence (*strī jita*), an impotent person (*klība*), a degraded (*patita*) and uncivilized person, a cruel person, one who is addicted to illicit activities, those who are about to die, from places where a recent death has taken place, those who are miserable, public enemies, prostitutes, public inns, gamblers or cunning people, and misers. One should never associate, eat, or drink with such people in the day or at night.

Note: During ancient times food was never a business commodity that was sold. It was the norm in society that no person should go hungry. Every family would regularly feed hungry people before having their food. The state would have free food-supply centers, where anyone could come and eat. The places of worship would also distribute free food. This can be seen today as well. The other two items that were never sold were medical care and education. These were always given free being supported by the state.

One may ask this question: "In the midst of describing *vihāra* (activities), why is diet being introduced?" This is because eating is also a *kriyā* (activity). As far as eating is concerned, there are two components: first is the activity of eating, and the second is what we are eating. Here the first aspect is being described, and so it does not contradict the flow of thought. The second aspect of eating will be described in chapters 5 and 6 in the second volume of this book.

Recommendations on physical activities practically end here. Now *Vāgbhaṭa* begins to describe how we should behave with others and cultivate a healthy mental attitude, which is of utmost necessity for health.

AH Sū. 2.21–22a

Occupation, friends, and others

सुखार्थाः सर्वभूतानां मताः सर्वाः प्रवृत्तयः ॥२१॥

सुखं च न विना धर्मात्तस्माद्धर्मपरो भवेत् ॥२१॥

भक्त्या कल्याणमित्राणि सेवेतेतरदूरगः ॥२२॥

sukhārthāḥ sarva bhūtānāṁ matāḥ sarvāḥ pravṛttayaḥ
sukhaṁ ca na vinā dharmāt tasmād dharma-paro bhavet //21//
bhaktyā kalyāṇa-mitrāṇi sevet-etara-dūragaḥ //22//

sukhārthāḥ – for the purpose of happiness; *sarva* – all; *bhūtānāṁ* – living beings; *matāḥ* – opined; *sarvāḥ* – all; *pravṛttayaḥ* – working, perform activities; *sukhaṁ* – happiness; *ca* – and; *na* – not; *vinā dharmāt* – without *dharma*; *tasmād* – therefore; *dharma* – virtuousness; *paraḥ* – subservient to, adhere to; *bhavet* – become; *bhaktyā* – sincerely; *kalyāṇa* – benevolent, virtuous, beneficial; *mitrāṇi* – friends; *sevet* – be served; *itara* – others; *dūragaḥ* – kept at a distance (abhorred)

Translation

It is opined that all living entities perform activities only for the purpose of attaining happiness. Happiness is not possible without *dharma*. Hence, one should always be adherent to *dharma*. One must serve benevolent or virtuous friends with sincerity and keep a distance from others.

Commentary

This means that one should reject so-called friends if they are not virtuous.

So in the beginning it was said, "*āyuḥ kāmayamānena dharma artha sukha sādhanam*," and here it has been said, "*sukham ca na vinā dharmāt.*" It is not possible to be happy without following *dharma*. The reverse is also true, that is, the path of *adharma* will bring only misery. What is *dharma*? This has already been discussed in chapter one. Many items of *dharma* are explained here in this chapter. Others may also be found in the other *dharma śāstras*.

All living beings in the world are searching for happiness from the beginning to the end of life. Very few are able to find it. Here is the secret of how to find happiness. One has to find *dharma* first, and happiness will follow. Among the four *puruṣārthas* (goals of life), *dharma* is the most important without which the others cannot be enjoyed.

The *dharma* of an *Āyurvedic* practitioner is to help people attain good health and happiness. If one performs this *dharma*, one will be able to find happiness in life.

Note that *Āyurveda* advises you to keep a safe distance from those who have negative feelings toward you, but not to take any revenge against or harm them. Better to just avoid them and intelligently move away.

The words *kalyāṇa mitrāṇl* have been used here. It means a friend who is helpful or who brings about goodness. One may ask, "Why should we say a friend who is helpful? A friend is always supposed to be helpful, isn't it? This adjective is redundant as far as a friend is concerned." The answer is that sometimes even friends can be harmful. There is a saying in English that it is better to have an intelligent enemy than a foolish friend. This implies that it is important to stay close to friends who are *kalyāṇa* (bring good results) and keep a distance from "foolish friends" who are *akalyāṇa* (don't bring good results).

It is said in *Cāṇakya Nīti* *śāstra* 6.13:

> *varam na rājyam na kurāja rājyam*
> *varam na mitram na kumitra mitram*
> *varam na śiṣyo na kuśiṣya śiṣyo*
> *varam na dārā na kudāra dārā*

"It is better to be without a kingdom than to rule a useless kingdom; it is better to not have any friends than to have a rascal as a friend; it is better to not have any disciple than to have a stupid disciple; It is better not to have a wife (or husband) than to have a bad one.

Āyurvedarasāyana: Often, the obstruction in our activities is due to not following the path of *dharma*. *Āyurveda* practiced according to the principles of *dharma* will result in *sukha* (happiness). Though good health is obtainable with the help of *ṣoḍaśātmaka cikitsa* (sixteen components of treatment – see note below), it is possible only in accompaniment of *dharma*.

The word *bhaktyā* has been emphasized and explained by *ācārya*. *Bhakti* is defined as work that is done out of a feeling of duty with no expectation of anything in return.

Note: The sixteen components of treatment are *vaidya* (physician), *dravya* (medicine), *upasthātā* (caregiver), and *rogī* (patient), which are again divided into four each as described in chapter 1.

Hence, it is important to know the activities that perpetuate *adharma*, and this is told in the next verse.

AH Sū. 2.22b–23

Ten sins to strictly avoid

हिंसास्तेयान्यथाकामं पैशुन्यं परुषानृते ॥२२॥
सम्भिन्नालापं व्यापादमभिध्यां दृग्विपर्ययम् ॥२३॥
पापं कर्मेति दशधा कायवाङ्मनसैस्त्यजेत् ॥२३॥

hiṁsā-steyānyathā-kāmaṁ paiśunyaṁ paruṣānṛte //22//
saṁbhinnālāpaṁ vyāpādam-abhidhyā dṛk-viparyayaṁ
pāpaṁ karmeti daśadhā kāya vāk mānasais tyajet //23//

hiṁsa – violence; steya – theft; *anyathā kāmaṁ* – infidelity; *paiśunyaṁ* – calumny, making false and defamatory statements in order to damage someone's reputation, slander; *paruṣa* – rude, violent, brusque, severe, grouchy, rough; *anṛta* – lying, cheating; *saṁbhinnālāpaṁ* – uttering rubbish (*sambhinna* – interrupted, *ālāpam* – speech); *vyāpādam* – having an evil intention to harm, malice; *abhidhyā* – longing for other's belongings; *dṛk viparyayaṁ* – to turn one's sight away from, turn face away, ignore someone (can also mean atheism); *pāpaṁ* – sinful; *karmeti* – these actions; *daśadhā* – ten in number; *kāya* – by body; *vāk* – by words; *mānasais* – mentally; *tyajet* – must give up, avoid

Translation

One should physically, mentally and verbally give up the following ten sinful activities: violence, theft, infidelity, defamation, rude behavior, lying or cheating, useless talk or interrupting others while talking, evil intentions to harm someone, desire for others belongings, and ignoring someone in an insulting manner.

Commentary

First three are physical, next four are verbal, and the last three are mental sins. One must give up sinful activity by mind, words, and body.

These ten forbidden activities are the *mithyā yoga* of *karma* (the third cause of diseases) explained in Ch. 12.39–42

It is amazing how all the sinful activities that one can ever commit have been condensed into ten items. This is the brilliance of *Ācārya Vāgbhaṭa*.

1. *Himsa* should be understood on physical, emotional and spiritual levels. *Himsa* on a spiritual level means to

obstruct the spiritual progress of another living entity by thought, word or action.

2. *Steya* - The definition of 'thief' is explained in *Bhagavad Gīta 3.12 – yo bhunkte stena eva saḥ*. Everything in the creation belongs to and is supplied by the Supreme Lord. To not acknowledge that, and enjoy everything claiming them to be one's own is called *steya* mentality on the spiritual level. *Vaidyas* should not utilize the medical profession as a means to extract unfair amount of money from clients. One should be careful of being victimized by greed.
3. *Anyathā kāmam* – lust is the greatest enemy of the living entity, stealing away his intelligence causing him to spiral down to lower and lower levels of existence. *Vaidyas* should be especially aware of this while dealing with the opposite sex. Due to the close proximity of the *Vaidya* and the client, there is always a risk of being victimized by lusty desires.
4. *Paiśunyam* – calumny is an example of *himsa* using words. Why would someone do such a thing? It is only out of envy for another person who is making progress. Envy ultimately leads to one's own downfall. The nature of the world is that whenever someone becomes successful, many people will become envious and inimical trying to malign him or her.
5. *Paruṣa* – One should not be rude to others and one should also not allow others to behave rudely with them. This is described in BG 16.4. *Vaidyas* should speak

kindly and compassionately with their clients. But if a client is too rude, a *Vaidya* should avoid them.

6. *Anṛta* – lying – This results in a loss of trust in the *Vaidya*. Trust is a very important aspect of healing and *Vaidyas* should never lie to their clients about their illness and all personal information should be kept confidential. Sometimes clients trust their *vaidyas* even more than their own family members and hence *vaidyas* should live up to that.
7. *Sambhinnālāpam* – this is also known as *prajalpa* and is one of the six items that are unfavourable for success in any activity. They are accumulating more than what is necessary, endeavouring more than what is necessary, talking excessively and uselessly, following the rules without understanding their purposes, associating with unfavourable people and being greedy.
8. *Vyāpādam* – wanting to harm due to malice. These are different grades of negativity described here. To ignore, to speak ill about, to be rude to, desire to take away what belongs to another and lying are external. But here we see the intention of actually wanting to harm the person. This is one of the extreme mental states of negativity. A *Vaidya* should never deliberately prescribe substances which will cause harm to a person.
9. *Abhidya* – desiring what belongs to others. Contentment is described as an austerity of the mind which should be practiced (BG 17.16). There is a quote by Mahātma Gāndhi – "the world has enough for everyone's need but

not enough for even a single person's greed". A *vaidya* should practice staying content. This does not mean that one should not endeavour to improve one's situation.

10. *Dṛk viparyayam* – *dṛk* means eye and the literal translation of the term is "avoiding eye contact" – this is a type of body language which is indicative of ignoring a person. *Dakṣa* ignored Lord *Siva* during his sacrifice and this resulted in the destruction of the whole sacrifice.

It is only out of ignorance that one commits these sinful activities. Even if one has knowingly or unknowingly committed these sins in the past, this is the time to repent and take a firm resolve to avoid them in the future. This will help one become a blessed *Vaidya*.

Kāma (uncontrolled and illicit desires) is described in all the *śāstras* as the greatest enemy. It is also described as a disease in *Āyurveda* that should be curbed. There is another *kāma* which is in line with the principles of *dharma*. (*dharmoviruddho bhūteṣu kāmosmi bharatarṣabha* BG 7.11) That is not condemned.

Nīti śāstra says:

> *nāsti kāma samo vyādhir nāsti moha samo ripuḥ*
> *nāsti kopa samo vahnir nāsti jñānāt param sukham*

"There is no greater disease than lust, no greater enemy than infatuation (illusion), no greater fire than anger, and no greater happiness than knowledge."

The *Bhagavad Gīta* 3.37 explains, "*kāma eṣa krodha eṣa rajoguṇa samudbhava...*" that "lust is born out of the *rajas* (mode of passion), burns like an all devouring fire, and is greatly sinful." Hence, it is important to control this insatiable fire of lust.

It is not only sufficient to just avoid sinful activities; one must also help those who are in need. Who are the people to be helped? This is described next.

Anyathā kāmam also means desiring what belongs to others.

AH Sū. 2.24

People who must be helped

अवृत्तिव्याधिशोकार्ताननुवर्तेतशक्तितः ॥२४॥

आत्मवत्सततं पश्येदपि कीटपिपीलिकम् ॥२४॥

āvṛtti vyādhi-śokārtān-anuvartet-aśaktitaḥ

ātmavat-satataṁ paśyed-api kīta-pipīlikam //24//

āvṛtti – not having support (those in poverty); *vyādhi* – disease; *śokā* – afflicted, grieving; *artān* – distressed; *anuvartet* – should attend to; *aśaktitaḥ* – those not having strength; *ātmavat* – as oneself; *satataṁ* – always; *paśyed* – should see; *api* – even; *kīta* – worms, insects; *pipīlikam* – ants

Translation

One should always help those in poverty and those without support, those who are afflicted with diseases and grief (mental agony). One should see even the insects, worms and ants as oneself.

Commentary

Three kinds of distressed people are mentioned here: those distressed due to poverty, due to disease, and due to mental agony. Seeing an ant or worm as equal to oneself is a sign of great humility. Humility is the most important of all virtues.

The beauty of *Āyurveda* is that the same knowledge can be said in a single line as well as through volumes and volumes of textbooks. It is the same message; the only difference being how much you expand it.

This is the essential instruction of how to judge or treat others. First put yourself in their shoes, and you will understand why they behave the way they do.

If a person in poverty comes to us requesting for help and we turn them away without any consideration, it can make our heart hard. Yet there are some categories of people who are to be rejected, and that list was given in chapter 1. So it is a fine line to discriminate and do the right thing at the right time. That is the reason why the path of *dharma* is described in the *kaṭhopaniṣad* 1.3.14 as a razor's edge. (…*kṣurasya dhārā niśitā duratyayā durgam patha*…)

To see other living beings as oneself is a sign of knowledge and humility. The *Bhagavad Gīta* 5.18 explains that "One who is endowed with knowledge and humility sees a scholar, cow, elephant, dog...as one and the same." This vision of oneness of all living beings is explained by *Vāgbhaṭa*. This vision of oneness means that a knowledgable person is able to see how every living being is a spirit soul inspite of having different outer coverings - their material bodies.

The people who are to be helped have been described here. These are people who are socially or physically less fortunate than us and are asking us for help. At the same time, there are people who are situated on a higher strata and those from whom we learn the lessons of life. These personalities should be worshipped. Who are they?

AH Sū. 2.25

Seven kinds of persons to be worshipped

अर्चयेद्देवगोविप्रवृद्धवैद्यनृपातिथीन् ॥२५॥

विमुखान्नार्थिनः कुर्यान्नावमन्येत नाक्षिपेत् ॥२५॥

arcayed-deva-go-vipra-vṛddha-vaidya-nṛpātithīṅ

vimukhān-nārthīnaḥ kuryāt-nāvamanyeta nākṣipet //25//

arcayed – to be worshipped, revered; *deva* – Lord; *go* – cows; *vipra* – brāhmaṇas (scholars); *vṛddha* – elderly; *vaidya* – physician; *nṛpa* – king; *atithīṅ* – guests; *vimukhān* – reject, refuse to meet, ignore (send back empty handed); *na* – never; *ārthīnaḥ* – one who is coming in expectation of receiving something; *kuryān* – to do; *na* – never; *avamanyeta* – insulted, disrespect; *nā* – never; *ākṣipet* – insult, disdain, accuse, scold

Translation

The Supreme Lord, cows, learned scholars, elderly, physicians, kings, and guests should always be revered. Never refuse or reject one who is coming in expectation of something. Never accuse or insult anyone.

Commentary

These are the seven kinds of personalities who should be respected or worshipped. It is interesting that among the seven, one of them is *cow*. Why is each one of them recommended for worship? This brings us to several questions: What is the meaning of worship? Why should anyone be worshipped in the first place? What is special about these personalities mentioned here? What has that got to do with good health?

These personalities are only representatives and others can also be included. The principle is to give respect to those who are contributing to the upkeep of ethical and moral principles in society. The cause of disease was defined in the first verse of *Aṣṭāṅga Hṛdayam* as being the distorted state of the mind (*rāgādi roga*). These are all practices to bring the mind back to its healthy state. Intake of food is not enough for health. Unless the mind is in a healthy state, one cannot assimilate the food that is consumed. A humble state of mind is a favorable situation to assimilate food and convert it into healthy components. The egoistic state of mind (*ahankāra*) is a pathological state of mind, which has to be transformed.

The *Vedic* culture is based on respect for all living beings. The personalities mentioned in this verse are especially to be respected because they contribute in a huge way for the betterment of the society. As we look closely, we can see that if they are not maintained properly, society as a whole may crumble and anarchy will result.

Each of these can be understood in detail. For example, *atithi* although commonly translated as "guest" has a deeper meaning. Literally it means one who comes without a *tithi* (date or prior appointment). In the *Vedic* society, there were wandering monks who would come to your home to ask for charity, and they would impart spiritual knowledge in return. They are allowed to come at any time, since they do not have any selfish motivations.

One who comes begging for help should never be rejected. Why?

In today's society those who beg or request for help are looked down upon. Most people do not want to associate with them. But there was a time when helping someone in need was considered a great honor and opportunity. This gives us some idea about the *Āyurvedic* culture. This is still the case in some households and communities where people go out in the street looking for anyone who may be hungry before themselves having a meal. The action of selflessly helping another person gives us a *sattvik* mental framework, which is the basis of knowledge and happiness. The highest and most respected section of society—the renounced *sannyasis*—lived by begging from house to house. It was for the pupose of giving the other sections of society an opportunity to purify their consciousness and make progress in life by giving charity.

To accuse or insult another person is an act of false pride. Even if the person has done something wrong, it should be rectified in a pleasant manner. This is the *sattvic* way of behavior. We can see that all the recommendations mentioned here are meant for those following the *sattvic* way of life. When one is engaged in a *rajasic* mode, some of these principles may not be applicable.

The cow is especially worshipped in *Vedic* culture as equal to the position of mother. The child is nourished by the milk of the mother and the cow during the early years. All the *Vedic* rituals and sacrifices require milk, yogurt, ghee, and so on, which are given by the cow. The *Vedic* system recognizes seven personalities to be given the respect of mother, and the cow is one of them.

ātma-mātā guroḥ patnī
brāhmaṇī rāja-patnikā
dhenur dhātrī tathā pṛthvī
saptaitā mātaraḥ smṛtāḥ (*Canakya Niti*)

The seven mothers are the original mother, the wife of the teacher or spiritual master, the wife of a *brāhmaṇa*, the king's wife, the cow, the nurse, and the earth.

The *Cāṇakya Nīti śāstra* (5.21–22) also explains in another context that there are five fathers and five mothers.

jānitācopanetāca yastuvidyām prayacchati

annadātā bhayatrātā pañcaite pitaraḥ smṛtāḥ

These five people are to be respected as father—your birth father, the one who initiates you into the study of the *Vedas* (*Āyurveda* included), he who teaches you, provides you with food, and protects you from fearful situations.

rājapatnī guroḥ patnī mitrapatni tathaiva ca

patnimātā svamātā ca pañcaitā mātaraḥ smṛtāḥ

The king's wife, the guru's wife, the friend's wife, your wife's mother, and your own mother are the five mothers.

Hospitality and warmly welcoming guests into homes, though they are strangers, are other specialties of *Vedic* culture. During *Vedic* times, people used to travel long distances on foot, and in many places, there would be no facility like hotels to stay in or for food. So one could go to any home in the village and ask for food and shelter, and it would be provided. It was considered a sacred duty to never disrespect a guest. Such a high level of faith and trust existed in the society that no one would try to exploit this principle unnecessarily.

There is another instruction that says a society where five personalities—women, children, elderly persons, *brāhmaṇas* (intellectuals), and cows—are not respected is on a course of self-destruction. This verse also reflects the same principle.

The lesson that is being conveyed here is the importance of being sensible and sensitive to others. *Āyurvedic* lifestyle teaches us to not hurt any living being physically, verbally, or even mentally and to offer respect to all. This brings purity and grace into our lives and that of others.

Whenever we see people better or higher than us, it is natural to feel envious. What to do about it?

AH Sū. 2.26

Helpfulness and envy

उपकारप्रधानः स्यादपकारपरेऽप्यरौ ॥२६॥

सम्पद्विपत्स्वेकमना, हेतावीर्ष्येत्फले न तु ॥२६॥

upakāra-pradhānaḥ syād-apakārapare 'pyarau

sampad-vipatsv-ekamanā hetāv-īrṣyet-phale na tu //26//

upakāra – help; *pradhānaḥ syād* – it is important to; *apakāra* – one who is causing harm; *paraḥ api* – comparatively also; *arau* – (ari) enemies; *sampat* – prosperity; *vipatsu* – and calamity; *ekamanā* – even minded; *hetāu* – the causes; *īrṣyet* – be envious of; *phale* – result; *na* – not; *tu* – but

Translation

It is important to help even enemies who are causing harm. One should be undisturbed in times of prosperity and calamity. Envy only the cause of the activity and never the result.

Commentary

Three basic principles of life are enumerated in this verse:

1. Always be helpful to all.
2. Be situated in equanimity.
3. Be inspired by the achievements of others.

There are two types of people: *upakāra paraḥ* and *apakāra paraḥ* (i.e., those trying to help you and those trying to harm you).

Āyurveda is a highly philosophical life science. Your understanding of the philosophy and way of life will influence your health on all levels.

Here we see that a culture based on helping even enemies who are in need is encouraged. What to speak of friends! This actually puts an end to the enmity and fosters love and friendship. Enmity can never be overcome by fighting with each other. It is especially recommended here to help the enemy. Mahātma Gandhi said that an "eye for an eye" will only make the whole world blind. Of course this does not encourage foolishness. One should intelligently apply these principles in all circumstances.

Envy the cause but not the result. It means that one should strike at the cause of a problem rather than trying to cover up the result. Treat the cause of the disease rather than the symptom. The nature of envy is that one wants to destroy the object of envy.

Sarvāṅgasundara: The definition of *envy* is "the inability to tolerate the progress of another person." When we see people getting good results, the tendency is to become envious of them and think, "Why am I not making as much progress as the other?" This is enviousness. This especially affects those who want to attain abundance without hard work. The formula given here is meant to help us overcome that. Envy cannot be dissolved into thin air. It is quite natural for this feeling to arise in the mind of a person. The solution is to redirect this feeling in a positive manner.

Progress is the result of hard work. Hard work is the cause of progress. Hence, it is recommended to direct the feeling of envy towards the cause (i.e., hard work) rather than the result. The nature of envy is that you want more of it than the other person. This will make the person work hard, which will in turn cause his own progress as well. The result is not in our control. It is only our effort (the cause) that we can control.

It is advised to be even minded in prosperity and calamity. How is this possible? This directly points toward spirituality. It is not possible to have equanimity without spiritual understanding of life.

Though one may be trying to harm a person all the time, it is not necessary that the effort should be successful. Sometimes though someone tries to harm you, they will not be successful. Sometimes a person may try to harm you, but the result, on the contrary, may turn out to be favorable to you. At other times a friend may try to help you, but eventually it may turn out to be harmful to you. An *ari* is a person who, by nature, has an intent to harm you just as the *doṣas* are by nature disease causing, but only when there is a favorable circumstance can they cause harm. This is the point to be understood. So there is no harm in helping an enemy as long as you avoid any situation where they can harm you.

Enemies (*ari*) are of two types:

1. *Upakara* (intending good but resulting in harm)
2. *Apakara* (intending harm and resulting in harm)

How can we direct our envy in the positive direction? The easiest way is to start glorifying the wonderful activities of the person we are feeling envious about. This is described in the next verse.

AH Sū. 2.27–28a

The art of speaking

कालेहितं मितं ब्रूयादविसंवादि पेशलम् ॥२७॥

पूर्वाभिभाषी, सुमुखः सुशीलः करुणामृदुः ॥२७॥

नैकः सुखी, न सर्वत्र विश्रब्धो, न च शङ्कितः ॥२८॥

kāle hitaṁ mitaṁ brūyād avisaṁvādi peśalam

pūrvābhibhāṣī sumukhaḥ suśīla karuṇā mṛduḥ //27

naikaḥ sukhī na sarvatra viśrabdho na ca śaṅkitaḥ //28//

kāle hitaṁ – relevant or beneficial to the context and time; *mitaṁ* – precise, in few words; *brūyād* – to speak; *avisaṁvādi* – non-contradictory speech, truthful; *peśalam* – soft, delicate, charming; *pūrvābhibhāṣī* – speak with a pleasant smile; *sumukhaḥ* – gracious, cheerful, favorable (having a beautiful mouth); *suśīla* – well mannered; *karuṇā* – compassionate; *mṛduḥ* – gentle; *na* – not; *ekaḥ* – selfishly; *sukhī* – enjoying; *na* – not; *sarvatra* – everything and everyone; *viśrabdho* – confiding, trusting; *na* – not; *ca* – and; *śaṅkitaḥ* – suspicious

Translation

Speak precisely, relevant to the context and time, without contradicting, in a delicate manner, and with a pleasant smiling look on the face. Be well mannered, compassionate, and gentle. Never enjoy selfishly. Neither trust or confide in everyone always nor be always suspicious.

Commentary

Learning to speak properly is one of the most important things in life. A wrong word spoken can seldom be taken back. Twelve principles of speech are mentioned in this verse.

1. Relevant to context and time
2. Precise and to the point
3. Noncontradictory
4. Soft
5. Speaking pleasantly with a smile
6. Favorable
7. Well mannered

8. Compassionate
9. Gentle
10. Not selfish
11. Not confiding everything
12. Not being suspicious of everyone

Think—before you speak (quotation adapted from the teachings of Socrates, the Greek philosopher)

- T—is it *true*?
- H—is it helpful?
- I—is it *inspiring*?
- N—is it *necessary*?
- K—is it *kind*?

Note that here the emphasis is not on always speaking the truth. Truth should be spoken, but it should be spoken in a palatable way. Speaking the truth in a way that causes antagonism and hurt is counterproductive.

The words *hitam* (beneficial) and *mitam* (appropriate quantity) are the golden words used in many instances. You will notice that the same words are used while describing the rules of eating in AH. Sū. 2.20.

Confidentiality is one of the most important aspects of medical practice, and here it is emphasized by the term *na sarvatra viśrabdho*.

Regarding speech it is said in the *Cāṇakya Nīti śāstra 2.5*:

parokṣe kārya hantāram pratyakṣe priya vādinam

varjayet tādṛśam mitram viṣa kumbham payo mukham

"Avoid him who speaks sweetly in front of you but tries to ruin you behind your back, for he is a pitcher of poison with milk on the top."

Yet another beautiful song from the *Cāṇakya Nīti śāstra* 2.13:

kāhi bhāra samarthānām kim dūram vyavasāyinām
kovideśa suvidyānām ko'priyaḥ priyavādinām

"What is too heavy for one who is capable? Which is the place too distant for a businessman? Which land is foreign for the learned? Who can be inimical to one who speaks in a pleasing manner?"

jale taila khale guhyam pātre dānam manāgapi
prājñe śāstram svayam yāti vistāram vastu śaktitaḥ
(*Canakya Niti* 14.5)

"Oil on water, a secret told to a man of low character, charity given to a worthy person, and scriptural knowledge given to an intelligent person spread out by virtue of their nature."

This is a description of how refined speech is the real decoration that makes a person attractive.

keyūrā na vibhūṣayanti puruṣam hārā na candrojjvalā
na snānam na vilepanam na kusumam nālankṛtā mūrdhajāḥ
vāṇyekā samalankaroti puruṣam yā samskṛtā dhāryate
kṣīyante khalu bhūṣaṇāni satatam vāgbhūṣaṇam bhūṣāṇam
- From *Nītiśataka* by King *Bhartṛhari*

A beautiful necklace shining like the moon, a bath, applicationof fragrant pastes, flowers or a crown will not decorate a person as much as refined speech does. All the other decoration will dwindle away to fine speech will always be present.

At the end of the last verse it was said that one should not reveal everything indiscriminately. What are the things that should not be revealed?

AH Sū. 2.28b–29a

Four things that should be concealed

न कञ्चिदात्मनः शत्रुं नात्मानं कस्यचिद्रिपुम् ॥२८॥
प्रकाशयेन्नापमानं न च निःस्नेहतां प्रभोः ॥२९॥

na kañcid-ātmanaḥ śatruṁ nātmānaṁ kasyacid-ripuṁ //28//
prakāśayen-nāpamānaṁ na ca niḥ-snehatāṁ prabhoḥ //29//

na kañcid – never unto anyone; *ātmanaḥ* – one's own; *śatruṁ* – enmity; *na* – neither; *ātmānaṁ* – unto oneself; *kasyacid* – any; *ripuṁ* – enmity; *prakāśayen* – reveal; *na* – not; *apamānaṁ* – experiences of insult; *na* – not; *ca* – and; *niḥ*-(*snehatāṁ*): – lack of love; *prabhoḥ* – for authorities

Translation

Never reveal one's enmity to another person nor another's hostility toward the self. Do not speak to anyone about insulting experiences or express lack of respect for senior authorities.

Commentary

Four activities to avoid while speaking are

1. revealing enmity toward any person;
2. revealing anybody's hostility toward yourself;
3. talking about experiences of insult; and
4. expressing lack of love/respect for authorities.

This advice means that one should not publicly declare these things. Here the principle of diplomacy is mentioned. What a profound instruction! Diplomacy in life is not such a bad thing when used constructively. There are some who believe that everything should be told straight to the face, and this is the meaning of being straightforward and honest. But this method of functioning is not encouraged here in *Āyurveda*, since it can produce adverse reactions.

The goal of *Āyurveda* is *sukha* or happiness. Anything that can disturb the happiness of a person is to be avoided. If one does not follow the advice in this verse, he or she could end up making many enemies in life.

The urge to speak (*vāco vegam*) is one of the most difficult to control according to the *Vedas*. This is one of the qualifications required to become a *guru*. And here we find that this is one of the qualifications to be a good *vaidya* too.

Some of the current psychologists advise that one should speak out for the sake of better health. This is true. But one should know the right time, place, and person to speak with. Or else it can be disastrous.

It is said in the *Cāṇakya Nīti śāstra* 2.7:

manasā cintitam kāryam vācā naiva prakāśayet
mantreṇa rakṣayet gūḍham kāryam cāpi niyojayet

"Do not reveal what you have thought of doing, keep it a closely guarded secret, being determined to carry it to execution."

And even when you speak, it all ultimately depends on how it is received by the person you are talking to. Hence it is important to understand the level and mentality of the person you are dealing with.

As explained in this verse, the world is replete with hostile and insulting people. If one is not suppose to reveal these things, how should one deal with them?

AH Sū. 2.29b–30a

How to deal with people in general: to please them

जनस्याशयमालक्ष्य यो यथा परितुष्यति ॥२९॥
तं तथैवानुवर्तेत पराराधनपण्डितः ॥३०॥

janasyāśayam-ālakṣya yo yathā parituṣyati //29//
taṁ tathaivānuvarteta parārādhana-paṇḍitaḥ //30//

janasya – of the people; *āśayam* – the intention, disposition of mind, perceptions; *ālakṣya* – understanding carefully; *yo* – one who; *yathā* – in that way; *parituṣyati* – is pleasing, making happy; *taṁ* – them; *tatha* – thus; *eva* – also; *anuvarteta* – follow along, deal accordingly; *para* – other people; *ārādhana* – propitiation of, respected; *paṇditaḥ* – learned or skilled person

Translation

Having understood the mentality of people very carefully, and knowing what makes each one happy, one who is skilled in propitiating people should behave favorably with each person in that particular manner.

Commentary

One should carefully understand the mentality of every person one is dealing with. Sometimes what one says or does is not what is intended. It is important to understand the intention behind what was spoken or done.

How to recognize a *paṇḍita* (learned person) is described here. Knowledge means one should know how to deal favorably with everyone. If one knows the simple formula of how to keep people happy, one will be successful in life. Having loads of information or academic qualifications is not a sign of knowledge. This verse emphasizes the principle of being personal in your dealings with everyone. The *Vaidya* should be skilled in keeping everyone happy and satisfied. At the same time, in an effort to try and be nice to all, one should not go to the other extreme and become duplicitous.

How to keep everyone happy without being duplicitous is the subject of the next verse.

AH Sū. 2.30b–31b

The golden mean

न पीडयेदिन्द्रियाणि न चैतान्यतिलालयेत् ॥३०॥

त्रिवर्गशून्यं नारम्भं भजेत्तं चाविरोधयन् ॥३१॥

अनुयायात्प्रतिपदं सर्वधर्मेषु मध्यमाम् ॥३१॥

na pīḍayed-indriyāṇī na-caitāny-atilālayet //30//

trivarga śūnyaṁ nārambhaṁ bhajettaṁ cāvirodhayan

anuyāyāt pratipadaṁ sarva dharmeṣu madhyamām //31//

na pīḍayed – do not strain; *indriyāṇī* – the senses; *na* – not; *ca* – and; *etāni* – of the senses; *atilālayet* – too much indulgence; *trivarga* – the three groups (*dharma, artha, kāma*); *śūnyaṁ* – devoid of; *nārambhaṁ bhajet* – do not start any endeavor; *taṁ* – among the *trivargas* (*dharma, artha, kāma*) ; *ca* – and; *avirodhayan* – there should not be conflict; *anuyāyāt* – always follow; *pratipadaṁ* – at every step; *sarva* – every; *dharmeṣu* – duty; *madhyamām* – the middle path

Translation

The sense organs should not be excessively strained or tortured and, at the same time, neither excessively pampered. All activities should be done in accordance with the *trivarga* (*dharma*, *artha*, *kāma*). At the same time, activities should be done in such a way that they do not produce a conflicting situation between the *trivargas* (*dharma*, *artha*, *kāma*). Always follow the middle path (or golden mean) in every duty, at every step.

Commentary

The most important instruction in life is given here in this verse—*always follow the middle path*. Too much or too little of anything is not good. These are also explained in AH Sū. 1.19 to be the only causes of disease. More details about excessive, deficient, and perverted engagements will be explained in chapter 12 of *Sūtra sthāna*.

The way how one should work is explained here. *Dharma*, *artha*, *kāma*, and *mokṣa* have been described in the last chapter as the goal of a long life, which is the purpose of *Āyurveda*. One should perform work in this world in such a way that there is no conflict between ethical principles, earning wealth, fulfillment of desires, and attaining liberation. Some people feel that earning money is bad. But here the *ācārya* is clearly saying that we should earn enough money to fulfill all our desires in an ethical manner. This will eventually lead us to liberation. On the other hand, compromising dharma to accumulate wealth or posessions is impractical. This is what we see in a consumeristic society today where we have people with houses full of things and empty dissatisfied minds. We have strong houses and cars but broken relationships. This is because, as we began to run after accumulating things, we compromised on *dharma*. The "things" accumulated at the expense of *dharma* will eventually fail to truly satisfy us, though they may give a false sense of temporary pleasure. At the same time, the things acquired without compromising the principle of *dharma* result in satisfying our desires and cravings. That is the art or secret of living a successful and satisfied life.

It refers to using the senses to interact with the external world, in such a way as not to indulge in excessive sense gratification. At the same time one should also be careful to avoid excessive sense deprivation. Both extremes can result in physical and mental imbalances. This is the recommendation of *Āyurveda*.

How to decide how much is too much and how little is too little? That is the million-dollar question. Each one of us has to decide that for ourselves by individual introspection, retrospection, and using the guidance of *Vedic* literature and learned personalities.

While trying to walk the middle path, it is important to dress and only then address. Now *ācārya* is going to tell us about the importance of external appearance and cleanliness. It is by your attire that the world is going to make their first impression about you. This is important for you to be able to perform your work and influence people in a satisfying manner.

AH Sū. 2.32–33a

Norms of personal appearance: hygiene

नीचरोमनखश्मश्रुर्निर्मलाङ्घ्रिमलायनः ॥३२॥

स्नानशीलः सुसुरभिः सुवेषोऽनुल्बणोज्ज्वलः ॥३२॥

धारयेत्सततं रत्नसिद्धमन्त्रमहौषधीः ॥३३॥

nīca roma nakha śmaśru nirmalānghri malāyanaḥ
snāna-śīla susurabhiḥ suveṣo 'nulbaṇojjvalaḥ //32//
dhārayet satataṁ ratna siddha-mantra mahauṣadhīḥ //33//

nīca – trim; *roma* – hair; *nakha* – nails; *śmaśru* – moustache/beard; *nirmala* – clean or hygenic; *anghri* – feet; *malāyanaḥ* – excretory orifices; *snānaśīla* – habit of bathing regularly; *susurabhiḥ* – applying fragrances; *suveṣo* – well dressed; *anulbaṇa* – not excessively; *ujjvalaḥ* – gaudy
dhārayet – wear; *satataṁ* – always; *ratna* – jewels; *siddha-mantra* – perfected sacred hymns; *mahauṣadhīḥ* – divine medicines (ginger is also called *mahauṣadhīḥ*)

Translation

One should regularly perform the following - trim hair, nails, and beard, clean the feet and excretory orifices (nine openings of the body), bathe, apply fragrances, and be well dressed. Avoid dressing in an excessively flashy manner. One must always wear jewels, mantras, and medicinal herbs on the body.

Commentary

Āyurveda advises to trim one's nails, hair and so on at least once in three weeks. The nine openings in the body are - two eyes, two nostrils, two ears, mouth, anal orifice, urinary orifice. In females there are three more orifices – the two breasts and vagina. All these openings should be cleansed regularly as part of *dinacaryā*.

This verse could indicate wearing of amulets with *mantras* for protection and *mantra kavaca* (a divine incantation placed inside an amulet).

Body odor is one the things that can repel people away from us. These days it is quite common for people to neither bathe in the morning nor bathe regularly. There are certain regions in the world where people who bathe once in a week or even once in a month and this could be due to the unique seasonal characteristics of a particular place. This is not approved by *Āyurveda*. Hence *ācārya* advises to bathe regularly and use pleasant fragrances which improves the presentability.

Dressing in a flashy manner may be suitable for people of certain professions that are more *rajasic* in nature but it is not befitting a *Vaidya*. One should dress in a simple and clean manner.

AH Sū. 2.33b–34a

Rules to be followed before going out at night

सातपत्रपदत्राणो विचरेद्युगमात्रदृक् ॥३३॥

निशि चात्ययिके कार्ये दण्डी मौली सहायवान् ॥३४॥

sātapatra padatrāṇo vicared-yugamātra-dṛk //33//

niśi cātyayike kārye daṇḍī maulī sahāyavān //34//

sa – along with; *ātapatra* – large umbrella or head protector (that which protects from the sun is called *ātapatra* – [*ātapa trāyate* iti *ātapatra*]); *padatrāṇo* – foot wear; *vicared* – going to walk; *yugamātra* – a visual field of (three meters approximately); *dṛk* – look at; *niśi* – in the night; *ca* – and; *ātyayike* – if very important; *kārye* – work; *daṇḍī* – with a stick; *maulī* – wearing a cap; *sahāyavān* – with a helper

Translation

One should walk outside with an umbrella, wear footwear, and have visibility up to a distance of one *yugamātra* (approximately three meters) ahead of the path. If it is for very important work, one can go out in the night with a stick, wearing a cap, and with a helper to accompany.

Commentary

Umbrella is to protect one from the sun and rain. Footwear is used for the purpose of preventing loss of *dṛkbala* (power of eyesight) and *śukla kṣaya* (loss of reproductive ability). There are two *nāḍis* (energy channels) going all the way from the feet to the eyes. Injury to these *nāḍis* can result in loss of vision. Having visibility ahead is to avoid snakes. While traveling at night, one should repeatedly keep striking the ground with the stick to drive away any snake that may be lying in the path. The cap is to protect from fog at night.

Note: *Ācārya Vāgbhaṭa* has spoken elaborately about things that should be done. Now he enumerates a few things that should be avoided.

From verse 34b to 44 is a list of items (about fifty-two items) to avoid.

AH Sū. 2.34b–35a

Eleven items to avoid

चैत्यपूज्यध्वजाशस्तच्छायाभस्मतुषाशुचीन् ॥३४॥

नाक्रामेच्छर्करालोष्टबलिस्नानभुवो न च ॥३५॥

caitya-pūjya-dhvajāśastac-chāyā-bhasma-tuṣāśucīn //34//

nā-krāmec-charkarā-loṣta-bali-snāna-bhuvo-na-ca //35//

caitya – sacrificial altar, the ; *pūjya* – worshipful personalities; *dhvaja* – flag post; *aśastat* – inauspicious things; *chāyā* – shadow; *bhasma* – ashes; *tuṣā* – chaff of grains; *aśucīn* – dirty things, remnants of food; *nā* – not; *krāmet* – walk over, trespass, step over; *śarkara* – gravel; *loṣta* – lump of earth, stone; *bali* – platform of sacrificial offerings; *snāna bhuva* – bathing place; *na* – not; *ca* – and

Translation

Do not walk over or trespass the sacrificial altar, worshipful personalities, flag posts, shadow (of uncivilized people), ashes, chaff, unclean things, gravel, lump of earth, sacrificial platform, and bathing place.

Commentary

To touch holy or worshipful items or such a person with one's feet is considered disrespectful. At the same time, to touch the feet of holy or senior persons, parents, and so on with one's hands is considered very respectful. Every institution usually has a flag post in front of it. The flag of the institution is considered highly respectable as it represents the values and principles of the institution.

It is said that one should avoid the shadow of wicked and uncivilized persons. This means that one should keep a safe distance from them. *Ucchiṣṭham* represents leftovers of food after eating, which are considered unclean. This is also described in the *Bhagavad Gīta* as food in the *tāmasic guṇa*. It is possible that one is advised to avoid stepping over small pebbles (*śarkara*) due to the risk of slipping and falling. Ashes and chaff are considered impure to touch. *Bhasma* that is left over after the *yajña* or sacrificial fire is considered holy and is often applied on the body for consecration.

The sacrificial altar described here especially refers to places where animal sacrifices are performed. These places are often filled with the constant cries of dying animals and blood flowing everywhere. It is not the best place for a *sattvik* person. This place also contains the energy of fear that is released by the animal as it is dying in pain. An example of such a place in modern times is the slaughterhouse.

The bathing place is not considered pure because we go there to wash away all the dirt on the body and our sins. This is explained earlier in the chapter while describing the benefits of bathing. Such places contain a lot of negative energy and we should avoid being there for a long time. This does not apply to rivers because the water is constantly flowing purifying everything.

Some of these things cannot be trespassed because they are too holy; some others, because they are too inauspicious; and others, because it is dangerous.

In the *Cāṇakya Nīti śāstra* 10.2, it is said:

> *dṛṣṭi pūtam nyaset pādam*
> *vastra pūtam pibet jalam*
> *śāstra pūtam vadet vākyam*
> *manaḥ pūtam samācaret*

We should carefully scrutinize the place upon which we step. In English there is a saying, “Look before you leap”; we should only drink water that has been purified through a cloth (the principle is to avoid contaminated water); our words should be purified by speaking only from *śāstra*; and any action should be performed only after careful consideration.

AH Sū. 2.35b–36a

Five more items to avoid

नदीं तरेन्न बाहुभ्यां, नाग्निस्कन्धमभिव्रजेत् ॥३५॥

सन्दिग्धनावं वृक्षं च नारोहेद्दुष्टयानवत् ॥३६॥

nadīṁ tarenna bāhubhyāṁ nāgni-skandham-abhivrajet //35//

sandigdha-nāvaṁ vṛkṣaṁ ca nārohed-duṣtayānavat //36//

nadīṁ – river; *taret* – go across; *na* – not; *bāhubhyāṁ* – with hands; *na* – not; *agni* – fire; *skandham* – aggregate; (*agni skandham*: remnants of a bonfire); *abhi* – begin to; *vrajet* – go towards; (*abhi vrajet*: – begin to advance toward); *sandigdha* – doubtful; *nāvaṁ* – boat; *vṛkṣaṁ* – tree; *ca* – and; *na* – not; *ārohed* – climb; *duṣta* – malfunctioning; *yānavat* – in a vehicle

Translation

Avoid swimming across the river, walking over ashes left behind after a bonfire, boarding a doubtful boat, climbing a tree, and getting into an improperly functioning vehicle.

Commentary

Duṣta yānavat can also mean an evil-minded or reckless driver. In the modern context, it is advice for safe driving. One should also check to see if the car is in the proper condition before getting into it.

These are all risky situations that can result in loss of life or accidents. The principle is that one should try to avoid any situation that is risky. The truth is that any situation in this world is risky. It is described in the *Vedas*, "*padam padam yad vipadam*" meaning that in this world there is danger at every step.

In his *Nīti śāstra 1.15*, *Cāṇakya Pandita* has said, "*nakhinām ca nadīnām ca śṛṅgiṇām śastra pāṇinām, viśvāso naiva kartavyam strīṣu rājakuleṣu ca.*" Here he says that one should never trust a river, an animal with nails or horns, a person holding weapons, a (cunning) member of the opposite sex, and a politician. Many such instructions are found in *Cāṇakya Nīti* and *Vidura Nīti*, and it is advised to read such books to understand moral instructions.

These are all examples of different situations that can endanger life. Only examples are given here. The principle is that any situation that is a risk for injury or loss of life should be avoided as much as possible.

AH Sū. 2.36b–37b

Seven more items to avoid

नासंवृतमुखः कुर्यात्क्षुतिहास्यविजृम्भणम् ॥३६॥

नासिकां न विकुष्णीयान्नाकस्माद्विलिखेद्भुवम् ॥३७॥

नाङ्गैश्चेष्टेत विगुणं, नासीतोत्कुटकश्चिरम् ॥३७॥

nāsaṁvṛta-mukhaḥ kuryāt-kṣuti-hāsya-vijṛmbhaṇam //36//

nāsikāṁ na vikuṣṇīyān-nākasmād-vilikhed-bhuvam

naṅgaiś-ceṣṭeta viguṇaṁ nāsītotkuṭakaś-ciram //37//

na – not; *asaṁvṛta* – with an uncovered; *mukhaḥ* – face, mouth; *kuryāt* – should be done; *kṣuti* – sneezing; *hāsya* – laughing; *vijṛmbhaṇam* – yawning; *nāsikāṁ* – the nose; *na* – not; *vikuṣṇīyān* – twisting with fingers; *na* – not; *akasmād* – without any reason; *vilikhet* – write; *bhuvam* – on the earth; *na* – not; *aṅgaiś* – of the body parts; *ceṣṭeta* – move; *viguṇaṁ* – awkwardly; *na* – not; *asīta* – is to be; *utkuṭakaś* – squatting; *ciram* – prolonged period of time

Translation

One should not sneeze, laugh, or yawn without covering the mouth. Avoid twisting the nose, writing on the earth (using hands or feet) without any reason, awkwardly moving the different body parts, or sitting for a prolonged period of time in the squatting position.

Commentary

What is the importance of not twisting the nose in particular or writing on the earth? All the sense organs should be given special protection. One should not unnecessarily stimulate or excessively manipulate any sense organ. For example, one should not put any pointed objects into the ears or eyes, and so on. Nor should one try to use the hands or fingers excessively in the eyes, ears, or nose. This can cause damage, as the sense organs are sensitive areas. Many people have the habit of removing the dirt from their nose excessively. Others have the habit of putting things in their ears trying to clean it.

Does *Āyurveda* prohibit the activity of sitting in meditation in squatting position for a long time? Yes, from the strictly *Āyurvedic* point of view of health, this is not recommended. The general principle is that the same activity should not be performed continuously over a long period of time. Everything should be given a break in between.

Moving the body parts excessively leads to aggravation of *cala guṇa* and thus *vāta* aggravation. Some people have the habit of shaking their legs constantly while sitting. It is commonly said that if one has this habit, then he or she will be poverty stricken, probably due to the fact that the restlessness of the mind will not give stability to the person in his or her life. This habit can cause aggravation of *vāta*.

Sitting for a long time (being sedentary) is explained as one of the causes of *prameha* (polyuria disorder), that is, *āsya sukhatva* (comfort of lying in bed) and even *arśas* (hemorrhoids). In the squatting position, there is stress on the knees, and hence, this should be avoided for excessive periods of time. This is the position assumed when using Indian-style lavatories.

Covering the mouth while sneezing is also a part of personal hygiene. It is explained that when one yawns, ghostly entities get an opportunity to enter the body through the open mouth. They are unable to do so during other times. Hence, one is advised to either close the mouth or snap the fingers to avoid this. The same is applicable to sneezing, laughing, and so on.

During earlier days, I have seen people in India covering their mouth with the hands while conversing as a sign of respect. One may have the habit of using the finger to clean the waste or snot from the nose. But to dig the finger deep inside is not advisable. There are certain vital sensitive *marma* points in that area, and if one unnecessarily engages in twisting the nose, it can result in injury to those *marmas*. It was commonplace to twist the ears of a student who was disobedient. But this kind of twisting should not be done over the nose, as it can result in the person becoming unconscious.

Sarvāṅgasundara: In *vikuṣṇīyān*, the *vi* indicates that twisting the nose in a certain manner or excessive cleaning of the snot (dirt in the nose) can result in injury. Drawing on the earth is not advised. The earth is also worshipped as mother in the *Vedas*. *Utkuṭakaściram* means one should not sit for long, because it produces diseases like hemorrhoids.

AH Sū. 2.38

When to stop activities, prolonged squatting, and places to avoid for night stay

देहवाक्चेतसां चेष्टाः प्राक् श्रमाद्विनिवर्तयेत् ॥३८॥

नोर्ध्वजानुश्चिरं तिष्ठेत् नक्तं सेवेत न द्रुमम् ॥३८॥

deha-vāk-cetasāṁ ceṣṭāḥ prāk śramād-vinivartayet

nordhva-jānuś-ciram tiṣṭhet naktaṁ seveta na drumam //38//

deha – body; *vāk* – words; *cetasāṁ* – of mind; *ceṣṭāḥ* – activities; *prāk* – before; *śramād* – fatigue; *vinivartayet* –

terminated; *na* – never; *ūrdhva* – upright position; *jānuś* – knees; *ciram* – long time; *tiṣṭhet* – keep; *naktaṁ* – in the night; *seveta* – take shelter; *na* – never; *drumam* – tree

Translation

Activities of the body, words, and mind should be terminated before reaching the point of fatigue. Never sit with the knees in upright position for an extended period of time or take shelter under a tree at night.

Commentary

The amount of work one should perform is explained here. Sitting with the knees bent in an upright position for a long time is a cause of *atiyoga* or stress on the knees causing degeneration.

Sarvāṅgasundara: It is recommended to avoid trees, because there may be insects and also to avoid the stool and urine, which may drop on us, of birds and other creatures residing in the trees.

Here it is recommended to avoid *ūrdhva jānu* position for a long time. The same was also said in the previous verse—*utkuṭakaś ciram*. Why is this being emphasized so much?

The significance of not sitting for a long time with knees bent can be understood in the present context in relation to what has been told just before this. The key phrase is *before reaching the fatigue point*. It is known that sitting for a long time in the squatting position can initiate pain in the knees. This can lead to faster degeneration of the knee joint causing osteoarthritis, and so on. Any position that is not comfortable should not be maintained for too long. At the same time an excessively comfortable position should not be accepted for too long as well. *Āyurveda* suggests the middle path in life.

AH Sū. 2.39

More places to be avoided in the day as well as night

तथा चत्वरचैत्यान्तश्चतुष्पथसुरालयान् ॥३९॥

सूनाटवीशून्यगृहश्मशानानि दिवापि न ॥३९॥

tathā catvara caityāntaś catuṣpatha surālayān

sūnāṭavī śūnya gṛha śmaśānāni divāpi na //39//

tathā – then; *catvara* – crossroads where three roads meet; *caityāntaś* – funeral place; *catuṣpatha* - junction of four roads; *surālayān* – place of the devas (Gods) i.e. temple; *sūna (vadha sthānam)* – place of slaughter; *āṭavī* – lonely place; *śūnya gṛha* – (*ujjaṭam bhavanam*) empty or vacant houses; *śmaśānāni* – cremation sites; *diva* – day time; *api* – also; *na* – not

Translation

One should also avoid crossroads where four or three roads meet, funeral places, and temples at night. Slaughterhouses, lonely places, empty or vacant houses, and cremation sites should be avoided during the daytime as well.

Commentary

This verse describes areas where there is a possibility of being attacked by ghosts and evil spirits. This is called *bhūta pratiṣedha* in *Āyurveda* and is described in more detail in *Uttara sthāna*. Many of the mental and personality disorders are explained to be due to this reason. There are methods to remove these spirits from the body too. Many of these techniques come under the *daiva vyapaāśraya cikitsa* (taking shelter of higher powers) category. Hence, it is advised to avoid these areas or places to prevent such consequences.

Sarvāṅgasundara: *Catvāra* is a junction where three roads meet, and *catuṣpada* is where four roads meet. It is also a place where the residents of the village meet to discuss various matters.

It is described in AH *Uttara sthāna* that for *bāla graha*, some *pujas* for exorcism of ghosts and spirits have to be performed at the *catvāra*. This means that ghosts and spirits have a tendency to congregate there.

Sleeping in a lonely house is described as one of the *nidāna* for *unmāda*. This is also due to the increased chances of possession by spirits.

All these are places where ghosts and spirits reside. One is at the risk of getting possessed or attacked by them at these locations.

AH Sū. 2.40

Looking at the sun, carrying weight, and protecting eyes

सर्वथेक्षेत नादित्यं, न भारं शिरसा वहेत् ॥४०॥

नेक्षेत प्रततं सूक्ष्मं दीप्तामेध्याप्रियाणि च ॥४०॥

sarvathekṣeta nādityaṁ na bhāraṁ śirasā vahet

nekṣeta pratataṁ sūkṣmaṁ dīpt-āmedhy-āpriyāṇi ca //40//

sarvatha – at all times; *īkṣeta* – looking; *na* – never; *ādityaṁ* – the sun; *na* – never; *bhāraṁ* – weight; *śirasā* – on the head; *vahet* – should carry; *na* – never; *īkṣeta* – look; *pratataṁ* – continuously; *sūkṣmaṁ* – minute; *dīpta* – bright; *amedhya* – dirty things; *apriyāṇi* – disliked; *ca* – and

Translation

One should never look directly at the sun, carry a heavy weight on the head, and look continuously at minute objects, bright light, dirty, and unpleasant items.

Commentary

The items described in this verse are examples for *atiyoga*. *Atiyoga* is one of the three subdivisions for the cause of diseases.

Here we can see that sun gazing is not encouraged in *Āyurveda*. It is advised not to continuously look at bright objects, and then special mention is made to not look at the sun, which is also bright. The sun is the brightest object in the universe.

***Sarvāṅgasundara*:** One should especially not gaze at the sun while it is rising and setting. Many people have a habit of enjoying the sunrise and sunset, and it is also done in several tourist places. This is probably because during the rising and setting of the sun, the rays which enter the eyes are increasingly towards the red part of the spectrum and could cause harm. It will be interesting to investigate why *Āyurveda* recommends against it.

The same example will be discussed in chapter 12 while explaining about *ati*, *hīna*, and *mithyā yoga*. Looking at the sun is *atiyoga* of eyes, and looking at a minute object for a long time is *hīna yoga*. Carrying heavy objects is *atiyoga* of the body.

AH Sū. 2.41

Dealing with alcohol and exposure to natural forces

मद्यविक्रयसन्धानदानपानानि नाचरेत् ॥४१॥

पुरोवातातपरजस्तुषारपरुषानिलान् ॥४१॥

madya vikraya sandhāna dāna-pānāni nācaret

purovāt-ātapa-rajas-tuṣāra paruṣānilān //41//

madya – alcohol; *vikraya* – selling, bartering (*vinimaya*); *sandhāna* – brewing; *dāna* – offering in charity; *pānāni* – consuming; *na* – never; *ācaret* – perform; *purau* – from the east;

vāta – the wind; *ātapa* – heat, sunlight; *rajas* – dust; *tuṣāra* – frost, snow, ice; *paruṣānilān* – storm

Translation

Selling, brewing, or offering alcohol in charity should not be done. One should also avoid the wind from the east, heat (sunlight from the east), dust, frost, and storm.

Commentary

Āyurveda discourages the practice of intoxicating oneself for pleasure. The inebriated state is another condition where ghosts and spirits have easy access to enter the body. Alcoholism is also addictive and the cause of many chronic health disorders.

This instruction about alcohol is especially meant for warm climates. In other parts of the world where the climate is extremely cold, a little alcohol is a part of the diet in order to maintain the heat in the body, and they also take a very *snigdha* diet in order to balance the *śīta rūkṣa* (cold and dry).

The recommendation to avoid the eastern breeze will again be mentioned in AH Ni. 1.21. The eastern breeze is said to be a cause for the aggravation of all the three *doṣa*s causing *sannipāta* (combination of all three doṣas) disease. Usually according to *vāstu*, the entrance of the home should be pointing toward the east or north. So it is interesting to note that the breeze coming in through the front door may not be so good for health.

We also see that the wind blowing from the east is generally more violent than that from the west. These are called the nor'easter winds, which create a lot of damage.

Sarvāṅgasundara: Five items including *purovāta* (eastern breeze) are to be given up.

AH Sū. 2.42
Avoid awkward body positions and five more items to avoid

अनृजुः क्षवथूद्गारकासस्वप्नान्नमैथुनम् ॥४२॥
कूलच्छायां नृपद्विष्टं व्यालदंष्ट्रिविषाणिनः ॥४२॥

anṛjuḥ kṣavathūdgāra kāsa svapnānna maithunam
kūlacchāyāṁ nṛpa dviṣṭam vyāla daṁṣtri viṣāṇinaḥ //42//

anṛjuḥ – crooked, perverted; *kṣavathu* – sneezing; *udgāra* – belching; *kāsa* – coughing; *svapna* – sleeping; *anna* – eating; *maithunam* – sexual intercourse; *kūla (vaprah)* – river bank, ditch, slope; *chāyāṁ* – shadow of; *nṛpa* – king; *dviṣṭam* – enemy of; *vyāla* – wild animals, mad, vicious; *daṁṣtri* – animal having sharp teeth; *viṣāṇinaḥ* – poisonous animals (eg. snake)

Translation

Avoid perversions in the acts of sneezing, belching, coughing, sleeping, eating, and sexual intercourse. Avoid ditches or slopes (shadows of river banks), enemies of the king, wild animals, animals with sharp teeth, and poisonous creatures.

Commentary

This is a random list of items that can cause harm to health. There does not seem to be any other relation between the items. In the section of *arśas nidāna* (AH Ni. Ch. 7), it is explained that hemorrhoids can be caused due to repeated, excessive, and abrasive intercourse. In one sense it refers to anal sex. This is an example of what is mentioned here as perverted sex. Another common example of perverted sex in today's world is pornography. Pornography destroys loving feelings, sanctity of the sexual union, and respect for your partner; it corrupts the mind, leads towards many mental disturbances, and eventually to other physical diseases.

An example of perverted sleeping is sleeping during the day when it is not recommneded. This increases *kapha*, causes *agni māndya*, and so on.

Perverted eating means eating that is excessive, deficient, untimely, incompatible, and so on. Detailed descriptions of this will come in the next volume of this series.

Perverted sneezing, belching, and so on means suppressing or artificially trying to produce these urges. We tend to suppress them when we are in a meeting or in public places due to etiquette. This can result in severe *vāta* aggravation. The same is the case with sleeping, eating, and so on. This will be explained in more detail in chapter 4 of this book.

The king's enemy should be avoided, because if one is seen closely associating with public enemies of the state, it can lead to legal entanglements, imprisonment, and so on. *Āyurveda* is advising these things in order to protect us in every way.

Shadows of river banks should be avoided, because the trees on the river banks are always at risk of falling off. In the *Cāṇakya Nīti śāstra*, it is said:

> *nadī tīre ca ye vṛkṣā parageheṣu kāminī*
> *mantrahīnāśca rājānaḥ śīghram naśyatyasamśayam* (2.15)
>
> Trees on a river bank, a woman staying in another man's house[5], and kings without advisors go without doubt to swift destruction.

AH Sū. 2.43

Association with different types of people and five activities to avoid during sandhya

हीनानार्यातिनिपुणसेवां विग्रहमुत्तमैः ॥४३॥

सन्ध्यास्वभ्यवहारस्त्रीस्वप्नाध्ययनचिन्तनम् ॥४३॥

hīnānāryātinipuṇa-sevāṁ vigraham-uttamaiḥ

sandhyāsv-abhyavahāra-strī-svapnādhyayana-cintanam //43//

hīna – low class, inferior; *anārya* – uncivilized; *atinipuṇa* – over smart, excessively calculative; *sevāṁ* – dependence upon; *vigraham* – quarrel with; *uttamaiḥ* – people with excellent behaviour, those who are more powerful; *sandhyāsu* – in the

[5] This is also applicable in the reverse manner. This refers to a married woman who is staying with a man other than her husband.

evening (during the transition periods) ; *abhyavahār* – taking food ; *strī* – woman (indicates sexual intercourse); *svapna* – sleeping; *adhyayana* – learning, studying; *cintanam* – thinking

Translation

One must avoid being dependent upon degraded, uncivilized, and oversmart people. One should not quarrel with those who are civilized. One should avoid eating, intercourse, sleeping, studying, and thinking about important matters during the transition periods of the day.

Commentary

Now Vāgbhaṭa comes to the discussion of more subtle energy shifts causing disease.

Why are some of these activities to be avoided in the evening? This is one of the *sandhis* (transition junction) during the day. Any time when there is a transition of energy state is a vulnerable period. This is applicable when the energy changes take place during the day, seasons, eclipses, and so on. During vulnerable periods it is recommended to avoid any stressful work, as our system is adapting to the change. So any activity that produces additional stresses is best avoided.

During these transitions the mind is also not stable. There is a possibility of *vāta* imbalances, and hence, it is better to sit quietly and meditate. In India we find the *brahmanas* chanting their *gayatri mantras* and other *mantras* during these times. Some others perform the *agni hotra* sacrifice during the sunrise and sunset. These practices can be adopted by *vaidyas*. It is also recommended not to conduct consultations during these times.

Those people who have a tendency to remain unclean and engage in uncivilized and despicable activities are considered to be of a low status. An uncivilized person will not hesitate to do anything for some personal profit. Such people cannot be relied upon.

> *durācārīs duṣṭa dṛṣṭir durāvāsī ca durjanah*
> *yanmaitrī kriyate pumsāstu śīghram vinaśyati*
> (*Canakya Niti* 2.19)

"He who befriends a man whose conduct is vicious, whose vision is impure, and who is notoriously crooked is rapidly ruined."

***Sarvāṅgasundara*:** *Hīna* can be in three ways: *kula* (lineage), *śīla* (habits), and *vitta* (wealth). *Anārya* means *asādhava* (one who is not honorable or respectable).

Five activities to be avoided during *sandhyā* are enumerated. The principle is that one should take it easy during the transitions, as the energy is changing, and the atmosphere and body are in a vulnerable state.

Atinipuṇaḥ means those people who are excessively calculative about everything. Avoid eating at an enemy's house, in public places, and sacrificial remnants (this refers to sacrifices performed with selfish intentions). Sometimes sacrifices are done to absolve one from sinful reactions or exorcise a person from ghosts and spirits. The sinful reactions or subtle living beings are invoked into the sacrificial offerings and then fed to someone else or animals of a lower species. In India it is commonplace to be extremely careful when accepting any kind of eatables from anyone. Another reason is that when someone wants to effect harmful black magic (a kind of voodoo) on another, it is often done using contaminated food articles. Though some of us may doubt this, I have seen increasing numbers of such cases in my practice. This should not be taken lightly.

Vigraham uttamaiḥ: It is recommended to avoid getting into a debate, quarrel, or fight with someone who is stronger than you because you may be severely beaten up or defeated. The intelligent thing to do is to avoid it.

AH Sū. 2.44

Where not to accept food from and avoiding making sounds using body parts

शत्रुसत्रगणाकीर्णगणिकापणिकाशनम् ॥४४॥

गात्रवक्त्रनखैर्वाद्यं हस्तकेशावधूननम् ॥४४॥

śatru-satra-gaṇākīrṇa-gaṇikā-paṇikāśanam

gātra-vaktra-nakhair-vādyaṁ hasta-keśāvadhūnanam //44//

śatru - enemy; *satra* – inns, restaurants, hotels; *gaṇa* – wandering actor or singer; *ākīrṇa* – in a crowded place; *gaṇikā* – prostitute; *paṇikā* – merchant; *aśanam* – food;
gātra – with the body; *vaktra* – with mouth; *nakhair* – with nails, *vādyaṁ* – produce sound; *hasta* – hands; *keśa* – hair; *āvadhūnanam* – shaking, agitating, flickering, vibrations, and tremors

Translation

One should avoid eating at an enemy's place, in a public place, in crowded places, and with prostitutes, accepting food from wanderers and business-minded people, and also activities causing excessive vibration to the hands and hair. Avoid making sounds using the body, mouth, nails, or agitating the hands and hair.

Commentary

Sarvāṅgasundara: *Paṇa* is trade, and *paṇika* is one who lives only for the sake of *paṇa*, that is, a sinful trader. *Paṇika* is a sinful person who does not hesitate to sell sinful things. The trader who is honest and sells things that are not sinful is not called *paṇika*. There are different categories of traders.

Vakreṇa nakha can be understood as overgrown and curved nails. This is not recommended for producing musical sounds. It is recommended in the *Caraka Samhita* that one should clip one's nails and cut the hair on the head and face at least once in three weeks.

Eating from an enemy's place (*śatravaśanam*), eating remnants of *yajña*, and eating food that is not seasonal are also to be avoided. It is said, *"Yajñānte tad-udbhūta pāpopaśamanīya prāyaścittam śrūyate,"* meaning that remnants of the *yajña* are the atonements performed for the performance of sinful activities. Hence, it is to be avoided.

The general principle about food is that one should avoid all food as far as possible from outsiders. Anyone who you cannot completely trust should not be cooking or serving you food. Along with the food also comes the consciousness of the person who is cooking and serving it. So if the person cooking or serving does not have a pure mind, the food can infect the one who is consuming it as well. This is the reason why in *Vedic* culture many of the spiritual persons prefer to cook their own food. In other words, food that is grown, harvested, cooked, and served with love and affection has a great nourishing and healing effect.

Akīrṇa means one who gives the wrong thing in charity to the wrong person at the wrong time *or* one who throws away wealth without due consideration. This is considered to be charity in *tāmasic guṇa* (mode of ignorance).

AH Ut. 7.2 says, "*śārīra mānasair duṣṭair ahitād annapānataḥ*" meaning that the mind and body get vitiated from consuming improper food. This is a cause for *unmāda* (mental disorders). How does the mind get *dūṣita* (vitiated) from the food? It is the subtle part of the food that affects the mind. The mind is connected to the body, and if the body becomes imbalanced, the mind will get affected as well.

In Arabia there is a kind of dance that is performed by the women by shaking the hair to and fro. This seems to be an example of *keśa avadhūnanam*. Probably activities like break dancing which involves perverted movements of the body and hands come under this category.

What is meant by *gātra vādyam*? Perhaps, it means using the body to make different kinds of movements. Is whistling discouraged in *Āyurveda*? Any unwanted twisting of a body part is discouraged in *Āyurveda*. What is *nakhair vādyam*? Rubbing the nails together was not considered a good omen. What is *hasta avadhūnanam? Hasta avadhunanam* could also mean masturbating. Excessive and perverted movement of body parts is *vāta* aggravating. For example, some people have the habit of shaking their legs constantly while sitting. These kinds of movements unconsciously disturb the stability of the mind.

As explained earlier, one should be extremely wary about where and from whom to accept food. This is because contaminated food can corrupt one's consciousness. One should also keep in mind the possibility of being poisoned. This will be discussed in greater detail in Chapter 7 in the second volume of this series.

It is explained in the *Cāndogya Upaniṣad* 7.26.2:

āhāra śuddhau sattva śuddhi
sattva śuddhau dhruva smṛti
smṛti lambe sarva granthinām vipramokṣaḥ

"If a person's food is pure, his mind will be pure. If the mind is pure, one can have good memory (i.e., remember that to achieve liberation is the ultimate goal of life). If one always remembers the real goal of life, one will achieve liberation."
So it all begins with pure food.

AH Sū. 2.45

Six more items to avoid

तोयाग्निपूज्यमध्येन यानं धूमं शवाश्रयम् ॥४५॥
मद्यातिसक्तिं विश्रम्भस्वातन्त्र्ये स्त्रीषु च त्यजेत् ॥४५॥

toyāgni-pūjya-madhyena-yānaṁ dhūmaṁ śavāśrayam
madyātisaktiṁ viśrambha-svātantrye strīṣu ca tyajet //45//

toya – water; *agni* - fire; *pūjya* – respectable personalities; *madhyena* – through the middle; *yānaṁ* – walking; *dhūmaṁ* – (inhaling) smoke; *śavāśrayam* – of funeral pyre; *madya* – alcohol; *atisaktiṁ* – excessive addiction; *viśrambha* – trust; *svātantrye* – freedom; *strīṣu* – to women; *ca* – and; *tyajet* – give up, avoided

Translation

Walking in between water, fire, and respectable personalities is prohibited. Inhaling the smoke of a funeral pyre, excessive addiction to alcohol, trusting and giving freedom to women should also be avoided.

Commentary

It has been mentioned for the third time to avoid addiction to alcohol. Earlier mention was in verse 40 of this chapter, and verse 38 advises that one should avoid liquor shops.

This recommendation regarding women is applicable only to men of principle and deep integrity and is never for the exploitation of women. Women also have the right to pursue their dreams in life. Here "not giving freedom to women" does not mean bondage or slavery. It means to give them protection, love, and care at all times. Women and children in the *Vedic* culture are always to be given full protection, because they are more vulnerable. Thus when a child's freedom is restricted in certain ways, it is only to give protection. The women were glad to be lovingly protected by such men of integrity. When the men gave up their responsibility to protect and care for women, it naturally gave rise to the present situation of rebellion and freedom movements from the side of women.

In the *Vedic* civilization, the difference between both the sexes was clearly understood and practiced. Unlike in the modern day, artificial equality of both sexes was not promoted. There was no competition between men and women to prove superiority over each other. Both men and women have their own unique strengths and weaknesses. It is known that women tend to have more hormonal fluctuations than men which tends to affect their moods as well. So, especially during those times, they need to be given physical rest and emotional protection.

The list of things to avoid ends here. Now the author gives general advice on how to conduct oneself and learn by carefully observing the world around us.

AH Sū. 2.46

आचार्यः सर्वचेष्टासु लोक एव हि धीमतः ॥४६॥

अनुकुर्यात्तमेवातो लौकिकेऽर्थे परीक्षकः ॥४६॥

ācāryaḥ sarva-ceṣṭāsu lokaeva hi dhīmataḥ

anukuryāt-tam-evāto laukike'rthe parīkṣakaḥ //46//

ācāryaḥ – teacher; *sarvaceṣṭāsu* – for all actions; *loka-eva* – the world itself (general norms of society); *hi* – is; *dhīmataḥ* – intelligent person; *anukuryāt* – imitate, follow; *tam* – that; *eva* – certainly; *ataḥ* – thus, therefore; *laukike* – in worldly matters (practical matters); *arthe* – for that purpose; *parīkṣakaḥ* – one who observes carefully, one who experiments

Translation

The world itself is the teacher in all activities for one who is intelligent. Therefore in all practical matters, such a person should follow the generally accepted societal norms by keenly observing them carefully (how things are going on around them).

Commentary

This verse says that one should intelligently experiment with one's actions based on the ethics, customs, and beliefs existing around him or her according to time, place, person, and circumstance.

Some of the important things about *sadācāra* (proper behaviour) have been mentioned by the *ācārya* in the previous verses, and then he says that you can learn the rest by carefully observing the people around you, because everything cannot be told. One must learn to observe carefully and use common sense. During the early days, the student would assist the teacher in his work and learn by observing the teacher. The teacher would not explain everything. The student was expected to observe and learn. Of course they could ask if something was not understood. *Āyurveda* is more caught than taught.

This verse emphasizes the need to learn by keenly observing the activities going on in the world around us. One should not isolate oneself from the world and live in an ivory tower. An intelligent person learns simply by observation. He does not have to be told each and everything. One who understands without needing to be told everything is a highly intelligent person. One who understands after being told is less intelligent person. One who does not understand even after being told is the least intelligent person. Here the *ācārya* is describing the most intelligent type of person who simply observes and understands.

We can see that many of the examples about life explained in the *śāstras* have come about through observing natural phenomena. Many of the diseases and symptoms have been named after flowers, animals, and other phenomena seen around us. This tells us about the power of observation of the great sages. *Vāgbhaṭa* is here indirectly instructing us to develop this power of keen observation, which is essential also for successfully examining clients to find out the cause and progression of disease.

Everything is already present in the creation. As is written in the book of Kohelet (Ecclesiastes) 1:9, "The thing that has been, it is that which shall be; and that which is done is that which shall be done; and there is no new thing under the sun."
It is up to us what we want to take—good or bad. Many lessons can be learned simply by carefully observing nature.

In the *Caraka Samhita*, it is said:

> *krtsno hi loke buddhimatām ācāryaḥ*
> *śatruśca abuddhimatām*

For one who is intelligent, the whole world is a teacher. One who is unintelligent sees everything and everyone as enemy. There are some people who say that life is frustrating, and the whole world is full of negative things. They cannot see anything positive in their life or others. Such people are called *abuddhimatām*. On the other hand there are others who always see only positive things everywhere. Such people are called *buddhimatām*.

Sometimes even if we observe that something is wrong in society or a person, we cannot abruptly and drastically change things. We will have to accept it temporarily and gradually work towards a change. That is more intelligent. This will be explained at the end of chapter 3.

AH Sū. 2.47

Definition of *sadvṛtti* (good behavior)

आर्द्रसन्तानता त्यागः कायवाक्चेतसां दमः ॥४७॥

स्वार्थबुद्धिः परार्थेषु पर्याप्तमिति सद्व्रतम् ॥४७॥

ārdra-santānatā tyāgaḥ kāya-vāk-cetasāṁ damaḥ

svārtha-buddhiḥ parārtheṣu paryāptam-iti sad-vratam //47//

ārdra – compassion; *santānatā* – melting of the mind or heart; *tyāgaḥ* – renunciation of the mentality of ownership; *kāya* – body; *vāk* – words; *cetasāṁ* – mentally; *damaḥ* – self restraint; *svārtha buddhiḥ* – considering as one's own need; *parārtheṣu* – the needs of others; *paryāptam* – sufficient; *iti* – these; *sat-vratam* – code of ethics

Translation

A heart melting with compassion; detachment (giving charity); control over the body, words, and mind; and considering other people's needs as one's own are the essential aspects of virtuous behavior.

Commentary

The author has so eloquently and concisely explained the essence of *sadvṛtta*. Considering another person's happiness and sorrow as one's own means to put ourselves in their shoes and understand their situation. It means to behave with others in a way we would like others to behave with us, if we would have been in a similar circumstance. That sums up the meaning of *dharma* in one line. Do unto others as how you would have them do unto you. This can be done only by a person who has control over body, mind, and words, along with a compassionate heart. This automatically defines *adharma* as "Doing unto others how you would not have others do unto you."

It is said in the *Nīti śāstra*:

mātravat paradāreṣu paradravyeṣu loṣṭravat
ātmavat sarva bhūteṣu yaḥ paśyati sa paṇḍitaḥ

"One who sees another's wife as one's own mother, another's wealth as stone, and all other living entities as oneself is truly learned."

Controlling the body is easier than controlling the speech, which is easier than controlling the mind. It is accepted in the *Bhagavad Gīta* that controlling the mind is more difficult than controlling a raging tornado. But it is possible by regular practice and detachment.

Cāṇakya Nīti says:

dāridrya nāśanam dānam śīlam durgati nāśanam
ajñāna nāśinī prajñā bhāvanā bhaya nāśinī

"Charity puts an end to poverty; righteous conduct to misery; discretion (intelligence) to ignorance; and scrutiny to fear."

AH Sū. 2.48

Benediction to one who follows the rules of *dinacaryā*

नक्तंदिनानि मे यान्ति कथम्भूतस्य सम्प्रति ॥४८॥

दुःखभाङ्ग न भवत्येवं नित्यं सन्निहितस्मृतिः ॥४८॥

naktaṁ dināni me yānti katham-bhūtasya samprati

duḥkha-bhāṅg na bhavaty-evaṁ nityaṁ sannihita-smṛtiḥ //48//

naktaṁ – nights; *dināni* – days; *me* – during; *yānti* – passes; *katham* – of whatsoever time; *bhūtasya* – one who; *samprati* – at present moment; *duḥkha* – grief; *bhāk* – afflicted by; *na* – not; *bhavati* – become; *evaṁ* – also; *nityaṁ* – at all times; *sannihita* – closely; *smṛtiḥ* – conscious, remembers, considers

Translation

For one who is thus situated in the present moment, and at all times consciously considers every action closely, the days and nights pass without becoming afflicted by grief.

Commentary

The root cause of misery is succinctly described here – to be unconscious of one's activities. The significant word is *samprati*. When we become conscious of what we think, speak, and do at every moment, we will automatically become aware of the pros and cons and thus avoid those activities that bring misery. This is called mindfulness. An example is eating. When we eat, we should be conscious of what, how, where, and how much we are eating. Most of us are not so conscious of that. This can later become troublesome. The same principle should be applied to all other activities, dealings and circumstances.

Āyurvedarasāyana: This refers to one who is conscious about the place, time, age, attitude, and activity. Such a person will never experience any misery.

There are only six questions to ask in any circumstance: why, when, where, who, what, and how. The answer to these questions will tell you everything about the situation. Keep asking these questions as often as possible.

AH Sū. 2.49

इत्याचारः समासेन, यं प्राप्नोति समाचरन् ॥४९॥

आयुरारोग्यमैश्वर्यं यशो लोकांश्च शाश्वतान् ॥४९॥

ityācāraḥ samāsena yaṁ prāpnoti samācaran

āyur-ārogyaṁ-aiśvaryaṁ-yaśo lokāṁśca śāśvatān //49//

ityācāraḥ – these etiquettes; *samāsena* – in brief; *yaṁ* – those who; *prāpnoti* – having received; *samācaran* – follows completely; *āyur* – longevity; *ārogyaṁ* – health; *aiśvaryaṁ* – good fortune; *yaśo* – fame; *lokāṁśca* – unto those people; *śāśvatān* – eternally

Translation

In short, those who follow these etiquettes completely will receive longevity, health, good fortune, and eternal fame.

Commentary

The word *samāsena* is very significant here. The etiquettes are only described in essence in this chapter. There are other books that describe them in detail, such as *Nīti śāstras, Manu samhita*, other *Purāṇas*, and so on. In this verse, the author is indirectly advising the student to refer to those books for knowing the details.

This is a very huge promise made by the author. We find people in the world who possess one or two of the items mentioned here. But to find someone who has longevity, health, good fortune, and fame, and that too eternally, is very difficult. But by following the principles of *dinacaryā* one can achieve it.

One may say, "If all the items mentioned in the chapter have to be practiced, it will probably take up the entire day." The answer is that when we enumerate the items of *dinacaryā* in a book, all the items have to be mentioned. But that does not mean that everything is for everyone. One must understand one's specific situation, and choose the items that are practical and useful for maintaining one's health.

इति श्रीवैद्यपतिसिंहगुप्तसूनु
श्रीमद्वाग्भटविरचितायामष्टाङ्गहृदयसंहितायां सूत्रस्थाने
दिनचर्या नाम द्वितीयोऽध्यायः ॥

iti śrī vaidyapati siṁhagupta sūnū vāgbhaṭa viracitāyām aṣṭāṅga hṛdaya samhitāyām sutra sthāne dinacaryā nāma dvitīyodhyāyaḥ

iti - this; śrī vaidyapati simhagupta sūnu - the son of Śri vaidyapati Simhagupta; Śrī Vāgbhaṭa viracitāyām - composed by Śrī Vāgbhaṭa; aṣṭāṅga-hṛdaya saṁhitāyāṁ - of the aṣṭāṅga hṛdaya samhita; sūtra-sthāne - of the sūtra sthāna; dinacaryā nāma - named dinacaryā; dvitīyodhyāyaḥ - the second chapter

Translation

Thus ends the second chapter of the *Sūtra sthāna* of the *Aṣṭāṅga Hṛdaya samhita*, composed by *Śrī Vāgbhaṭa*, the son of *Śrī Vaidyapati Simhagupta.*

Topics in the Chapter

1. Waking up—1
2. *Śauca* (Cleaning bowels)—1
3. *Danta dhāvanam* (Cleaning teeth)
    a. Items used—2
    b. Size of brush—2

27. Benefits of following all the rules of *dinacaryā*—48, 49

Chapter 3

ऋतुचर्या

Ṛtucaryā

Seasonal Regimen

Summary of the chapter:

The *dinacaryā* (daily regimen) described in the last chapter will vary according to the change of seasons. Hence, *ṛtucaryā* is described next. So *ṛtucaryā* is the modification of *dinacaryā* according to seasonal changes. In the beginning, time is divided into two sections based on the movement of the sun towards the north and south. Each of these is again divided into three parts depending on the change of seasons. The diet and lifestyle for each of the seasons is described to help keep the body in balance. And then the regimen to be followed at the intersection, during the change of seasons is also described.

Sections in the chapter

Seasons – Verse numbers

I. Early winter (*Hemanta*)—7 to 16
II. Late winter (*Śiśira*)—17
III. Spring (*Vasanta*)—18 to 25
IV. Summer (*Grīṣma*)—26 to 41

V. Rainy (*Varṣa*)—42 to 48

VI. Autumn (*Śarad*)—49 to 57

Key *Sanskṛt* words in this chapter

hemanta, śiśira, vasanta, grīṣma, varṣa, śarad, uttarāyaṇa, dakṣiṇāyana, ādāna, visarga, svādu, amla, lavaṇa, kaṭu, tikta, kaṣāya

Introduction

The *ṛtucaryā* in this chapter is designed for a *svastha* (healthy person) based on the changes that take place in a healthy body as the seasons keep changing from one to another (AS Sū. 3.62). The regular *Ṛtucaryā* described here is not meant for sick people (though these principles can obviously be used in treatment). They require a separate regimen according to their disease, which will be described later.

Kāla (time) has been described as one of the three exclusive causes of disease in AH Sū 1.19. In this chapter, the seasonal aspect of *kāla* and how to prevent the imbalances that can arise as a result of the movement of *kāla* is discussed.

Time in *Āyurveda*, has been divided predominantly into hours, days, fortnights, months and years based on the movement of the sun and the moon. The twenty-four hours are divided into day and night; a month, into approximately two fortnights of the waxing and waning moon; and a year is divided in two six monthly intervals called *ayana*— *uttarāyaṇa* and *dakṣiṇāyana*, where the sun moves in the north and south of the equator, respectively. Apart from the movement of the sun, the year was also seasonally divided into three parts based on rains, cold, and heat seen during the course of the year, called *ṛtu.*[1] These three climates were again subdivided into two each, thus forming the six seasons comprising of two months each. This division of two months for a season was more applicable to the areas situated north of the River Ganges and south of the Himalayas. It needs to be modified and used for other climatic zones.

In the past, the *Āyurveda ācāryas* studied the *ṛtu*s or seasons (and *ṛtucaryās*—seasonal regimens) in different parts of India and modified the *ṛtucaryās* based on changes in the amount of rains, heat, and cold. For example, the area south of the Ganges River has less of snow and more of rain. The people who lived in that area eliminated *śiśira ṛtu* (late winter) from the list and rearranged the seasons by creating a new season called *prāvṛt.* Those living in the extreme south of India, for example, Kerala, modified this further because in this region the rainy season is split into two parts and lasts for about six months a year.

Accordingly it behooves the practitioners of *Āyurveda* living in different parts of the world to understand the symptoms of climatic changes in their respective zones and classify the duration of the climates accordingly. This is the first and most important exercise a practitioner must undertake for the practical application of *ṛtucaryā.* This will enable us to understand the application and implications of the principles of *ṛtucaryā* explained in this chapter for each and every specific region of the world.

Unless we understand how to recognize the change of seasons and are able to map the duration and variation of the seasons in comparison with the symptoms of seasons described in the ancient texts, we will not be able to practically utilize the information given here to make seasonal lifestyle and diet recommendations. The descriptions given in this chapter are more applicable to the regions lying north of the Ganges River. Broad and general principles are also outlined along the way. One should not superimpose the recommendations given for a particular region on another.

The first thing is to be able to identify the *ṛtus* (seasons).

How do we recognize the changing of seasons?

There are three ways the seasonal calendar is recognized (AS Sū. 3.63):

1. *Māsi* by the calendar months
2. *Rāśi* by observing the astronomy—movement of planets and stars
3. *Svarūpa* by observing the characteristic features of the season

The third one, *svarūpa*, is the most reliable and practically used in *Āyurveda*. The change of seasons should be understood by the change of the *guṇa*s in the atmosphere which can be seen through the blooming of the flowers, coming of the dark clouds, filling up of the rivers and so on. This also brings about corresponding *guṇa* changes in the human body.

We can use *uṣṇa* (hot), *śīta* (cold), *rūkṣa* (dry), and *snigdha* (unctuous) to map the characteristics of each climate and their variations in different parts of the world.

How to identify the seasons according to heat, cold and rain? A simple method is described below. If the temperature is:

- Hot in the day and hot at night: *grīṣma* ṛtu (summer)
- Hot in the day and cold at night: *vasanta* ṛtu (spring)
- Cold in the day and cold at night: *śiśira* and *hemanta* ṛtu (winter)
- Increased and continuous rain: *varṣa* (rains)
- Intermittent rain: *śarad ṛtu* (autumn)

Note: It is important to understand the *Āyurvedic* concept of each of the seasons. Each season has got specific characteristics. Unless the environment and human body manifest these characteristics, technically we cannot say that the season has come. Conventionally we may call a warm climate in a cold region like Arctic as summer. But technically it is not summer (*grīṣma*) unless the temperature and humidity are sufficient to manifest the environmental and bodily changes according to the description in the *Āyurvedic* texts. By the same understanding, *Āyurvedically* we will say that the Arctic region has no summer season at all.

In a world where the climate is changing rapidly due to changes in the ozone layer and other environmental factors, there are differences in the pattern of seasons in every single year as well.

So a student of *Āyurveda* should learn to adapt the principles according to changing paradigms.
This is of paramount importance since the human body is a microcosm of the macrocosm in which we reside, and our health is closely connected to the change of seasons in our habitat. You will learn in the chapters ahead that one of the three primary causes for all disease is *kāla* or time, of which one representation is the changing of seasons.

Another practical utility of *ṛtucaryā* is explained in the chapter 14 of *Sūtra sthāna* for treatment of various disorders.

graiṣmaḥ prāyo marut-pitte vāsantaḥ kapha-mārute
maruto yogavāhitvāt kapha-pitte tu śāradaḥ //14//

"The summer seasonal regimen can usually be recommended in *vāta-pitta* disorders; spring seasonal regimen, in *kapha-vāta* disorders; and *śarad* (autumn) regimen, in *kapha-pitta* disorders. *Vāta* has got a *yogavahi* property (carrying and enhancing the properties of another).

This is because the *ṛtus* (seasons) are not restricted to the external environment. There is a change of *ṛtu* (season) going on inside the human body too. We can also say that the modification of the *dinacaryā* according to the *ṛtus* (seasons) is called *ṛtucaryā*. One should not blindly implement the ṛtucarya without considering the other factors. According to sūtra sthāna there are 10 factors to be considered to determine a balance or imbalance and "kāla" or time is one among them. The ṛtucarya is a generalized understanding of one of the aspects of the concept of kāla. One should understand the principles given in this chapter and implement them in an individual according to the status of the other 9 factors. Eg. Not everybody will require an udvartana in vasanta ṛtu.

It is noteworthy how all the principles of *rtucarya* (seasonal regimen) in *Āyurveda* do not describe how to manipulate mother-nature to suit our life style but rather how we can change our diet and lifestyles to adapt to the changes occurring in mother-nature. Modern science and technology attempts to do the opposite.

Title verse

अथात ऋतुचर्याध्यायं व्याख्यास्यामः

इति ह स्माहुरात्रेयादयो महर्षयः

athāta ṛtucaryādhyāyām vyākhyāsyāmaḥ

iti ha smāhur ātreyādayo maharṣayaḥ

athātaḥ – then and therefore; *ṛtucaryā* – seasonal regimen; *adhyāyām* – chapter; *vyākhyāsyāmaḥ* – described; *iti* – this; *ha smāhur* – now; *ātreyādayo* – son of Atri and others; *maharṣayaḥ* – sages

Translation

Therefore as advised/spoken by the great hermit *Ātreya* and the group of sages is described the chapter on seasonal regimens.

AH Sū. 3.1

The division of the year into seasons

मासैर्द्विसंख्यैर्माघाद्यैः क्रमात् षड्तवः स्मृताः ॥१॥

शिशिरोथ वसन्तश्च ग्रीष्मो वर्षाशरद्धिमाः ॥१॥

māsair-dvisankhyair-māghādyaiḥ kramāt ṣaḍ ṛtavaḥ smṛtāḥ

śiśiro'tha vasantaśca grīṣma-varṣā-śaraddhimāḥ //1//

māsair – of the months; *dvisankhyair* – two in number (in pairs of two); *māghādyaiḥ* – beginning with the month of māgha; *kramāt* – in the order; *ṣaḍ* – six; *ṛtavaḥ* – seasons; *smṛtāḥ* – known as; *śiśiraḥ* – extreme winter; *atha* – now; *vasanta* – spring; *ca* - and; *grīṣma* – summer; *varṣā* – rains; *śarad* – autumn; *himāḥ* – early part of winter (*hemanta*)

Translation

Two months each, beginning with the month of *māgha*, comprise each of the six seasons—*śiśira, vasanta, grīṣma, varṣa, śarad*, and *hima* in that same order.

Commentary

There is no *prakopa* (aggravation) of any of the *doṣa*s in the *grīṣma ṛtu* (summer season). Though it is hot outside, it does not cause *pitta* aggravation because *kapha* is undergoing *praśamana* (pacification) and thus neutralizes the heat caused due to summer. There is no obvious *prakopa* (aggravation) of any *doṣa* in *śiśira*. There is no obvious *sañcaya* (accumulation) of any *doṣa* in *vasanta* (spring).

This is the scenario in a healthy person (refer to definition of health according to *Suśruta* as discussed in chapter 1), but these changes will not happen in the same way in an unhealthy person. These changes happen in the atmosphere as well as in a healthy person. Hence, a healthy person is advised to take precautions accordingly. Similar changes as in the environment also happen in the body. For example, just as snow melts from the mountains in the spring, *kapha* melts in the body and flows down.

To understand the reasons for the *caya* (accumulation), *kopa* (aggravation), and *śama* (pacification) of the *doṣa*s in the different seasons, please refer to AH. 12.18–21. It is important to understand that the *sañcaya* (accumulation), *prakopa* (aggravation), and *praśama* (pacification) of the *doṣa*s described with respect to the seasons is not for the human body but for the atmosphere. The changes of the *doṣa*s in the atmosphere can surely have an influence on the *doṣa*s of the human body. Many other factors also influence the *doṣa* of the human body.

Why is there *sañcaya* (accumulation) of *pitta* in *varṣa ṛtu* (rainy season)? What are the factors that support this?

Earth generates *amlatva* (sourness), but the aggravation is stopped by the cold of *varṣa* (rainy season). *Suśruta* mentions that *varṣa* (rainy season) is *tridoṣa kṛt* (causes the aggravation of all the three *doṣa*s)

Usually *vāta* is pacified by application of heat, but here we find that in summer there is *sañcaya* (accumulation) of *vāta*. How does this happen?

In summer in its classical *grīṣma* definition, which is hot during day and night, there is dryness, which increases *vāta*. Heat initially pacifies *vāta*, but excess heat results in *ruksha* (dryness), which aggravates *vāta*.

Here the name of the first month in the *Vedic* calendar, *māgha*, is mentioned. The *Vedic* calendar consists of twelve months, which is how long it takes the earth to move around the sun and twenty-eight days in each month according to the rotation of the moon around the earth. Time has been mapped in two ways: (1) by the movement of the sun and (2) by the movement of the moon. Both are done using the earth as the reference point.

The sky (360°) has been divided into compartments in two different ways:

1. Into twelve sections of 30° each (the twelve zodiac houses)—to map solar movement
2. Into twenty-seven sections of 13°20′ each (the twenty-seven stars)—to map lunar movement

The seasons change according to solar movement.

There are twelve months in the *Vedic* calendar. Each month of the lunar calendar (lunar month or synodic month) is completed when the moon traverses the horizon, which is divided into twenty-seven sections (the stars).

The names of the months do not correspond with the English (Gregorian) calendar. The twelve *rāśis* (the houses in the *Vedic* astrological chart) also do not exactly correspond with the twelve months. There is a little bit of overlap.

The approximate correspondence of the twelve months with the Gregorian calendar is as follows:

#	Vedic	Gregorian
1	*Chaitra*	March–April (begins first day after new moon)
2	*Vaiśākha*	April–May
3	*Jyeṣṭha*	May–June
4	*Āshāḍa*	June–July
5	*Śrāvaṇa*	July–August
6	*Bhādrapada*	August–September
7	*Aświna*	September–October
8	*Kārtika*	October–November
9	*Mārgaśīrṣa*	November–December
10	*Pauṣa*	December–January
11	*Māgha*	January–February
12	*Phālguṇa*	February–March

If the transits of the sun through various *rāśi* (constellations of the zodiac) are used, then we get solar months, which do not shift with reference to the Gregorian calendar. When sun enters the zodiac sign called *Makara*, it is celebrated as *Makara sankrānti* (approximately January 14 or 15, when there is the transition of the sun into *Makara rāśi*). This is the point when the sun ends the *dakṣiṇāyana* (movement toward the south) and starts the *uttarāyaṇa* (movement toward the north).

The twelve *rāśis* (zodiac signs) are

1. *Meṣa* (Aries);
2. *Vṛṣabha* (Taurus)
3. *Mithuna* (Gemini)
4. *Karkaṭaka* (Cancer)
5. *Simha* (Leo)
6. *Kanya* (Virgo)
7. *Tulā* (Libra)
8. *Vṛścika* (Scorpio)
9. *Dhanu* (Sagittarius)
10. *Makara* (Capricorn)
11. *Kumbha* (Aquarius)
12. *Mīna* (Pisces)

There are two fortnights in a month, each having fifteen days. From the first day of *śukla pakṣa* onward, the size of the moon goes on increasing till it reaches full moon. From the first day of *kṛṣṇa pakṣa* onward, the size of the moon goes on decreasing till it reaches new moon (*amāvasya*).

	Śukla Pakṣa ***(full moon fortnight)***	***Kṛṣṇa Pakṣa*** ***(new moon fortnight)***
1.	*Prathama*	*Prathama*
2.	*Dvitīya*	*Dvitīya*
3.	*Tṛtīya*	*Tṛtīya*
4.	*Caturthi*	*Caturthi*

5.	*Pañcami*	*Pañcami*
6.	*Ṣaṣti*	*Ṣaṣṭi*
7.	*Saptami*	*Saptami*
8.	*Aṣṭami*	*Aṣṭami*
9.	*Navami*	*Navami*
10.	*Daśami*	*Daśami*
11.	*Ekādaśi*	*Ekādaśi*
12.	*Dvādaśi*	*Dvādaśi*
13.	*Trayodaśi*	*Trayodaśi*
14.	*Caturdaśi*	*Caturdaśi*
15.	*Purnima*	*Amāvasya*

Note: One may ask, "So why is this important in *Āyurveda*? Why did *ācārya* include this?" As explained before, the change of seasons are understood in three different ways. This is the first method. So one must know how time is quantified in the *Vedic* system. Since *Āyurveda* is a *Vedic* system, it is helpful to know how it was done using this system. Correlation with the western calendar may be attempted once you properly understand the *Vedic* system.

AH Sū. 3.2

***Uttarāyaṇa* (*Ādānakāla*)—verses 2 to 4**

शिशिराद्यास्त्रिभिस्तैस्तु विद्यादयनमुत्तरम् ॥२॥

आदानं च, तदादत्ते नृणां प्रतिदिनं बलम् ॥२॥

śiśirādyais-tribhis-taistu vidyād-ayanam-uttaram

ādānaṁ ca tad-ādatte nṛṇāṁ pratidinaṁ balam //2//

śiśirādyais – consecutive seasons starting from winter (*śiśira* [snowy extreme winter], *vasanta* [spring], *grīṣma* [summer]); *tribhis-taistu* – three in number; *vidyād* – known as; *ayanam* – movement, journey; *uttaram* – north (of equator); *ādānaṁ* – period of extraction (of strength); *ca* – and; *tad* – that; *ādatte* – is accepted; *nṛṇāṁ* – of men (people); *pratidinaṁ* – day by day; *balam* – strength

Translation

It is known that during the three consecutive seasons beginning with *śiśira*, the journey (of the sun) is toward the north. It is recognized as the period of extraction of the strength of people, day after day.

Commentary

What does it mean when it says, "Sun is traveling in the north of equator during *śiśira*, *vasanta*, and *grīṣma*"?

It means that the northern hemisphere of the earth is beginning to receive increasing duration of sunshine, since it is facing more toward the sun. The *Vedic* astronomical system is a geocentric system and charts the movement of the sun with the earth as reference point as experienced from the earth. This is why we hear words like "sun moving to the north" or "sun moving to the south."

When sun is moving in the north of equator, why does the earth (land) reduce in moisture content?

Much of the land area of the earth is situated in the northern hemisphere. When the sun rays fall more on the land (earth) rather than water, it makes it *uṣṇa* (hot) and *rūkṣa* (dry).

Does that have anything to do with the northern journey of the sun being a weakening time for the earth? When the sun rays fall more on the land area of the planet where we live, the scorching rays of the sun drain the energy from the earth, plants, and animals. This is why it is said to be a *ādāna kāla* (weakening time) for all the animals and plants.

Due to the peculiar tilt of 23.5° in the axis of rotation and the movement of the earth in its orbit around the sun, the sun rays fall more on the northern hemisphere during the *ādāna* period.

Please know that this is mainly in relation to the Indian subcontinent and areas lying on the same latitude around the globe. For other parts of the globe, the *ādāna* period can be a different time of the year.

To get a better idea of the effect the movement of the earth has on the amount of sun rays falling on the land in different parts of the globe, you can see

http://astro.unl.edu/naap/motion1/animations/seasons_ecliptic.swf

AH Sū. 3.3–4

Description of *ādāna kāla* (sun travels toward the north)

तस्मिन् ह्यत्यर्थतीक्ष्णोष्णरूक्षा मार्गस्वभावतः ॥३॥

आदित्यपवनाः सौम्यान् क्षपयन्ति गुणान् भुवः ॥३॥

तिक्तः कषायः कटुको बलिनोत्र रसाः क्रमात् ॥४॥

तस्मादादानमाग्नेयम्.............................॥४॥

tasmin-hy-atyartha-tīkṣṇoṣṇa-rūkṣā mārga-svabhāvātaḥ

āditya-pavanāḥ saumyān kṣapayanti guṇān bhuvaḥ //3//

tiktaḥ kaṣāyaḥ kaṭuko balino'tra rasāḥ kramāt
tasmād-ādānam-āgneyaṁ ....

tasmin – indeed during that *uttarāyaṇa*; *hy* – certainly; *atyartha* – increased to the maximum; *tīkṣṇa* – sharp; *uṣṇa* – hot; *rūkṣā* – dry; *mārga* – path of; *svabhāvātaḥ* – due to the natural; *āditya* – sun; *pavanāḥ* – and wind; *saumyān* – gentle nature; *kṣapayanti* – weakens; *guṇān* – qualities; *bhuvaḥ* – of the earth; *tiktaḥ* – bitter; *kaṣāyaḥ* – astringent; *kaṭuko* – pungent; *balino* – strength of; *atra* - indeed; *rasāḥ* – tastes; *kramāt* – in that order; *tasmāt* – hence, therefore; *ādānam* – period of extraction; *āgneyaṁ* – is fiery

Translation

During the same period (i.e., *uttarāyaṇa*), due to the natural movement of the sun (in the northern hemisphere), the sun and wind cause an excessive increase in the sharp, hot, and dry qualities of the earth while weakening its gentle qualities. Bitter, astringent, and pungent tastes become, stronger. Thus the period of extraction, called *ādāna*, is fiery in nature.

Commentary

Note that the special feature of *uttarāyaṇa* is the excessive increase of *uṣṇa*, *tīkṣṇa* and *rūkṣa guṇas* which weaken the *saumya guṇas* of the earth (and the inhabitants as well).

Here the word *kramāt* indicates that *tikta* (bitter) taste becomes stronger in *śiśira* (late winter); *kaṣāya* (astringent) taste becomes stronger in *vasanta* (spring); and *kaṭu* (pungent) taste becomes stronger in *grīṣma* (summer). What is the meaning of saying that a particular taste is strong in a particular season? Out of the six tastes, it has been explained that *madhurā* (sweet), *amla* (sour), and *lavaṇa* (salty) are strengthening and the last three, that is, *kaṭu* (pungent), *tikta* (bitter), and *kaṣāya* (astringent) are weakening. So when there is a weakening effect on the body (as it happens during the *ādāna* period), it is natural that this is a period where the last three tastes (pungent, bitter, astringent) are strong.

Though *kaṣāya* (astringent) is the most weakening taste of all, why is *kaṭu* (pungent) taste the most prominent and strongest in the summer, which is the most weakening of all the seasons? This is because though *kaṣāya* (astringent) is the most weakening, it is a cooling taste. *Kaṭu* (pungent) is also weakening, but it is a heating taste. Summer is a heating weather, and hence, a heating and weakening taste will be prominent during this time.

Since the *tikta, kaṣāya*, and *kaṭu rasas* become strong during the late *śiśira* (winter), *vasanta* (spring), and *grīṣma* (summer), these tastes should be reduced during these seasons, respectively. The opposite taste should be used to prevent weakening of the body. This is also explained in verse 55 of this chapter.

Vasanta is predominant in *kaṣāya* (astringent) taste, while *śiśira* is prominent in *tikta* (bitter) taste. But they don't create much *balakṣaya* (loss of strength), since both these are *kapha*-dominant seasons. But in *grīṣma* (summer), along with *kaṭu rasa* (pungent taste), *vāta caya* (accumulation of *vāta)* causes a greater harm to the strength (*balahāni*), since there is no opposing factor.

Tikta (bitter), *kaṣāya* (astringent), and *kaṭu* (pungent) *rasa* (tastes) have an affinity to degenerative processes, and in a case where there is already a degenerative process going on, these tastes get even more strength and defeat the protective barriers of the earth.

AH Sū. 3.4b–5a

Dakṣiṇāyana (visarga kāla)—sun travels to the south

……………………ऋतवो दक्षिणायनम् ॥४॥
वर्षादयो विसर्गश्च यद्बलं विसृजत्ययम् ॥५॥

…………………………………… *ṛtavo dakṣiṇāyanam //4//*
varṣādayo visargaśca yad-balaṁ visṛjatyayam

ṛtavaḥ – seasons; *dakṣiṇāyanam* – movement in the south (of equator); *varṣādayo* – rainy season etc (*varṣa* [rainy], *śarad* [autumn], *hemanta* [early winter]); *visargaḥ* – period of discharge; *ca* – and; *yat* – that which; *balaṁ* – strength; *visṛjatyayam* – releases, discharges

Translation

The seasons during the movement of the sun in the southern hemisphere are rainy, autumn, and early part of winter. This is called a period of discharge, as it releases energy into the earth.

Commentary

This period sees less sunlight falling on the land and thus less drying effect.

AH Sū. 3.5b–6

Strength of the moon and sun during *dakṣiṇāyana*

सौम्यत्वादत्र सोमो हि बलवान् हीयते रविः ॥५॥

मेघवृष्ट्यनिलैः शीतैः शान्ततापे महीतले ॥६॥

स्निग्धाश्चेहाम्ललवणमधुरा बलिनो रसाः ॥६॥

saumyatvād-atra somo hy balavān hīyate raviḥ //5//

megha-vṛṣṭy-anilaiḥ śītaiḥ śāntatāpe mahītale

snigdhāścehāmla-lavaṇa-madhurā balino rasāḥ //6//

saumyatvād – in a way that gives prominence to cooling; *atra hy* – during *dakṣiṇāyana*; *somo balavān* – moon is stronger; *hīyate raviḥ* – sun is weaker; *megha* – clouds; *vṛṣṭi* – rain; *anilaiḥ* – and wind; *śītaiḥ* – cooling; *śānta* – pacifies; *tāpe* – the burning heat of; *mahītale* – of the earth; *snigdha* – unctuousness; *ca* – and; *iha* – here; *amla* – sour; *lavaṇa* – salt; *madhurā* – sweet; *balino* – of strength; *rasāḥ* – tastes

Translation

During the period of *dakṣiṇāyana* (southward movement of the sun), due to the increasing strength of the moon and decreasing strength of the sun, the gentle qualities (*saumyatvād*) become stronger. When the cool clouds, rain, and winds pacify the heat of the earth, the unctuous tastes—sweet, sour, and salty—become strong.

Commentary

The sun becoming weak and the moon becoming strong only mean that it becomes cooler and the heat reduces. *Dakṣiṇāyana* (southward movement of the sun) begins with the coming of the rainy season. The sky is usually covered with dark clouds. Due to rains and the winds, the heated earth cools down. When the earth cools down, the tastes that have prominent *snigdha* (unctuous) *guṇas* become strong—*madhurā* (sweet), *amla* (sour), and *lavaṇa* (salty). In the *varṣa* (rainy) season, *amla* (sour) taste becomes prominent; in the *śarad* (autumn) season, *lavaṇa* (salty) taste becomes prominent; and during the early *hemanta* (winter), *madhurā* (sweet) becomes prominent. It would be better to say that the earth becomes *snigdha* (unctuous) rather than cool. The word *mahītale* indicates that it is the outer crust of the earth that becomes cool, while the inner core is still hot.

The passage of heat from the inner core to the outer crust of the earth reduces the cooling effect of the rainy season, and the sun rays that appear at the end of the rainy season make the body hotter. It could be due to this, though not as unctuous as the *amla* (sour) taste, *lavaṇa* (salty) taste, which is hotter than *amla* (sour), becomes strong in the *śarad* (autumn) season.

The above verses that describe the changes in *guṇas* due to the movement of the sun in the *uttarāyaṇa* and *dakṣiṇāyana* is the background upon which we will be able to understand *ṛtucaryā*.

AH Sū. 3.7a

Bodily strength in the different seasons

शीतेऽग्र्यं वृष्टिघर्मेऽल्पं बलं मध्यं तु शेषयोः ॥७॥

śīte'gryaṁ vṛṣṭi-gharme'lpaṁ balaṁ madhyam tu śeṣayoḥ

śīte – in the winter (*śiśira* and *hemanta*); *agryaṁ* – is maximum; *vṛṣṭi* – rainy season; *gharme* – in summer; *alpaṁ* – minimal; *balaṁ* – bodily strength; *madhyaṁ* – moderate; *tu* – but; *śeṣayoḥ* – remaining

Translation

Bodily strength is maximum during early and late winter, minimal during rainy and summer, and moderate during the remaining seasons (spring and autumn).

Commentary

Here we find an apparent contradiction to the earlier description that the earth gains strength during *dakṣiṇāyana* (southern movement of the sun) and that the earth loses strength during *uttarāyaṇa* (northern movement of the sun). *Varṣa* (rainy) season is in the *dakṣiṇāyana* group of seasons, but is still a time of minimal bodily strength. Similarly, late winter is under *uttarāyaṇa*, but still gives maximum bodily strength. Why? Rainy season begins where the *uttarāyaṇa* ends or *dakṣiṇāyana* begins, from where the strength starts increasing. *Śīśira* is the end of *dakṣiṇāyana* when the strength reaches a peak from where it begins to decline. *Uttarāyaṇa* begins at the end of *śiśira* and beginning of *vasanta* (spring).

Why are *hemanta* and *śiśira* the strongest seasons?

Both these seasons are *śīta* (cool) and *snigdha* (unctuous), and hence, strong—end of *dakṣiṇāyana* and beginning of *uttarāyaṇa*.

Why are summer and rainy seasons the weakest seasons?

Both these seasons are end of *uttarāyaṇa* and beginning of *dakṣiṇāyana*, respectively.

The remaining two seasons are in the middle, and hence, of moderate strength.

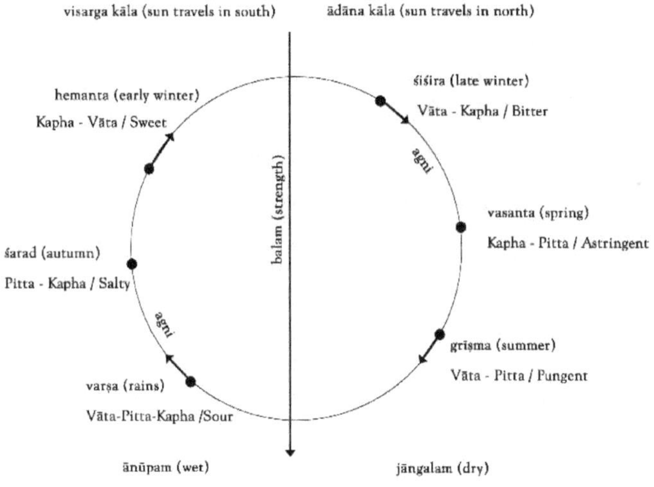

(diagram contributed by Dr Rajmohan, Asst. Prof. Dept. of Rasaśāstra and Bhaiṣajya, Govt. Ayurveda College, TVM)

This picture depicts the movement of the *ṛtus* (seasons) along with the change of *agni*, *balam* (strength), *doṣās* and *rasa* (taste).

हेमन्त ऋतुचर्या

Hemanta ṛtucaryā

Early winter seasonal regimen

Key points to remember

- *Doṣa*: *Kapha sañcaya* (accumulation of *kapha*) + *Pitta praśama* (pacification of *pitta*)
- *Agni*: *Prabala* (very strong), withdrawn internally
- *Guṇa*: *Madhyama śīta* (moderate cold) + *Utkṛṣṭa snigdha* (excessive unctuousness)
- *Āhāra* (food) – heavy, unctuous, nourishing, sweet, sour and salty foods
- *Dwelling* – underground, heated with embers
- *Activities* - Wrestling, foot massage, powder massage, fumigation of body, sun bathing, regular use of footwear
- *Diseases* – *Kapha Vāta* diseases

AH Sū. 3.7b–8

बलिनः शीतसंरोधाद्धेमन्ते प्रबलोनलः ॥७॥

भवत्यल्पेन्धनो धातून् स पचेद्वायुनेरितः ॥८॥

अतो हिमेस्मिन्सेवेत स्वाद्वम्ललवणान् रसान् ॥८॥

balinaḥ śīta-saṁrodhād hemante prabalo'nalaḥ //7//

bhavaty-alpendhano dhātūn sa paced-vāyuneritaḥ

ato hime'smin seveta svādvamla lavaṇān rasān //8//

balinaḥ – in strong persons; *śīta* – the cold; *saṁrodhād* – due to blockage by; *hemante* – during winter; *prabalaḥ* – is very strong; *analaḥ* – the digestive fire;
bhavati – becomes; *alpa* – inadequate; *indhno* – if the fuel (food); *dhātūn* – of body tissues; *sa* – that will; *pacet* – digest; *vāyuneritaḥ* – persuaded by vāyu (*vāta*) (*īritaḥ* – set in motion); *ataḥ* – therefore; *hime* – in winter; *asmin* – in this; *seveta* – (advisable to) consume; *svādu* – sweet; *amla* – sour; *lavaṇān* – salty; *rasān* – tastes

Translation

In strong persons, the cold of the winter obstructs the escape of heat. This makes the digestive fire very strong inside. In case of inadequate fuel for the fire, it will digest body tissues, persuaded by *vāta*. Hence in winter one should consume sweet, sour, and salty tastes.

Commentary

Is the internal body heat in winter increasing due to the blocking of heat dissipation or due to an increase in the body's metabolism?
It is the blockage of dissipation of heat (due to lack of sweating and closure of the pores of the body) that is causing the increase in the body's metabolism.

In case of healthy people with strong *agni*:

Cold of the winter causes the reduction of sweat and closure of the body pores

↓

Lack of dissipation of heat from the body to the outside and *srotorodha* (obstruction in the channels) of the flow of *vāta*

↓

Vāta becomes *viguṇa* (distorted in quality)

↓

Increases the *jaṭhara agni* (digestive fire)

It is very important to have proper food intake during the winter seasons to prevent digestion and depletion of body tissues. This is applicable to *balinaḥ* (healthy people) only. In case of those who are weak, the *agni* will also be weak. Due to the cold, the *agni* will become even more weak and thus present with symptoms of indigestion. Both these situations can be prevented by using *madhurā* (sweet), *amla* (sour), and *lavaṇa* (salty) tastes appropriately.

Though *amla* (sour) taste causes *agni dīpti* (ignition of digestive fire), it is still used here, since it pacifies *vāta.*

AH Sū. 3.9–10

Bodily strength in the different seasons

दैर्घ्यान्निशानामेतर्हि प्रातरेव बुभुक्षितः ॥९॥

अवश्यकार्यं सम्भाव्य यथोक्तं शीलयेदनु ॥९॥

वातघ्नतैलैरभ्यङ्गं मूर्ध्नि (मूर्ध) तैलं विमर्दनम् ॥१०॥

नियुद्धं कुशलैः सार्धं पादाघातं च युक्तितः ॥१०॥

dairghyān-niśānām-etarhi prātareva bubhukṣitaḥ
avaśyakāryaṁ saṁbhāvya yathoktaṁ śīlayedanu //9//
vātaghna-tailair-abhyaṅgam mūrdha-tailam vimardanam
niyuddhaṁ kuśalaiḥ sārdhaṁ pādāghātaṁ ca yuktitaḥ //10//

dairghyān – are very long; *niśānām* – the nights; *etarhi* - during this time; *prātareva* – in the morning itself; *bubhukṣitaḥ* – one will feel hungry; *avaśya kāryaṁ* – necessary duties like going to toilet, and so on; *saṁbhāvya* – after completing; *yathoktaṁ* – according to the prescribed routine; *anu* – after that; *śīlayed* – one should practice; *vātaghna tailair* – with *vāta* reducing oils; *abhyaṅgam* – massage; *mūrdha-tailam* – oil application on head; *vimardanam* – strong massage of the whole body; *niyuddhaṁ* – wrestling (for exercise); *kuśalaiḥ* – expert wrestlers; *sārdhaṁ* – along with; *pādāghātaṁ* – foot massage; *ca* – and, along with; *yuktitaḥ* – according to requirement

Translation

During this time, the nights are very long, and one can feel hungry (early) in the morning rather than later in the day. After having completed the necessary duties as prescribed, one should practice strong massage of the body and head with *vāta*-reducing oils. One should then engage in wrestling with expert wrestlers along with foot massage according to requirement.

Commentary

An example of oil that can be used on the head at this time is *asana vilvādi tailam* (name of a formulation). The wrestling and foot massage will help to reduce *staimitya* (rigidity of the body). The wrestling is meant to be a form of exercise. Foot massage is mentioned here specifically because it is stronger than the hand massage. The sequence has been described in the previous chapter.

Abhyaṅga means just application of oil. This is done for the pacification of *vāta*, which accumulates in the cold *hemanta* (early winter). Then it is also advised to do *pādāghata* (hard foot massage) as per requirement. This is meant for melting the *kapha* that accumulates under the skin during the cold season. Melting of *kapha* requires hard massage, which is done with the feet. Here we can see that foot massage is especially suitable for cold countries. *Vāta*-reducing oils are recommended, thereby, indicating that there is a tendency for *vāta* increase in *hemanta* (early winter) season as well.

The feeling of hunger in the morning is significant. This is due to the long night and thus enough time available for the *agni* to digest the food and become active again. This is also a sign of *hemanta ṛtu* in the body (*ṛtu* can be identified inside and outside the body). If one feels hungry in the morning, it is important to eat something or else the digestive fire will digest the healthy body tissues.

AH Sū. 3.11

Removing the excess oil after oil massage

कषायापहृतस्नेहस्ततः स्नातो यथाविधि ॥११॥

कुङ्कुमेन सदर्पेण प्रदिग्धोगुरुधूपितः ॥११॥

kaṣāyāpahṛta-snehas-tataḥ snāto yathāvidhi

kuṅkumena sadarpeṇa pradigdho'garu-dhūpitaḥ //11//

kaṣāya – astringent (herbal powder); *apahṛta* – to remove; *snehas* – the (excess) oil; *tataḥ* – thereafter (the wrestling and massage); *snāto* – take bath; *yathāvidhi* – as per rules and regulation; *kuṅkumena* – with saffron; *sa-darpeṇa* – with musk (*darpa* – musk); *pradigdho* – (made into a paste and) fully anointed; *agaru* – agar; *dhūpitaḥ* – fumigate with

Translation

Thereafter (having completed the massage and exercise) according to the regulation, one should remove the oil on the body using astringent (herbal powders), take a bath, and anoint the body with a paste of saffron and musk. Fumigate the body with herbal smoke of *agaru*.

Commentary

Agaru is a type of wood which is *kapha* reducing. Musk is produced from a gland situated in the rectal area of musk deer. It is one of the most expensive animal products in the world. The musk deer has to be killed in order to obtain the gland. About thirty deer are required to get one kilogram of musk grains. In the present day, it is illegal to kill a musk deer to obtain musk. Astringent is a taste that can reduce the oiliness by absorbing *kapha*. Green gram powder is a common example of *kaṣāya* (astringent) powder used to remove oil from the body. Saffron and musk are also astringent in quality.

Sarvāṅgasundara: *Rodhrādi*[2] is the name of a group of herbs that have *kaṣāya* (astringent) taste and can be used to remove the oil. *Kunkuma* mentioned here is *kāśmīra* (*Corcus sativus*).

Note: It is sometimes believed that *Āyurveda* is a vegetarian science. But it is not true. There are several animal products used in *Āyurveda* including meat, bones, blood, semen, and so on. For the sake of saving a human life it is sometimes necessary to kill another animal or bird. This has to be done with discretion and respect. Human life is the highest form of life on earth according to the *Vedas*. The *Vedic* injunction is that to save a higher form of life, a lower life can be sacrificed (lower in terms of evolution of consciousness). It is also a principle that one living being subsists on another (*jīvo jīvasya jīvanam*).

AH Sū. 3.12

Diet for *hemanta* (early winter)

रसान् स्निग्धान् पलं पुष्टं गौडमच्छसुरां सुराम् ॥१२॥

गोधूमपिष्टमाषेक्षुक्षीरोत्थविकृतीः शुभाः ॥१२॥

rasān snigdhān palaṁ puṣṭaṁ gauḍam-acchasurāṁ surām

godhūma-piṣṭamāṣekṣu-kṣīrottha-vikṛtīḥ śubhāḥ //12//

rasān snigdhān – meat soups that are prepared using ghee; *palaṁ puṣṭaṁ* – with the meat of strong animals; *gauḍam-accha-surāṁ surām* – alcoholic drinks made from jaggery and rice powder; *godhūma-piṣṭa-māṣa-ikṣu-kṣīra-uttha-vikṛtīḥ* – food items prepared using wheat, black gram, sugar cane, milk (*vikṛtiḥ* - transformation, cooking); *śubhāḥ* – of good quality and tasty

Translation

Meat soups prepared using ghee from the meat of healthy animals, alcoholic drinks made from jaggery and rice powder, different types of food articles made from wheat, rice powder, sugarcane, and milk of good quality (should be consumed).

Commentary

These are some examples of nourishing foods given in the verse:

1. *Rasān*: liquids (soups); *snigdhān*: made in unctuous manner (with ghee etc.)
2. *Palaṁ*: meat; *puṣṭaṁ*: of healthy animals
3. *Gauḍam*: from molasses; *acchasurāṁ*: pure, clear; *surām*: beverages
4. *Godhūma*: wheat; *māṣa* – black gram; *piṣṭamāṣ*: pastries made of or mixed with flour
5. *Ikṣu*: sugarcane
6. *Kṣīrottha*: produced from milk, fresh butter; *vikṛtīḥ*: transformed; *śubhāḥ*: auspicious, are recommended

These are all highly nourishing foods, which are required to be eaten during winter, since the digestive fire is very strong. Winter is the best time to improve one's health.

Sarvāṅgasundara: There are two types of alcohols that can be prepared: *surā* and *acchasurā.* Those made out of *amla* (sour) substances and those made out of *kaṣāya* (astringent) substances are both called *surā* (strong alcohol). *Acchasurā* (a type of mild alcohol) can be taken at all times.

AH Sū. 3.13

Diet, cleansing, and clothing during winter

नवमन्नं वसां तैलं, शौचकार्ये सुखोदकम् ॥१३॥

प्रावाराजिनकौशेयप्रवेणीकौचवास्तृतम् ॥१३॥

navam-annaṁ vasāṁ tailaṁ śaucakārye sukhodakam

prāvārājina-kauśeya-praveṇī-kauthapāstṛtam //13//

navam-annaṁ – fresh rice (from new paddy); *vasāṁ* – animal fat; *tailaṁ* – sesame oil; *śaucakārye* – for toiletry purposes; *sukhodakam* – pleasantly warm water; *prāvāra* – cotton clothes; *ajina* – animal fur; *kauśeya* – silk cloth; *praveṇī* – braided or stitched garment; *kaucavaṁ* – deer skin; *āstṛtam* – spread on the floor

Translation

Use of fresh rice, animal fat, and sesame oil are recommended. For the purposes of cleansing (e.g., washing hands, bathing, toilet, etc.), pleasantly warm water should be used. The clothes or blankets made of *prāvāra, ajina, kauśeya, praveṇi*, and *kauthapa* are spread on the floor (contd. in next verse). The special property of these clothes are that they are very warm at the same time light in weight.

Commentary

Usually it is recommended to eat grains that have been stored for up to one year. Fresh grains are heavy to digest and after storing for an year the grains become light. This is one of the rare instances where we see that fresh rice is recommended for consumption, because the capacity to digest is high during this season.

1. *Prāvara* (*kārpāso romavān ghanaā paana*): thick furry cotton cloth
2. *Ajinah* (*sukha sparśa roma carma*): animal fur that is soft to touch
3. *Kauśeya* (*paśey vasanan*): silk cloth
4. *Praveha* (*sūcī bācīhany vastra viśeran*): a type of stitched cloth (woollen)
5. *Kaucava* (*rācavan vastra bhedaa*): a type of fur made from deer skin (*rāinaan*)

These are all different types of warm clothes that were used during ancient times to cover the body and also spread on the floor. The newly harvested rice has got a property of *vidāhitvam* or causing burning sensation. Sesame oil can be consumed as well as applied on body. In extremely cold situations, animal fat is very much used to keep the body warm. According to the principle of similars (*vṛddhi samānaiḥ sarveṣāṁ - AH Sū 1.14*), consumption of animal fat is the best way to increase body fat, which will keep the cold away. The Āyurvedic properties of most of the substances described in this chapter will be detailed in volume 2 of this series which will further illustrate the reasons why they are recommended in their respective seasons.

AH Sū. 3.14

Sleeping, sunbathing, and wearing footwear in winter

उष्णस्वभावैर्लघुभिः प्रावृतः शयनं भजेत् ॥१४॥

युक्त्यार्ककिरणान् स्वेदं पादत्राणं च सर्वदा ॥१४॥

uṣṇa-svabhāvair-laghubhiḥ prāvṛta-śayanaṁ bhajet

yuktyārka-kiraṇān svedaṁ pādatrāṇaṁ ca sarvadā //14//

uṣṇa-svabhāvair – warm type of; *laghubhiḥ* – and lightweight; *prāvṛtas* – well wrapped or covered; *śayanaṁ* – sleeping, taking rest on bed; *bhajet* – is done; *yuktyā* – according to logic, as per requirement and availability; *arka-kiraṇān* – (warm) with the sun rays (sunbathing); *svedaṁ* – sweating using dry or wet heat; *pādatrāṇaṁ* – footwear; *ca* – and; *sarvadā* – all these

Translation

...to be used for sleeping, with warm and light material for covering the body. Expose the body to sunshine (sunbath) as per requirement, and one should use footwear at all times.

Commentary

Why is the use of footwear especially emphasized for the winter season? In the winter season, there is the risk of feet becoming too cold. This should be avoided, as it can cause *vāta* aggravation, since the feet are already a home for *vāta*. Sunbathing is recommended for the winter when possible.

Āyurvedarasāyana: In CS Sū. 6.14, a type of heating treatment called *jentāka* is advised for the winter. *Jentāka* is similar to sauna that is done in the modern day. Different types of *svedana* are described in volume 5 of this series.

AH Sū. 3.15

Utilization of body heat to keep warm

पीवरोरुस्तनश्रोण्यः समदाः प्रमदाः प्रियाः ॥१५॥

हरन्ति शीतमुष्णाङ्ग्यो धूपकुङ्कुमयौवनैः ॥१५॥

pīvaroru-stana-śroṇyaḥ samadāḥ pramadāḥ priyāḥ

haranti śītam-uṣṇāṅgyo dhūpa-kumkuma-yauvanaiḥ //15//

pīvara – plump, thick, voluptuous; *uru* – thighs; *stana* – breast, bosom; *śroṇyaḥ* – hips, buttocks; *samadāḥ* – intoxicated and excited with passion; *pramadāḥ* – young provocative women with large bosom and pleasing curves; *priyāḥ* – loving embraces; *haranti śītam* – eliminates the cold; *uṣṇāṅgayo* – warm bodied; *dhūpa* – fumigated; *kumkuma* – saffron; *yauvanaiḥ* – and youthful

Translation

Loving embraces by young, provocative women with plump breasts, voluptuous thighs, and prominent hips, intoxicated with passion, their warm bodies, anointed all over with the paste of saffron and fumigated with scented herbs, eliminates the cold (of the season).

Commentary

In today's social milieu, this verse can be misunderstood as promiscuity or chauvinism. But this is not the case. According to the *Tantra Sārasangraha*, the female body is described to be predominantly *āgneya*, and the male body to be predominantly *śīta*. Hence, females are prone to be hotter than males.

Unlike the modern day, where being thin and slim is advertised as attractive and desirable, during the *Vedic* times as we can see that women with plump breasts, voluptuous thighs, and prominent hips were considered more attractive. We can appreciate how the perception of beauty varies according to many factors like culture, climate, purpose and so on. The concept of *thin is beautiful* has actually led many women to undergo depression due to self-perception of their external appearance as obese. On the contrary women who are too thin develop many physical imbalances due to the lack of body fat. The Āyurvedic concept of obesity is not based only on external appearance.

The concept of *āgneya* shows that the female body has a greater ability to produce, absorb, store, and retain heat in comparison to the male body. Implied here is also a gift of nature to the mother to enable her to protect the child with her warmth. This verse is not meant to encourage illicit sexual activity. The importance of body fat in conserving heat has already been mentioned, and hence, the same is mentioned here once again. One may wonder if this advice is for men what should women do in winter? The answer is that since the men are advised to embrace the women, there is no need to separately tell what the women should do.

Probably these recommendations were for the royalty and aristocracy who had a lot of female companions to fulfil these requirements.

AH Sū. 3.16

Underground residence regulates temperature

अङ्गारतापसन्तप्तगर्भभूवेश्मचारिणः ॥१६॥

शीतपारुष्यजनितो न दोषो जातु जायते ॥१६॥

aṅgāra-tāpa-santapta-garbha-bhūveśma-cāriṇaḥ

śīta-pāruṣya-janito na doṣo jātu jāyate //16//

aṅgāra – burning embers; *tāpa* – heat; *santapta* – fully warmed by; *garbha-bhūveśma* – inside underground room, underground cellars; *cāriṇaḥ* – one who inhabits; *śīta* – cold; *pāruṣya* – severity; *janito* – caused due to (born from); *na* – will not; *doṣo* – of the adverse effects; *jātu* – at any time; *jāyate* – become affected

Translation

One who lives in an underground home (room), heated with burning embers, will never at any time be affected by the adverse effects caused by severe cold.

Commentary

Here the heat-retaining benefits of living under the ground are described. Those in extremely cold regions can take this advice and build their residences accordingly with an underground room to help beat the winters. Underground homes are more stable in terms of temperature all round the year, ecofriendly, have a lower building cost, are resistant to severe weather, cold, rain, wind, and natural abrasions. The energy consumption is kept down to a minimum. In Switzerland, by building the house underground, the architects were able to almost completely eliminate the need for heating in winter or cooling in summer months. In Iran there are homes that are carved out from rock and situated under the ground. In Vrindavan and other holy places in India, I have seen many underground caves and holes dug into the ground, which were used by sages to perform their *bhajans* (prayers) that would go on for years, and one reason was that it was temperature friendly throughout the year, where the temperatures vary between 50°C (122°F) in the summers and 2°C (35.6°F) in the winters.

Cāriṇaḥ means one who inhabits, just as the word *dehacāri* means one who inhabits the body. The word *carya* is a variation of the word *cāri*.

शिशिर ऋतुचर्या

Śiśira ṛtucaryā

Seasonal regimen in extreme winter

Similar to *hemanta*

Key points to remember

- *Doṣa*: *Kapha sañcaya* (accumulation of *kapha*)
- *Agni*: *Prabala* (very strong)
- *Guṇa*: *Utkṛṣṭa śīta* (excessively cold) + *Utkṛṣṭa rūkṣa* (excessively dry)

AH Sū. 3.17

अयमेव विधिः कार्यः शिशिरेपि विशेषतः ॥१७॥

तदा हि शीतमधिकं रौक्ष्यं चादानकालजम् ॥१७॥

ayameva vidhiḥ kāryaḥ śiśire'pi viśeṣataḥ

tadā hi śītam-adhikam raukṣyam cādāna-kālajam //17//

ayam – similar; *eva* – certainly; *vidhiḥ* – regimen; *kāryaḥ* – activities; *śiśire* – in winter; *api* – also; *viśeṣataḥ* – characteristic; *tadā hi* – because at that time; *śītam-adhikam* – of extreme cold; *raukṣyam* – dryness; *ca* – and; *ādāna-kālajam* – caused due to period of extraction

Translation

The same regimen is to be adopted during the *śiśira* (later part of winter) as well, because at that time the characteristic features are those of extreme cold and dryness caused due to *ādāna kāla* (movement of the sun to the north).

Commentary

Hemanta is the end of *visarga* and *śiśira* marks the beginning of *ādāna*. Since *śiśira* (late winter) is part of *ādāna* period, dryness is a marked feature of the season compared to *hemanta* (early winter). During *hemanta*, coldness is only due to the fog. But in *śiśira* the earth as well as the sky becomes cold. The earth becomes covered with snow due to constant snowfall. Thus, the intensity of cold increases. This is the reason why this part of the winter is recognized as a different season.

The difference between *hemanta* (early winter) and *śiśira* (late winter) is that the former is predominantly *śīta snigdha* (cold and unctuous) and the latter is predominantly *śīta rūkṣa* (cold and dry). These are the two specific qualities of *śiśira* season (late winter). The reason why ācārya *Vāgbhaṭa* started the description of the seasons with *hemanta* is in order to illustrate and clarify the transition taking place at this junction.

Sarvāṅgasundara: *Snigdha rasa* (unctuous tastes) is to be practiced in *hemanta* (early winter). In *śiśira* (late winter) it is to be practiced even more. The same regimen as for *hemanta* (early winter) is to be practiced but with even more intensity. *Rūkṣa* (dry) is the feature of *ādāna kāla* (weakening time), which becomes manifest in *śiśira* (late winter). The difference in the dryness in *śiśira* (late winter) and *grīṣma* (summer) is that the dryness in summer is due to heat and the sharp penetrating quality of *grīṣma* (summer) while that in the winter is due to the extreme cold.

So there are two causes for *rūkṣatva* (dryness): one is extreme cold, and the other is extreme heat.
Thus end the recommendations of the regimen to be followed during the winter season.

वसन्त ऋतुचर्या

Vasanta ṛtucaryā

Spring seasonal regimen

Key points to remember:

- *Doṣa*: *Kapha prakopa* (aggravation of *kapha*)
- *Agni*: *Hatva agni* (very weak *agni*)
- *Guṇa*: *Alpa uṣṇa* (mild heat) + *Madhyama snigdha* (medium unctuousness)
- *Āhāra (food)* – pungent, bitter, astringent, sharp, penetrating, light, rough, barley and wheat preserved for one year, alcoholic beverages, wine, honey, mango flower juice, ginger water, kino, musta, honey water

- *Dwelling* – island, flowing stream, southern breeze, moderate sun, fragrant flowers, exotic locales, melodious birds
- *Activities* – emesis, nasal drops, interactive discussions, avoid day sleeping, exercise, strong massage, anoint body with camphor, agar etc.
- *Diseases – Kapha Pitta (*the *kapha* here is aggravated *kapha. Kapha* in an aggravated state is always associate with *pitta.* The role of *vāta* is as *yogavāhi* – a carrier*)*

AH Sū. 3.18

कफश्चितो हि शिशिरे वसन्तेर्कांशुतापितः ॥१८॥

हत्वाग्निं कुरुते रोगानतस्तं त्वरया जयेत् ॥१८॥

kaphaścito hi śiśire vasante'rkāṁśu-tāpitaḥ

hatvā'gniṁ kurute rogānantastaṁ tvarayā jayet //18//

kaphaścito (*kapha* + *citaḥ*) – *kapha* that increased and accumulated [*citaḥ* – heaped or piled up]; *hi* – certainly; *śiśire* – in the late winter; *vasante* – in the spring; *arkāṁśu* – due to sunshine; *tāpitaḥ* – is heated (liquefied); *hatvā'gniṁ* – kills the digestive fire; *kurute* – gives rise to; *roga-anantas* – unlimited diseases; *taṁ* – due to that reason the *kapha* ; *tvarayā* – should be quickly; *jayet* – pacified

Translation

The *kapha* that increased and accumulated in the later part of winter melts due to the sunshine in spring season and destroys the digestive fire giving rise to many diseases. Hence, the *kapha* should be quickly pacified.

Commentary

According to this verse, springtime is a time of unlimited diseases. *Agni* is the immune strength of the body, and any season where *agni* is muffled, the body will be susceptible to many diseases which originate from *agni māndya*. The quickest way of *kapha* pacification is to perform a *vamana* (emesis). In fact it is common in certain parts of India to practice *vāsantika vamana* (emesis in spring), where people in the community come to a common place and perform *vamana* (emesis) in groups. This is especially beneficial in those who have chronic affliction with *kapha* diseases like certain types of bronchial asthma or skin diseases.

The analogy of snow accumulating on the peaks of mountains, which melts and flows down in the summer as rivers is given. This is because the *kapha* solidifies and accumulates at the top part of the body (head) during the winter, melts in the summer, and flows down to cause *kapha*-related complications.

The word *tvarayā* is very important here. The *kapha* aggravation should be controlled *immediately* otherwise there is a possibility of it getting out of control. We must inform the clients about this – especially those suffering from or prone to *kapha* diseases.

AH Sū. 3.19–23a

Nasal drops, massage, bath, diet, and drinks in spring season

तीक्ष्णैर्वमननस्याद्यैर्लघुरूक्षैश्च भोजनैः ॥१९॥

व्यायामोद्वर्तनाघातैर्जित्वा श्लेष्माणमुल्बणम् ॥१९॥

स्नातोनुलिप्तः कर्पूरचन्दनागुरुकुङ्कुमैः ॥२०॥

पुराणयवगोधूमक्षौद्रजाङ्गलशूल्यभुक् ॥२०॥

सहकाररसोन्मिश्रानास्वाद्य प्रिययार्पितान् ॥२१॥

प्रियास्यसङ्गसुरभीन् प्रियानेत्रोत्पलाङ्कितान् ॥२१॥

सौमनस्यकृतो हृद्यान्वयस्यैः सहितः पिबेत् ॥२२॥

निगदानासवारिष्टसीधुमार्द्वीकमाधवान् ॥२२॥

शृङ्गबेराम्बु साराम्बु मध्वम्बु जलदाम्बु च ॥२३॥

tīkṣṇair-vamana-nasyādyair-laghu-rūkṣaiśca bhojanaiḥ
vyāyām-odvartan-āghātair-jitvā śleṣmāṇam-ulbaṇam //19//
snāto'nuliptaḥ karpūra-candanāgaru-kuṅkumaiḥ
purāṇa-yava-godhūma-kṣaudra-jāṅgala-śūlya-bhuk //20//
sahakāra-rasonmiśrān-āsvādya priyayā'rpitān
priyāsya-saṅga-surabhīn priyā-netrotpalā'ṅkitān //21//
saumanasya-kṛto hṛdyān vayasyaiḥ sahitaḥ pibet
nigadān-āsavāriṣṭa-sīdhu-mārdvīka-mādhavān //22//
śrṅga-verāmbu sārāṁbu madhvambu jaladāṁbu vā

Word for word translation (verse 19)

tīkṣṇair – sharp; *vamana* – emesis; *nasya* – nasal drops/ errhines; *ādyair* – etc; *laghu* – light; *rūkṣaiśca* – and rough; *bhojanaiḥ* – foodstuffs; *vyāyāma* – exercise; *udvartana* – upward powder massage; *āghātair* – by hard massages with hands and feet; *jitvā* – cures; *śleṣmāṇam* – of *kapha*; *ulbaṇam* – excessive

Translation (verse 19)

Using therapeutically induced emesis and nasal drops with sharp, penetrating substances; food with light and rough qualities; exercise; and hard (deep tissue) massage (with hands and feet); the accumulated excess *kapha* should be conquered.

Commentary

Note that especially *vamana* (emesis) of *tīkṣṇa* (sharp) variety is mentioned here. This is the practical application of the verse *caya eva jayed doṣām* mentioned in AH Sū 13.15. The word *tīkṣṇa* indicates that it is *kapha doṣā* that is being targeted here. An example of a sharp and penetrating nasal drop is garlic oil.

We can see how the food pattern changed from *snigdha* (unctuous), *guru* (heavy) and *madhura* (sweet in *hemanta* / *śiśira*) to *Laghu* (light) and *rūkṣā* (dry) type of foods that are specifically meant to pacify *kapha doṣā*. Some examples of *laghu* (light) and *rūkṣa* (dry) or *khara* (rough) food is popcorn, puffed rice, flat rice, barley, broken wheat, steamed salads, vegetables, and so on.

Note that *abhyaṅga* is not mentioned here unlike in *hemanta* and *śiśira* because this is a season where *kapha* aggravates. Here *udvartana* is emphasized instead.

Word for word translation (Verse 20)

snāto – after bath; *anuliptaḥ* – anointed; *karpūra* – camphor; *candana* – sandalwood; *agaru* – agar (Aquilaria agallocaha); *kuṅkumaiḥ* – saffron; *purāṇa-yava-godhūma* – old barley and wheat; *kṣaudra* – with honey; *jāṅgala* – (animals of) arid regions; *śūlya* – roasted on spear (barbequed); *bhuk* – eat

Translation (verse 20)

After bath, the body should be anointed with a mixture of camphor, sandalwood, agaru, and saffron (as perfume). Barley and wheat that have been preserved for long (more than a year) and barbeque of animals living in arid regions may be consumed along with honey.

Commentary

Note that all the substances mentioned here are *laghu* and *rūkṣa* which are *kapha-pitta* pacifying in nature. Anointing the body with sweet-smelling substances after bath was a part of the culture just as we use perfumes today. It is to be noted that perfumes can be of *kapha*, *pitta* or *vāta* pacifying varieties. The ones recommended here are the perfumes having *kapha-pitta* pacifying qualities. Here we see the example of *laghu* (light) and *rūkṣa* (dry) food described. In *hemanta* and *śiśira*, *navam annam* (freshly harvested rice) was recommended but here we see the transition to *purāṇa yava* (old barley or grains) and *purāṇa guḍā* (old jaggery). In the description of the seasons, we can also clearly see the poet in *Vāgbhaṭa*.

Word for word translation (Verses 21-22)

sahakāra-rasa – juice of mango flowers; *unmiśrān* – mixed with; *āsvādya* – that which has been sipped; *priyayā* – offered by the lover; *arpitān* – and offered by; *priyāsya saṅga* – in the lover's association or company; *surabhīn* – aromatic; *priyā* – of lover; *netra* – eyes; *utpalā* – lotus like; *aṅkitān* – marked (decorated) *saumanasya* – giving pleasure to be; *kṛto* – to do; *hṛdyān* – charming; *vayasyaiḥ* – girl friends, companions; *sahitaḥ* – along with; *pibet* – to drink, sip; *nigadān* – old (brewed for long); *āsava-ariṣṭa* – alcoholic beverages and wines; *sīdhu* – liquor distilled from molasses (sugarcane); *mārdvīka* – wine made of grapes; *mādhavān* – made of honey; *śṛṅga-verāmbu* – water boiled with ginger; *sārāṁbu* (sara + ambu) – water boiled with *Pterocarpus marsupium*; *madhvambu* (madhu + ambu) – water mixed with honey; *jaladāṁbu* (*jalada* + *ambu*) – water boiled with Cyperus rotundus or *musta;* vā – and

Translation (verses 21–22)

Alcoholic beverages like *āsava* and *ariṣṭa*, liquor distilled from molasses, wine made from grapes (*mardvika*), and honey mixed with the juice of mango flowers offered by the lover, aromatically flavored by the touch of the lips of the beloved, and decorated with glances of her lotus-like eyes should be pleasantly consumed in the company of friends. Water boiled with ginger, *sāra* (East Indian kino) and/or *musta* should be taken. Honey water may also be consumed.

Note: *Arista* is stronger variety of alcoholic drink and cannot be consumed regularly. But *mardvika* which is a milder variety of alcohol and can be taken regularly.

Commentary

Here it is advised to drink water boiled with different herbs rather than plain water. Ginger tea with honey is good. It is a common practice in places that are *kapha* predominant (called *ānūpa deśa*)—for example, Kerala, India—for people to always drink only warm water boiled with herbs like ginger, cumin, and so on. Water becomes light and easy to digest when boiled. *Sāra* or *vijaysār* is a herb that is *kaṣāya* (astringent) in taste, *laghu* (light) and *khara* (rough) in quality, *kapha-pitta* pacifying with *kaṭu* (pungent) *vipāka*. *Musta* or *jalada* is a variety of grass having *kaṭu* (pungent), *tikta* (bitter), and *kaṣāya* (astringent) taste; *laghu* (light) and *khara* (rough) quality; *kaṭu* (pungent) *vipāka*; cold *vīrya*; and *kapha-pitta* pacifying. *Musta* has a *prabhāva* (special quality) of being *agni dīpana* (ignition of digestive fire) and cooling at the same time, but ginger and honey are heating. Honey has a special property of being *madhurā* (sweet), *kapha* pacifying, and heating at the same time.

The presence of the lover is for the purpose of giving pleasure to the mind. Sexual intercourse in optimal quantity is also mentioned as a way to pacify *kapha* aggravation in the body.

Kapha aggravation tends to make the mind dull, and the presence of the lover will help keep the alertness at a high level. *Sahakāra rasa* described here is not mango juice, because mangoes have not begun to produce fruit in spring but only begun to flower. So it is the juice of the flowers.

Sarvāṅgasundara: *Sāraḥ* refers to *asana*, *candana*, and so on. The *asanādi* group of plants are explained in AH Sū. 15.19–20.

AH Sū. 3.23b–26a

Dwelling, activities, and diet in spring season

दक्षिणानिलशीतेषु परितो जलवाहिषु ॥२३॥

अदृष्टनष्टसूर्येषु मणिकुट्टिमकान्तिषु ॥२४॥

परपुष्टविघुष्टेषु कामकर्मान्तभूमिषु ॥२४॥

विचित्रपुष्पवृक्षेषु काननेषु सुगन्धिषु ॥२५॥

गोष्ठीकथाभिश्चित्राभिर्मध्याह्नं गमयेत्सुखी ॥२५॥

dakṣiṇā'nila-śīteṣu parito jalavāhiṣu //23//

adṛṣṭa-naṣṭa-sūryeṣu maṇikuttima-kāntiṣu

parapuṣṭavighuṣṭeṣu kāmakarmānta-bhūmiṣu //24//

vicitra-puṣpa-vṛkṣeṣu kānaneṣu sugandhiṣu

goṣṭī-kathābhiś-citrābhir-madhyāhnam gamayet sukhī //25//

Activities to be avoided in spring season

गुरुशीतदिवास्वप्नस्निग्धाम्लमधुरांस्त्यजेत् ॥२६॥

guru-śīta-divāsvapna-snigdhāmla-madhurāms-tyajet

dakṣiṇā'nila – southern breeze; *śīteṣu* – cooling; *parito* – surrounded on all sides; *jalavāhiṣu* – by flowing streams; *adṛṣṭa* – invisible; *naṣṭa-sūryeṣu* – hidden sun; *maṇi* – precious gems; *kuttima* – ground paved with small stones; *kāntiṣu* – radiant, bright; *parapuṣṭa* – Indian female cuckoo bird; *vighuṣṭeṣu* – reverberating; *kāma-karmānta* – conclusion of romantic activities (love making); *bhūmiṣu* – areas for; *vicitra* – exotic; *puṣpa* – flowers; *vṛkṣeṣu* – in the trees; *kānaneṣu* – in the forests; *sugandhiṣu* – fragrant; *goṣṭī-kathābhiś* – interactive discussions; *citrābhir* – animated, lively; *madhyāhnam* – during midday hours; *gamayet* – are to be spent; *sukhī* – happily

guru – heavy; *śīta* – cold; *divāsvapna* – sleeping in daytime; *snigdha* – unctuous; *amla* – sour; *madhurām* – sweet; *tyajet* – give up, avoid

Translation

On an island surrounded by flowing streams, cooled by the southern breeze; with moderate amount of sun and the melodious cooing of the cuckoo birds; surrounded by exotic locales of fragrant flowers, trees, radiant-looking grounds paved with precious gems, and areas suitable for lovemaking; one should spend the midday hours in enjoyable, animated, and interactive discussions.

Heavy, cold, unctuous, oily, fatty, sour, and sweet foods and sleeping during the daytime should be avoided.

Commentary

In short, one should accept *kapha-pitta* reducing and avoid *kapha-pitta* aggravating activities. This sounds like the description of a heavenly resort in the present context. It seems like these kinds of areas were commonly found in the ancient times but have become a luxury in the present day with the violent exploitation and destruction of nature and natural resources.

It is the responsibility of the government and/or community to make sure that there are a sufficient number of gardens, trees, and flowers in residential localities and work environments. Work schedules should include breaks given to the staff during the midday hours (midday break) to sit in the gardens and engage in discussions sipping *kapha*-reducing beverages to stimulate the appetite and improve digestion. The implementation of *dinacaryā* and *ṛtucaryā* in all schools and offices will ensure good health of the population and reduce health expenditure overall. The logic behind recommendations to have interactive discussions in the midday hours is to prevent the person from sleeping in the day, which aggravates *kapha*. This may not be applicable to someone who is working hard during the day but more to one who is relaxing at home.

Note that in the case of spring season, it is not just about doing the activities opposite to *kapha* qualities (e.g., to heat oneself). Here we can see that heat is the cause of the problem, but the advice is given to avoid cold. This is because we need to see what is happening inside the body as a result of what is happening in the atmosphere. In the case of spring season, the heat is causing a melting of the *kapha*. *Kapha kopa* (*kapha* aggravation) is already taking place in the body, and cold applications will cause more *kapha kopa* (*kapha* aggravation). Hence, it is to be avoided.

The foods that are heavy to digest are avoided, because the *agni* is weak during this time.

Sarvāṅgasundara: Heavy and cold foods are not recommended in order to avoid *kapha* accumulation. *Lavaṇa* (salty) taste also causes *kapha* accumulation, but why is this not prohibited? *Lavaṇa* (salty) taste is *kapha* increasing as *madhurā* (sweet) and *amla* (sour) tastes. *Lavaṇa* (salty) is normally not used in large quantity in the diet in the same way as *madhurā* (sweet) and *amla* (sour) tastes. *Lavaṇa* (salty) taste in small quantities also helps to melt the *kapha* that has been accumulated in the past and make it flow out. But the same *lavaṇa* in larger quantities can cause *kapha* accumulation. Thus end the recommendations for the regimen to be followed during the *vasanta* (spring) season.

---

1. The word *ṛtu* comes from the root word *ṛt*, which means "to pursue" or *ṛ*, which means "to go."
2. AH Sū. 15. 26–27.

ग्रीष्म ऋतुचार्या

Grīṣma ṛtucaryā

Summer seasonal regimen

Key points to remember

- *Doṣa*: *Kapha praśama* + *Vāta sañcaya*
- *Agni*: Strong but not as strong as in winter (since sweet and fatty foods are recommended)
- *Guṇa*: *Utkṛṣṭa uṣṇa* + *Madhyama rūkṣa*
- *Āhāra* (food) – sweet, light, fatty, cool, liquid, *hṛdya* (pleasing), *vṛṣya* (aphrodisiac), *rucikara* (tasty)
- Dwelling – soft beds, cooling atmosphere, away from the sun, sheets of clothes sprayed with cool scented water, bunch of flowers and creepers hanging, fountains
- Activities – wear garlands, play with children, associate with beautiful pleasing women, moon bathing, sleeping on soft beds
- Diseases – Vāta Pitta

AH Sū. 3.26b–27a

Weakening effect of summer

तीक्ष्णांशुरतितीक्ष्णांशुर्ग्रीष्मे संक्षिपतीव यत् ॥२६॥

प्रत्यहं क्षीयते श्लेष्मा तेन वायुश्च वर्धते ॥२७॥

tīkṣṇāṁśur-atitīkṣṇāmśu grīṣme saṁkṣipatīva yat //26//
pratyahaṁ kṣīyate śleṣmā tena vāyuśca vardhate

tīkṣṇāṁśur – sharp & powerful (this is a synonym for the sun); *ati* – extremely; *tīkṣṇāṁśu* – powerfully; *grīṣme* – in the summer season; *saṁkṣipati* – completely squeezing; *iva* – as if; *yat* – that which (the sun); *pratyahaṁ* – day by day; *kṣīyate* – weakens (*praśama*), dries up; *śleṣmā* – *kapha*; *tena* – of that; *vāyuśca* – and *vāta*; *vardhate* – increases (*sañcaya*)

Translation

In the summer season, the sun becomes extremely sharp and feels as if it is completely squeezing or wringing (the body). This weakens *kapha* day by day and increases *vāta*.

Commentary

Since it is the heat that is aggravating the *vāta* here, one should know that cold applications will reduce the aggravation of *vāta* in this condition. It is important to understand that heat initially pacifies *vāta*, but continued application of heat causes expansion and aggravates *vāta* due to the increase of *rūkṣa* (dry), *laghu* (light), *khara* (rough), *sūkṣma* (subtle), and *cala* (mobile) qualities (AH Sū. 1.11).
This is the last part of the *ādāna kāla* and most weakening. The other two seasons of *ādāna kāla* are not so weakening, because there is *kapha* predominance. But in the summer, there is *vāta* accumulation causing more weakness.

AH Sū. 3.27b

What to avoid in the summer season

अतोऽस्मिन्पटुकट्वम्लव्यायामार्ककरांस्त्यजेत् ॥२७॥

ato'smin-paṭu-kaṭvamla-vyāyāmārka-karāṁs-tyajet //27//

ataḥ – therefore; *asmin* – in this season; *paṭu* – salty; *kaṭu* – pungent, acrid; *amla* – sour; *vyāyāma* – exercise; *arka karāṁs* – exposure to sun; *tyajet* – to be avoided

Translation

(In the summer, *kapha* decreases day by day, while *vāta* increases day by day.) Therefore in this season, eatables that are salty, pungent, and sour in taste should be avoided. One should also avoid physical exercise and exposure to sunlight.

Commentary

kaṭu (pungent) aggravates *vāta* while lavaṇa (salty) and *amla* (sour) aggravate *pitta*. In the summer, it is a *vāta-pitta* atmosphere that is prevalent.

Note that it is advised to avoid physical exercise during the summer. But in some cold countries like Scandinavia, the summer is a time when people get out in the open and do a lot of exercise and sunbathing, but there the summers are very mild. Technically we can say that these countries do not have a summer season at all. The advice regarding exercise given here is for places that have very hot summers that drain your energy.

In addition to the draining of energy, these days we also run the risk of exposure to UV radiation when out in the sun.

Note the shift in the diet pattern again. The change is from light and dry foods in the spring to light and unctuous foods in summer. From *tikta* (bitter) taste – *laghu* and *rūkṣa* is bitter taste – in the spring to *madhura* (sweet) but *laghu* (light) in the summer. It should also be *snigdha* (unctuous) as compared to rūkṣa (dry) in spring. In the summer it should also be *hima* (cool) and *drava* (liquid) while in spring it was not too cool and dry.

AH Sū. 3.28

Qualities of foods consumed in summer

भजेन्मधुरमेवान्नं लघु स्निग्धं हिमं द्रवम् ॥२८॥

सुशीततोयसिक्ताङ्गो लिह्यात्सक्तून् सशर्करान् ॥२८॥

bhajen-madhuram-evānnaṁ laghu snigdhaṁ himaṁ dravam

suśīta-toya-siktāṅgo lihyāt-saktūn saśarkarān //28//

bhajet – to be used; *madhuram* – sweet; *eva* – certainly; *annaṁ* – food; *laghu* – light (easy to digest); *snigdhaṁ* – unctuous (fatty); *himaṁ* – cold; *dravam* – liquid; *suśīta* – refreshingly cool; *toya* – water; *sikta* – sprinkled; *aṅgo* – on the body; *lihyāt* – licked; *saktūn* – powder of parched paddy, rice and barley; *saśarkarān* – with sugar

Translation

Eatables that are sweet, light, fatty (oily), cold, and liquid could be taken during the summers. One can lick *saktu* flour mixed with water and sugar after taking bath in cool water.

Commentary

Sweet is to protect the strength; light is to produce strength; *snigdha* (unctuous or fatty) is to pacify *vāta*; *śīta* (cold) is to pacify *pitta*; and *dravam* (liquid) is to prevent *kapha* depletion. *Saktu* is a combination of the powdered barley, rice, and puffed rice (CS Sū. 27.263). It is light to digest and, at the same time, very strengthening, and hence, ideal for this time. During the summer, digestion and strength are both weak. So foods like *saktu* are recommended.

Spraying the body with water is a good way to keep cool in the summer and takes away the tiredness.

AH Sū. 3.29

Consumption of alcohol in summer

मद्यं न पेयं, पेयं वा स्वल्पं, सुबहुवारि वा ॥२९॥

अन्यथाशोषशैथिल्यदाहमोहान् करोति तत् ॥२९॥

madyaṁ na peyaṁ peyaṁ vā svalpaṁ subahuvāri vā

anyathā śopha śaithilya dāha mohān karoti tat //29//

madyaṁ – alcoholic beverages; *na peyaṁ* – do not drink; *peyaṁ* – drink; *vā* – if necessary; *svalpaṁ* – little quantity; *subahuvāri* – diluted with a lot of water; *vā* – also; *anyathā* –

otherwise; *śopha* – edema; *śaithilya* – slackness of body; *dāha* – burning; *mohān* – fainting; *karoti* – will cause; *tat* – that

Translation

Alcoholic beverages should not be consumed during summer. If necessary, they could be taken in a very small quantity after diluting with excess amounts of water. Otherwise it will cause edema, laxity of the body (debility), burning sensation, and delusion or fainting (in large doses).

Commentary

The qualities (*guṇa*) of alcohol are *pittāsra dussaham (*not tolerated by those who have *rakta pitta*[6] disease*), tīkṣṇa* (sharp)*, uṣṇa* (hot)*, rūkṣam* (dry), as described in chapter 5 of *Sūtra sthāna*. These are not favorable in the summer season. One should be careful while prescribing *ariṣṭam* to clients during the summer season. If it is unavoidable, it should only be given in low doses and high dilution with a lot of water. Remember that alcohols were prescribed to be taken during the winter and spring seasons but are to be avoided here.

***Sarvāṅgasundara*:** Alcohol in high dilution is appropriate for those having *pitta-kapha* constitution. Alcohol is recommended for reducing *kapha* and excess dilution is recommended to prevent *pitta* aggravation. For the reduction of *kapha-vāta*, it is

[6] Cause of rakta pitta will be discussed in nidāna sthāna of aṣṭāṅga hṛdayam

recommended in other seasons. If absolutely necessary in this season, it should be given after excessively diluting with water.

AH Sū. 3.30

Different foods consumed in summer

कुन्देन्दुधवलं शालिमश्नीयाज्जाङ्गलैः पलैः ॥३०॥

पिबेद्रसं नातिघनं रसालां रागखाण्डवौ ॥३०॥

kundendu-dhavalaṁ śālim-aśnīyājjāṅgalaiḥ palaiḥ

pibed-rasaṁ nātighnaṁ rasālāṁ rāga-khāṇḍavau //30//

kunda – jasmine flower; *indu* – moon; *dhavalaṁ* – as white as; *śālim* – śāli type of rice; *aśnīyāt* – one should eat; *jāṅgalaiḥ* – of dry lands; *palaiḥ* – meat of animals; *pibed* – drink; *rasaṁ* – meat soup, juice; *na atighnaṁ* – not excessively thick; *rasālāṁ* – see below[1]; *rāga* – soft drink made of sweet, sour and salty tastes; *khāṇḍavau* – soft drink made of all *rasas* except *kaṭu* (pungent)

Translation

During the summer, boiled rice, white like the jasmine flower and the full moon should be eaten along with meat of animals of arid regions. Meat juice which is not very thick (watery meat soup), yoghurt churned and mixed with pepper powder (*rasāla*), a syrup called *rāga* and a drink called *khāṇḍava* can be taken.

Commentary

The *rasālā* here indicates spiced yogurt and has the qualities of *bṛmhaṇa* (nourishing), *balya* (strengthening), *snigdha* (unctuous), *vṛṣya* (aphrodisiac), and *rucipradā* (appetizer), and it is *pratiśyāyaghni* (prevents running nose). Though yogurt is heating, it is recommended to be consumed in the summer, because it pacifies *vāta*. *Rasālā* is described to be *lassi* (a drink made out of yogurt) or grapes in other texts.

Some descriptions about the drinks

Rāga (*sitā-madhvādi-madhurā*)—a syrup that is sweet, sour and salty

Khāṇḍava (*peyāśca amśuka gālitā amlāḥ*): *praleha* (a kind of broth) *gālitā* (melted)—a drink that has all the tastes except bitterness

The properties of drinks like *rāga* and *khāṇḍava* are *hṛdya, vṛṣya,* and *rucikarā grāhiṇo* (pleasing, nourishing all tissues, tasty). These are the kinds of foods most suitable for summer.

What is important to understand here is that the foods and drinks recommended in summer are cooling, pleasing, nourishing, tasty, and enhance digestive functions.

AH Sū. 3.31–32a

Different beverages used during summer

पानकं पञ्चसारं वा नवमृद्भाजने स्थितम् ॥३१॥

मोचचोचदलैर्युक्तं साम्लं मृन्मयशुक्तिभिः ॥३१॥

पाटलावासितं चाम्भः सकर्पूरं सुशीतलम् ॥३२॥

pānakaṁ pañcasāraṁ vā nava mṛdbhājana sthitam

moca-coca dalairyuktaṁ sāmlaṁ mṛnmaya-śuktibhiḥ /31//

pāṭalā-vāsitaṁ cāmbhaḥ sakarpūraṁ suśītalam

pānakaṁ – drink; *pañcasāraṁ* – named *pañcasāram*; *vā* – also; *nava* – new; *mṛd-bhājana* – in the clay pot; *sthitam* – kept for long time; *moca* – banana fruit; *coca dalair* – fleshy edible part of jackfruit; *yuktaṁ* – along with; *sāmlaṁ* – made sour (fermented); *mṛd-maya śuktibhiḥ* – clay mugs or shells; *pāṭalā* – *Bignonia suaveolens* (trumpet flower); *vāsitaṁ* – spiced and scented with; *ca* – and; *ambhaḥ* – water; *sakarpūraṁ* – with camphor; *suśītalam* – pleasantly cool

Translation

Syrups made with several substances (*pānakaṁ*) and *pañcasāraṁ* (five substances, viz., *drākṣa, madhūka, kharjūra, kāśmarya*, and *parūṣaka*), all in equal quantities; cooled and added with the powders of *patra*, *tvak*, *elā*, and the like; kept inside a freshly made mud pot, along with leaves of plantain and coconut trees; and fermented can be drunk in mugs of mud or shell.

Pleasantly cool water kept in mud pots along with flowers of *pāṭalā* and *karpūra* (camphor) should be used for drinking purposes during this season.

Commentary

These were different drinks that were used in the early days instead of the coffee and cocoa that we drink today. Several kinds of *pānakas* (drinks) can be made using fruit juices—*rāgi*, yogurt, and so on.

There are elaborate descriptions of these cuisines available in *Bhāva Prakāśa* (the *Bhāva Prakāśa* mentioned here is a separate text that deals with descriptions of herbs and cuisines). Especially in the western countries now, we are seeing a resurgence of a lot of herbal teas and fruit teas that are in vogue. This is a very good trend and approved by *Āyurveda* if used intelligently.

Pañcarasam

- *Drākṣā* (grapes)
- *Madhūka* (honey)
- *Kharjūra* (dates)
- *Kāśmarya* (*Gmelina arborea* [*gambāri*])
- *Parūṣaka* (*Grewia asiatica*)

This combination is *madhura* (sweet), *śīta* (cooling), and *bṛṁhaṇa* (nourishing).

***Pāṭala* (*Stereospermum suaveolens*)—trumpet flower tree**

The flower of this herb is especially mentioned here. It is one of the herbs of the *daśamūla* group (a group of ten herbs that is effective in pacifying *vāta*). It is neuroprotective and hepatoprotective used in snake bites, scorpion bites, and so on. The flower is red or yellow in color, astringent-sweet (*kaṣāya-madhura)* in taste, cooling (*śīta*), and *pitta kapha* reducing. *Caraka* classifies it among the anti-inflammatory group of herbs. It is advised to drink water kept in a clay pot with camphor and *pāṭala* flowers.

AH Sū. 3.32b–33a

Summer nights—diet

शशाङ्ककिरणान् भक्ष्यान् रजन्यां भक्षयन् पिबेत् ॥३२॥

ससितं माहिषं क्षीरं चन्द्रनक्षत्रशीतलम् ॥३३॥

śaśāṇka-kiraṇān bhakṣyān rajanyāṁ bhakṣayan pibet //32//
sasitaṁ māhiṣaṁ kṣīraṁ candra nakṣatra śītalam

śaśāṇka-kiraṇān – called by this name; *bhakṣyān* – a certain dish; *rajanyāṁ* – in the night; *bhakṣayan* – is eaten; *pibet* – is drunk; *sasitaṁ* – with rock sugar; *māhiṣaṁ kṣīraṁ* – buffalo milk; *candra* – moon; *nakṣatra* – stars; *śītalam* – cooled by

Translation

In the night, after having had a dish called *śaśāṅka kiraṇa*, one must drink buffalo milk with sugar cooled by the moonlight and stars.

Commentary

śaśāṇka-kiraṇa: According to *Govindan vaidya*, this is a dish made by condensing milk and sugar. *Hṛdayabodhika* says that wheat is also added to it. It is a *vaṭaka* (round balls fried in oil) prepared with *tālīsapatra cūrṇa, sitopala*, and camphor (AH Ci. 5.49). *Śaśāṅka* means *karpūra* (camphor) according to *Āyurvedarasāyana*.

This appears to be a very heavy dish to be had at night. Why is it advised in the summer? This is because there is *vāta* accumulation in summer, and this kind of food is *vāta* pacifying. This conforms to the kind of food advised for the summer in AH Sū. 3.28. One should of course take into consideration the strength of *agni* as well.

We can see that everything mentioned here is cooling in nature – buffalo milk, moon light, night time and so on.

AH Sū. 3.33b–37a

Recommendations for dwellings during the summer season

अभ्रङ्कषमहाशालतालरुद्धोष्णरश्मिषु ॥३३॥

वनेषु माधवीश्लिष्टद्राक्षास्तबकशालिषु ॥३४॥

सुगन्धिहिमपानीयसिच्यमानपटालिके ॥३४॥

कायमाने चिते चूतप्रवालफललुम्बिभिः ॥३५॥

कदलीदलकल्हारमृणालकमलोत्पलैः ॥३५॥

कोमलैः कल्पिते तल्पे हसत्कुसुमपल्लवे ॥३६॥

मध्यंदिनेऽर्कतापार्तः स्वप्याद्धारागृहेऽथवा ॥३६॥

पुस्तस्त्रीस्तनहस्तास्यप्रवृत्तोशीरवारिणि ॥३७॥

abhraṅkaṣa-mahā-śāla-tāla-rūddhoṣṇa-raśmiṣu //33//

vaneṣu mādhavī-śliṣṭa-drākṣā-stabaka-śāliṣu

sugandhi-hima-pānīya-sicyamāna-paṭālike //34//

kāyamāne cite cūta-pravāla-phala-lumbibhiḥ

kadalīdala-kalhāra-mṛṇāla-kamalotpalaiḥ //35//

komalaiḥ kalpite talpe hasat-kusuma-pallave

madhyaṁ-dine'rka-tāpārtaḥ svapyād-dhārā-gṛhe'thavā //36//

pusta-strīstana-hastāsya-pravṛttośīra-vāriṇī

abhraṅkaṣa – touching the skies; *mahā* – big, tall; *śāla tāla* – (trees like) *śāla* and *tāla*; *rūddha* – block; *uṣṇa* – hot, scorching; *raśmiṣu* – rays (of the sun); *vaneṣu* – in the forests; *mādhavī* – jasmine flowers; *śliṣṭa* – clinging to, embracing; *drākṣā* – grapes; *stabaka* – cluster of; *śāliṣu* – lustrous, praise worthy *sugandhi* – scented; *hima* – cool; *pānīya* – water; *sicyamāna* – sprinkled; *paṭālike* – partitions made of cloth; *kāyamāne* – in a hut made of grass (thatch); *cite* – covered with; *cūta* – mango; *pravāla* – young sprouts of (mango); *phala* – fruits; *lumbibhiḥ* – bunches of;

kadalī – plantain; *dala* – petal, leaf; *kalhāra* – white esculent water lily (*saugandhika* flower); *mṛṇāla* – filament of lotus; *kamala* – of lotus; *utpalaiḥ* – of water lily; *komalaiḥ* – soft, which is not wilted; *kalpite* – well arranged; *talpe* – bed; (*komala kalpite talpe* – well-arranged soft bed); *hast* – like smiling teeth; *kusuma* – flower; *pallave* – of the petals; (*hasat-kusuma pallave* – of flower petals appearing like smiling teeth);

madhyaṁ – middle ; *dine* – of the day (*madhyaṁ dine* – mid-day); *arka* – sun; *tāpa* – heat; *ārtaḥ* – afflicted; *svapyād* – one should sleep;

dhārā gṛhe – in a shower house; *athavā* – or alternatively; *pusta* – statues of; *strī* – women; *stana* – breasts; *hasta* – hands; *āsya* – mouths; *pravṛtta* – coming out from; *uśīra vāriṇī* – water scented with *uśīra* (cuscus grass)

Translation

In forests with tall trees that appear to touch the skies, such as *śāla, tāla*, and so on, which obstruct the scorching rays of the sun, one should spend time in houses around which bunches of flowers and grapes are hanging from their creepers, looking praiseworthy. Sheets of cloth sprayed or sprinkled with cool scented water, and bunches of tender leaves and fruits of mango, hang all around a thatched house. One who is exhausted due to the heat of the midday sun should spend the long summer days sleeping on well-arranged soft beds, made with petals or leaves of *kadalī, kalhāra, mṛṇāla, utpala*, and fully blossomed flowers, white as the smiling teeth and red as lips, or alternatively in a shower house cooled by water fountains with *uśīra* scented water emerging out of the well-shaped breasts, hands, and mouth of statues.

Note: Here seems to be an apparent contradiction to the advice of avoiding sleeping during the day, which aggravates *kapha*. However, in the summer there is excessive *kapha* depletion, and sleeping during the day will replenish the *kapha* and compensate for the depletion.

Commentary

This is the description of a beautiful and natural summer house. Contrary to the spring season, sleeping in the day time is recommended in the summer season. Many arrangements are made inside the summer house to reduce the heat. It is recommended to take a shower with medicated water in which *uśīra* grass roots (*cuscus*) have been added. Similar medicated water can be made from other herbs depending on requirement and used. These are all natural ways of keeping cool and calm.

AH Sū. 3.37b–38

Moon bathing during summer nights

निशाकरकराकीर्णे सौधपृष्ठे निशासु च ॥३७॥
आसना स्वस्थचित्तस्य चन्दनार्द्रस्य मालिनः ॥३८
निवृत्तकामतन्त्रस्य सुसूक्ष्मतनुवाससः ॥३८॥

niśākara-karākīrṇe saudha-pṛṣṭhe niśāsu ca //37//
āsanā svastha-cittasya candanārdrasya mālinaḥ
nivṛtta-kāma-tantrasya susūkṣma-tanu-vāsasaḥ //38//

niśākara – the moon (night maker); *kara* – caused by; *ākīrṇe* – surrounded, spread, filled, flooded with; *saudha* – a fine house; *pṛṣṭhe* – terrace of; *niśāsu ca* – and in the nights; *āsanā* – sit, stay; *svastha cittasya* – with a relaxed mind; *candana* – sandal wood; *ārdrasya* – wet, fresh, anointed; *mālinaḥ* – wearing flower garlands; *nivṛtta* – staying away from; *kāma* – sexual activities; *tantrasya* – by a general rule or doctrine; *susūkṣma* – very thin; *tanu* – body; *vāsasaḥ* – of attire, clothes

Translation

In the nights, one should stay on the terrace of a fine house, flooded with moonlight, in a relaxed mood, body anointed with wet sandalwood paste, abstaining from any sexual activity as a rule and clothed in ultra-thin attire.

Commentary

The literal meaning of *niśākara kara* is that which is caused by the moon, which is *moonlight*. It is recommended to avoid sexual activity in summer to prevent further draining of the body.

In the nights, stay on the terrace of a fine house—*saudha-pṛṣṭhe niśāsu ca āsana*—surrounded or filled with moonlight (*niśākara karākīrṇe*).

Here moon bathing is specially advised for cooling and nourishing the body. Sunbathing is advised in the winter and moon bathing in the summer. There are many recommendations given in the verses and every one of them may not be possible in the present day. One should try to understand the principle and follow those that are within one's geographical, financial, and practical capacity with necessary modifications.

AH Sū. 3.39–41

More recommendations for the summer

जलार्द्रास्तालवृन्तानि विस्तृताः पद्मिनीपुटाः ॥३९॥
उत्क्षेपाश्च मृदूत्क्षेपा जलवर्षिहिमानिलाः ॥३९॥
कर्पूरमल्लिकामाला हाराः सहरिचन्दनाः ॥४०॥
मनोहरकलालापाः शिशवः सारिकाः शुकाः ॥४०॥
मृणालवलयाः कान्ताः प्रोत्फुल्लकमलोज्ज्वलाः ॥४१॥
जङ्गमा इव पद्मिन्यो हरन्ति दयिताः क्लमम् ॥४१॥

jalārdrāstālavṛntāni vistṛtāḥ padminī-puṭāḥ
utkṣepāśca mṛdūtkṣepā jalavarṣi himānilāḥ //39//
karpūra-mallikā mālā hārāḥ saharicandanāḥ
manohara kalālāpāḥ śiśavaḥ sārikāḥ śukāḥ //40//

mṛṇāla valayāḥ kāntāḥ protphulla kamalojjvalāḥ
jaṅgamā iva padminyo haranti dayitāḥ klamam //41//

jalārdrā – wet and fresh; *tāla-vṛntāni* – stalk of palm leaves; *vistṛtāḥ* – broad; *padminīpuṭāḥ* – lotus leaves; *utkṣepāḥ* – fanning; *ca* – and; *mṛdū* – slowly and softly; *utkṣepā* – yak tail whisks; *jalavarṣi* – by showering water droplets; *himānilāḥ* – cool breeze; *karpūra* – camphor; *mallikā* – jasmine; *mālā* – garlands; *hārāḥ* – necklaces; *saharicandanāḥ* – with sandal wood beads; *manohara* – enchanting; *kalālāpāḥ* – speaking in broken childish manner; *śiśavaḥ* – small children; *śārikāḥ* – talking birds (parakeets); *śukāḥ* – parrots; *mṛṇāla* – filament of lotus; *valayāḥ* – bangles; *kāntāḥ* – lovely women, beloved, wife; *protphulla* – full blooming; *kamala* – lotus; *ujjvalāḥ* – dazzling; *jaṅgamā* – moving; *iva* – just like; *padmini* – a specific type of woman with soft sweet voice and swan like gait; *haranti* – removing; *dayitāḥ* – beloved darling, wife; *klamaṁ* – fatigue

Translation

Soft and gentle fanning with fresh and wet palm leaves, yak -tail whisks, and large lotus leaves, spraying water droplets, making a cool breeze is recommended. Wear garlands made of camphor, jasmine, and necklaces of sandalwood. Small children speaking in an attractive manner; parrots and parakeets talking; and beloved women (*padmini*) with sweet voices moving with a swan-like gait, dazzling, and wearing lotus bangles and blooming lotuses take away the fatigue due to the intense heat.

Commentary

Fanning done commonly with peacock feathers or yak-tail whisk has the *prabhāva* of cooling the air. Another common practice noticed in hot climates is people wearing pearl necklaces, which cools the body. From this description we can also understand that speaking in different ways has a cooling or heating effect on the body and mind.

The water cooler used in India during the summer works by the technology of spraying water droplets to make a cool breeze. This is better than the air conditioner, because it is environment friendly, consumes less energy, and does not dry up the body.

There are four types of women described in *kāmasūtra*—*padmini, citriṇi, śaṅkhini* and *hastini*. It is also mentioned by *Kalyāṇa Malla* in his book *Anaṅgaraṅga.*

Her face is pleasing as the full moon, her body well covered with flesh, soft as the mustard flower, her skin is fine, tender and fair as the yellow lotus and never dark colored. Her eyes are bright and beautiful as the eyes of a young deer, well shaped and reddish corners. Her bosom is hard, full and high, she has a good neck, her nose is straight and lovely and three folds or wrinkles cross her middle – the umbilical region. Her external genitalia resembles the opening lotus bud and her secretions is like a perfumed lily that has just blossomed. She walks with a swan like gait, her voice is low and musical like that of a cuckoo bird, she loves white decorative clothes and fine jewels. She eats little, sleeps lightly, respectful, religion, clever and courteous. She is always anxious to worship the Gods and enjoys the conversations of the brahmanas.

Padmini is the most *rakta sāra, sattvik*, soft and spiritual woman whose actions are exactly what is pleasing to the man (just like chandānuvartini dārā – a wife who does according to the tune of the man)

Thus end the recommendations for the regimen to be followed during the summer season.

वर्षा ऋतुचर्या

Varṣā ṛtucaryā

Rainy seasonal regimen

Key points to remember

- *Doṣa*: *Pitta sañcaya* + *Vāta prakopa* + *kapha utkleśa*
- *Agni*: *Glāna* agni (weak agni)
- *Guṇa*: *Alpa śīta* (minimal cold) + *Utkṛṣṭa rūkṣa* (excessive dryness) in beginning...*alpa snigdha* (minimal oiliness) in the end, low *bala*
- *Āhāra* – sweet, sour, salty, unctuous, old grains, wines, whey with salt, pañcakola, boiled water, light, dry, combined with ghee and honey, meat soup, green gram soup

- Dwelling – upper floor of mansion, free from
- Activities – vamana, virecana, asthāpana vasti, body scented with perfumes, clothes fumigated with smoke, avoid the following - walking without footwear, sleeping in day, exposure sun, exertion
- Diseases – *Vāta Pitta Kapha*

AH Sū. 3.42–44

Vitiated water, *agni*, *doṣas*, and *dūṣyas*

आदानग्लानवपुषामग्निः सन्नोऽपि सीदति ॥४२॥

वर्षासु दोषैर्दुष्यन्ति तेऽम्बुलम्बाम्बुदेऽम्बरे ॥४२॥

सतुषारेण मरुता सहसा शीतलेन च ॥४३॥

भूबाष्पेणाम्लपाकेन मलिनेन च वारिणा ॥४३॥

वह्निनैव च मन्देन, तेष्वित्यन्योन्यदूषिषु ॥४४॥

भजेत्साधारणं सर्वमूष्मणस्तेजनं च यत् ॥४४॥

ādāna-glāna-vapuṣām-agni sanno'pi sīdati
varṣāsu doṣair-duṣyanti te'mbulambāmbude'mbare //42//
satuṣāreṇa marutā sahasā śītalena ca
bhūbāṣpeṇāmlapākena malinena ca vāriṇā //43//
vahninaiva ca mandena teṣvity-anyonya dūṣiṣu
bhajet sādhāraṇaṁ sarvam-ūṣmaṇas-tejanaṁ ca yat //44//

ādāna – period of extraction; *glāna* – deteriorated; *vapuṣām* – of the body; *agni* – digestive fire; *sannaḥ* - weak ; *api* – also; *sīdati* – sinks further down; *varṣāsu* – in the rainy season; *doṣaiḥ* – due to the *doṣa*s; *duṣyanti* – being vitiated; *te* – they; *ambulambāmbude* – when the dark clouds full of water gather (*ambu* – water; *ambude* – in the dark clouds); *ambare* - in the sky; *satuṣāreṇa* – with water droplets (like a spray), thin shower or rain; *marutā* – winds; *sahasā śītalena ca* – and due to fast and cold; *bhūbāṣpeṇa* – due to the vapors rising from the earth; *amlapākena* – generates *amlapāka*;
malinena – dirty, turbid; *ca* – and; *vāriṇā* – of water; *vahnina* – of the digestive fire; *eva* – certainly, also; *ca* – and; *mandena* – weak; *teṣu* – of that; *iti* – it; *anyonya* – reciprocally; *dūṣiṣu* – vitiate; *bhajet* – adopt practices; *sādhāraṇaṁ* – which are beneficial to all the three *doṣas*; *sarvam* – all; *ūṣmaṇas* – digestive fire; *tejanaṁ* – ignites, intensifies; *ca* – and; *yat* – that

Translation

The weak digestive fire, of those whose bodies have been weakened during the *ādāna kāla*, are further weakened during the rainy season, due to vitiation of the *doṣas*, though it is a part of *visarga kāla*.

The *doṣas* are vitiated due to the low digestive fire caused due to turbid or contaminated water, vapours arising from the earth which produce *amla pāka*, the sudden cold winds containing droplets of water as the dark clouds saturated with water hang over the horizon.

In this atmosphere, as the *doṣas* reciprocally vitiate each other, it is advised to adopt practices that pacify all the three *doṣās* and increase digestive fire.

Commentary

The first factor described here is the nature of the water that arises from the earth during the rainy season. It is unhealthy to drink that water because it has the quality of *amla pāka* (sour postdigestive effect), which can vitiate the *doṣas*. How *amla pāka* vitiates the *doṣa*s is a separate discussion, which will be done later.

What is it that vitiates the water? It is the vitiated earth. What makes the earth *amla pāka*[2]? Hot crust of the earth + water droplets in the atmosphere = *amla pāka.*[3] Imagine what will happen if we sprinkle water over a red hot iron plate. A similar phenomenon occurs when the rain falls on the earth at the end of the summer.

The second factor described here is the status of *agni* in the body during the rainy season. According to the two divisions of the year as per the movement of the sun (or earth around the sun), the rainy season belongs to *visarga kāla*, which is a strengthening period. But practically because it is only the beginning of *visarga kāla*, and we are entering into *visarga* after a long period of weakening (*ādāna*), the digestive fire that is already weak is slowly beginning to kindle and strengthen. At the same time, it is further challenged by the fast and cold winds. The above factors become a working equation:

Weak digestive fire in body + vitiated *amla pāka* water from the earth = vitiation of all *doṣas.*

The vitiated *doṣas* and *dūṣyas* further vitiate each other. This is explained in a linear way for the ease of understanding only. In reality, it forms a complicated network of *doṣas, duṣyas, agni*, and *malas* disturbing each other progressively, which is further fed by the continuous inflow of the vitiating factors.

It was mentioned earlier that *vāta* increases in the summer, but it does not aggravate due to the presence of heat. With the coming of rains, as the atmosphere becomes cold, *vāta* suddenly aggravates. How does it occur? The heated earth combines with the water of the rains to undergo *amla pāka* and produce *amla pitta*. The use of this water, which has undergone *amla pāka* and contamination, also causes the aggravation of *kapha*. This is due to the increase in *jala mahābhūta* (water element). It causes *srotorodha* (obstruction of channels) and aggravates *vāta*. The aggravated *vāta* moves in abnormal directions uncontrollably everywhere in the body, aggravating *pitta* and *kapha* in return.

In this season we can see that all the three *doṣa*s vitiate each other. After that, the vitiated *doṣa*s and weak *agni* vitiate each other. Hence, this is the worst climate as far as health is concerned. This is the reason why many viral fever epidemics (like dengue hemorrhagic fever, chikungunya fever etc.) occur in this season. They are usually *sannipāta* (involving all three doṣas) – Ref. AH Sū 1.12 – in nature, spread very quickly and difficult to control.

If the *agni* is strong and body is kept warm, it will be possible to prevent and correct the *doṣa* imbalances. Hence, one should take special care and adopt all practices – diet and lifestyle – to keep the digestive fire burning in a healthy manner and prevent disturbance of all the three *doṣās*.

What is described here is the picture we should have in our minds as we imagine the body transitioning from the summer to the rainy season. The picture is that of *pitta sañcaya*, *vāta prakopa*, *kapha utkleśa*, low *agni*, low strength and so on.

All the practical adivses that can be given in order to keep the digestive fire burning optimally and prevent the disturbance of any of the doṣās should be enlisted.

AH Sū. 3.45–47a

Recommendations for rainy season

आस्थापनं शुद्धतनुर्जीर्णं धान्यं रसान् कृतान् ॥४५॥

जाङ्गलं पिशितं यूषान् मध्वरिष्टं चिरन्तनम् ॥४५॥

मस्तु सौवर्चलाढ्यं वा पञ्चकोलावचूर्णितम् ॥४६॥

दिव्यं कौपं शृतं चाम्भो भोजनं त्वतिदुर्दिने ॥४६॥

व्यक्ताम्ललवणस्नेहं संशुष्कं क्षौद्रवल्लघु ॥४७॥

āsthāpanaṁ śuddhatanu-jīrṇaṁ dhānyaṁ rasān kṛtān

jāṅgalaṁ piśitaṁ-yūṣān madhvariṣṭaṁ cirantanam //45//

mastu sauvarcalāḍhyaṁ vā pañcakolāvacūrṇitam
divya kaupaṁ śṛtaṁ cāmbho bhojanaṁ tvatidurdine //46//
vyaktāmla-lavaṇa-snehaṁ saṁśukaṁ kṣaudravallaghu

āsthāpanaṁ – decoction enema (*kaṣāya* or *āsthāpana vasti*); *śuddhatanu* – body purified by cleansing (*vamana* and *virecana*) *jīrṇaṁ* – old; *dhānyaṁ* – grains; *rasān* – soups; *kṛtān* – made of; *jāṅgalaṁ* – of arid regions; *piśitaṁ* – meat; *yūṣān* – soups made of green gram; *madhu* – wines; *ariṣṭaṁ* – alcoholic beverages; *cirantanam* – old, ancient; *mastu* – whey; *sauvarcala āḍhyaṁ* – adding a lot of sauvarcala type of salt (*sochal*); *vā pañcakola* – or a mixture of black pepper, long pepper, *cavya*, *citraka* and dry ginger; *avacūrṇitam* – powdered; *divya* – rain water; *kaupaṁ* – from the well; *śṛtaṁ* – boiled; *ca* – and; *ambho* – of the water ; *bhojanaṁ* – food; *tu* – but; *atidurdine* – during these very bad days (when there is absolutely no sunlight due to heavy rains and clouds); *vyakta* – in a way that can be clearly tasted; *amla* – sour; *lavaṇa* – salty; *snehaṁ* – oily, fatty; *saṁśukaṁ* – not too wet, dry; *kṣaudravat* – honey; *laghu* – light (and easy to digest)

Translation

After having cleansed the body (with *vamana* and *virecana*) one should practice decoction enemas (to pacify *vāta*). Old grains, meat soups made from the flesh of animals living in dry lands, green gram soup, wines and alcoholic beverages that have been stored for long are used. Whey should be consumed with more amount of rock salt or *pañcakola* powder. Rainwater and well water should be boiled. However, the food on very bad days (when sun is not visible and there is lot of rain) should be light (easy to digest), dry, and prepared with a strong, sour, and salty taste, combined with ghee and honey.

Commentary

It is especially told here that the water in the rainy season should be drunk only after boiling. Boiling balances the *doṣa*s in the water and makes it easily digestible. Usually rain water is considered pure, but here that is also vitiated.

Days during which the sun is not visible are considered to be unhealthy. *Pañcakola* is a powder mixture that is very popular and strongly enhances digestion. Green gram is the lightest and the most easily digestible among the legumes (called *śimbī dhānya* in *Āyurveda*). Note that *āsthāpana vastis* (decoction enemas[4]) have been recommended after having cleared the *kapha* and *pitta* imbalances. We can see that procedures for pacifying all the three *doṣas* are being adopted. Though *asthāpana vasti* is advised here, we should know that it is always accompanied with *anuvāsana vasti* as well. Whey also has very good *agni*-kindling property. In essence, all the foods should be easy to digest and mixed with *agni*-kindling substances.

Although honey increases *vāta*, it is recommended here in order to remove the *kleda* and toxic wastes in the alimentary canal (*koṣṭha*). It reduces *kapha* and opens the *srotas*. Since it possesses the property of *yogavāhi* and is involved in the

movement of the bowels, honey, used in combination with the food articles, will hardly cause *vāta* aggravation.
This verse indicates that animals living in the same region should not be consumed during the rainy season.

Based on these principles we should be able to design a proper diet that can be followed during the rainy season.

AH Sū. 3.47b–48
More recommendations for rainy season

अपादचारी सुरभिः सततं धूपिताम्बरः ॥४७॥

हर्म्यपृष्ठे वसेद्बाष्पशीतशीकरवर्जिते ॥४८॥

नदीजलोदमन्थाहःस्वप्नायासातपांस्त्यजेत् ॥४८॥

apādacārī surabhiḥ satataṁ dhūpitāmbaraḥ //47//
harmya pṛṣṭhe vased-bāṣpa-śīta-śīkara-varjite
nadījaloda-manthāhaḥ svapnāyāsātapāṁs-tyajet //48//

apādacārī – avoid walking with exposed feet (i.e. wear shoes); *surabhiḥ* – scented, perfumed; *satataṁ* – always; *dhūpita* – fumigated; *ambaraḥ* – clothes; *harmya* – a big mansion; *pṛṣṭhe* – on the upper floor; *vaset* – must live, reside; *bāṣpa* – moisture; *śīta* – cold; *śīkara* – mist; *varjite* – free from; *nadījalod* – of river water; *manthāhaḥ* – powder of popped rice churned with water; *svapna* – sleeping (during the daytime); *āyāsa* – strain, exertion; *ātapāṁs* – sun bathing, exposure to the sun; *tyajet* – must be avoided

Translation

Walking without footwear, river water, *mantha*, sleeping in the day, exertion, and exposure to the sun should be avoided. The body should be always scented with perfumes and clothes fumigated with herbal smoke. One should reside on the upper floor of a mansion free from moisture, cold, and mist. River water, a drink made out of mixing popped rice in water, sleeping during daytime, hard work and exposure to the sun should be avoided.

Commentary

After describing the *āhāra* (diet) during the rainy season, now *Vāgbhaṭa ācārya* describes the *vihāra* (lifestyle). It was recommended to build an underground dwelling for the winter season. We can see that this principle is spontaneously followed by many other living beings in nature to escape the onslaught of the severe winter and summer. There is a possibility of many insects and reptiles that come out of their hibernation deep down in the ground and actively moving about during this season. Hence, the recommendation to protect the feet by wearing shoes. *Apādacārī* also means to avoid going out as far as possible during this time – especially in the night. Note that these recommendations are tailored for people who lived in a natural habitat.

One must fumigate the clothes to prevent bug infestation as the clothes may not be completely dry and thus susceptible to develop fungal infestation, and live on the top floor of the house to be free from moisture, cold, and mist. Moisture, cold and mist are heavy and tend to gravitate towards the ground and the ground floor has a greater tendency to gather moisture. Daytime sleeping aggravates *kapha* and will further dampen the digestive fire. Bodily strength is diminished during this season and hence hard work is avoided to conserve strength. Exposure to the sun should be avoided because it can cause more heat and increase the *amlatva* (sour effect). Thus ends the description of regimen for the rainy season.

शरद् ऋतुचर्या

Śarad ṛtucaryā

Autumn seasonal regimen

Key points to remember

- *Doṣa*: *Pitta prakopa* + *Vāta praśama*
- *Agni*: Moderate
- *Guṇa*: *Madhya uṣṇa* + *Alpa snigdha*
- *Āhāra (food)* – bitter, sweet, astringent, light, ghee with bitter herbs, śāli, green gram, rock sugar, gooseberry, snake gourd, honey and meat of the animals in dry regions, hamsodakam
- *Dwelling* – under silvery white moonlight
- Activities – purgation, blood letting, anoint body in the night with camphor, sandal wood, cuscus, wear pearl necklaces, brilliant clothes,
- Diseases – Pitta Kapha

AH Sū. 3.49

How *pitta* aggravates in autumn

वर्षाशीतोचिताङ्गानां सहसैवार्करश्मिभिः ॥४९॥

तप्तानां सञ्चितं वृष्टौ पित्तं शरदि कुप्यति ॥४९॥

varṣā śīto citāṅgānāṁ sahasaivārka raśmibhiḥ

taptānāṁ sañcitaṁ vṛṣṭau pittaṁ śaradi kupyati //49//

varṣā – in the rainy season; *śīto* – the cold; *cita* – is accumulated; *aṅgānāṁ* – in the body; *sahasā* – abruptly, suddenly; *eva* – certainly; *ārka raśmibhiḥ* – due to the sun rays; *taptānāṁ* – heat of the; *sañcitaṁ* – that which was accumulated; *vṛṣṭau* – in the rainy season; *pittaṁ* – *pitta*; *śaradi* – in the autumn; *kupyati* – aggravates

Translation

In the rainy season, the body has accumulated the cold atmosphere (hence, the accumulated *pitta* does not aggravate). When the sun's rays become hot in the autumn season, the body heats up suddenly, and the *pitta* that had accumulated in the rainy season aggravates.

Commentary

The body which had acclimatized to the cold of the rainy season, is now being confronted by the heat of the sun in the autumn as the climate changes. Now it has to acclimatize to the heat of autumn.

Observe how the accumulated pitta was lying dormant in the body waiting for a favourable season to aggravate. If the accumulated pitta is expelled from the body by suitable *virecana* at the end of the rainy season, the aggravation of pitta in the autumn can be avoided. This is the science of preventive health in *Āyurveda*.

AH Sū. 3.50–51a

Treatment for aggravated *pitta* in autumn

तज्जयाय घृतं तिक्तं विरेको रक्तमोक्षणम् ॥५०॥

तिक्तं स्वादु कषायं च क्षुधितोऽन्नं भजेल्लघु ॥५०॥

शालिमुद्गसिताधात्रीपटोलमधुजाङ्गलम् ॥५१॥

tajjayāya ghṛtaṁ tiktaṁ vireko raktamokṣaṇam
tiktam svādu kaṣāyaṁ ca kṣudhito 'nnaṁ bhajellaghu //50//
śāli-mudga-sitā-dhātrī-paṭola-madhu-jāṅgalam

tad – that *pitta*; *jayāya* – to cure; *ghṛtaṁ* – *ghee*; *tiktaṁ* – bitter; *virekaḥ* – purgation; *rakta mokṣaṇam* – blood letting; *tiktam* – bitter; *svādu* – sweet; *kaṣāyaṁ* – astringent; *ca* – and; *kṣudhitaḥ* – when hungry; *annaṁ* – food; *bhajet* – eat, use; *laghu* – light (easy to digest); *śāli* – a type of rice; *mudga* – green gram; *sitā* – rock sugar; *dhātrī* – (*āmla*) gooseberry; *paṭola* – snake gourd; *madhu* – honey; *jāṅgalam* – (meat) of arid regions

Translation

To conquer that *pitta*, use ghee with bitter herbs, purgation and blood letting. When hungry, eat foods having bitter, sweet and astringent tastes which is light such as śāli, green gram, rock sugar, gooseberry, snake gourd, honey and meat of the animals in dry regions.

Commentary

The choice of food articles to effect *śamana* of *pitta* are advised here.

AH Sū. 3.51b–53a

Haṁsodakam—an elixir that pacifies all *doṣas*

तप्तं तप्तांशुकिरणैः शीतं शीतांशुरश्मिभिः ॥५१॥
समन्तादप्यहोरात्रमगस्त्योदयनिर्विषम् ॥५२॥
शुचि हंसोदकं नाम निर्मलं मलजिज्जलम् ॥५२॥
नाभिष्यन्ति न वा रूक्षं पानादिष्वमृतोपमम् ॥५३॥

taptaṁ taptāṁśu kiranaiḥ śītaṁ śītāṁśu-raśmibhiḥ //51//
samantādapy-ahorātram agastyodaya nirviṣam
śuci haṁsodakaṁ nāma nirmalaṁ malajijjalam //52//
nābhiṣyandi na vārūkṣaṁ pānādiṣv-amṛtopamam

taptaṁ – heated by; *taptāṁśu kiranaiḥ* – the scorching rays of sun; *śītaṁ* – cooled by; *śītāṁśu raśmibhiḥ* – cooling rays of the moon; *samantād* – at all times and sides; *api* – also; *ahorātram* – during the day and night; *agastyodaya* – during the rising of the star named *Agastya*; *nirviṣam* – is detoxified; *śuci* – pure; *haṁsodakaṁ* – a divine elixir by this name (*hamsa* – swan;

udakam – drink); *nāma* – named as; *nirmalaṁ* – pure; *malajit* – pacifying the *doṣas*; *jalam* – water; *na* – not; *abhiṣyandi* – secretory; *na* – not; *vā* – also; *rūkṣaṁ* – dry; *pānādiṣu* – different drinks; *amṛtopamam* (*amṛta* – *upamam*) – like divine elixirs

Translation

Water that is heated by the scorching rays of the sun during the day and cooled by the cooling rays of the moon during the night from all sides, during the rising of the *Agastya (Canopis)* star constellation, is detoxified, clean, pure, pacifies all the three *doṣas*, is neither secretory nor dehydrating, and is said to be a divine nectarine elixir called *hamsodakam*.

Commentary

The swan is known to separate milk out of a mixture of milk and water, drink the milk, and leave the water behind. Hence those who are like swans are capable of taking only the essence. *Hamsodakam* is a nourishing drink. During this season the swans arrive in *Mānsarovar* (lake in the Himalayas) in the Himalayas to drink this water. The swans will not drink water of the autumn, which has *doṣas*.

***Agastya* star:**

Agastya, a bright yellow-colored star, remains visible from September to April every year from almost all places falling south of 37° latitudes. In the western world, this is called as *Canopus*; this is located at S 75°49′ latitude and S 52°41′ declination. *Varāhmihira* says, “A learned astrologer should always calculate its rising well in advance and should foretell its effects for the remaining months of the *samvatsara* (year)." In the classics of Vedic astrology, worshipping the star *Agastya* was a convention after its annual rising. The *Agastya* star sets around April and rises in the south in September. With the rising of *Agastya*, groundwater and the rivers naturally start their purification. During rains, particularly when the sun transits in the houses of *karka* (Cancer) and *simha* (Leo), all rivers become untouchable and the earth is considered to be undergoing her menstrual period. Therefore, drinking river water and swimming or making dips into rivers are only recommended after the rise of *Agastya*. The rising of *Agastya* is known as the concluding sign of the rainy season for the year. After the rise of *Agastya*, in the south immediately following dawn or dusk, the star should be worshipped by offering *arghya* (sacred water).

Note: Here we can see that the human body and the earth are one and the same in terms of their functioning. The human body cleanses itself by menstruation, and the same is the process of the earth, which does it through the turbulent and muddy flow of the rivers in the autumn season. A healthy female body – from menarche to menopause - goes through all the six *ṛtus* from one menstrual cycle to the next. The duration of menstrual bleeding corresponds to *śarad ṛtu* in its qualities and behaviour.

AH Sū. 3.53b–54a

Herbs and lifestyle for autumn nights

चन्दनोशीरकर्पूरमुक्तास्रग्वसनोज्ज्वलः ॥५३॥

सौधेषु सौधधवलां चन्दिकां रजनीमुखे ॥५४॥

candanośīra-karpūra muktā-srag-vasanojjvalaḥ //53//

saudheṣu saudha dhavalāṁ candrikāṁ rajanī-mukhe

candana – sandalwood; *uśīra* – cuscus grass; *karpūra* – camphor; *mukta* – pearl (necklaces); *srag* – wearing; *vasana* – clothes; *ujjvalaḥ* – brilliant; *saudheṣu* – like silver; *saudha* – on the mansion; *dhavalāṁ candrikāṁ* – white moon light; *rajanī* – the night; *mukhe* – during the initial part of, dawn of

Translation

During the initial part of the night, the body should be anointed with pastes of sandalwood, cuscus grass, and camphor. One should wear necklaces of pearls, brilliant clothes and stay in the mansion under the silvery-white moonlight.

Commentary

It is in most parts similar to the lifestyle recommendation for summer. The difference is that in summer it was *vāta-pitta* pacifying but in autumn it is *pitta-kapha* pacifying. All these are meant for reducing the heat.

AH Sū. 3.54b–55a

Some things to avoid in the autumn

तुषारक्षारसौहित्यदधितैलवसाऽऽतपान् ॥५४॥

तीक्ष्णमद्यदिवास्वप्नपुरोवातान् परित्यजेत् ॥५५॥

tuṣāra kṣāra sauhitya dadhi taila vasā "tapān //54//
tīkṣṇa madya divā svapna purovātān parityajet

tuṣāra – (exposure to) fog; *kṣāra* – a type of *Āyurvedic* medicine that is sharp, hot, light, dry, and burning in quality; *sauhitya* – eating to a full stomach; *dadhi* – yogurt; *taila* – sesame oil; *vasā* – animal fat; *ātapān* – sunshine; *tīkṣṇa* – strong; *madya* – alcoholic beverages; *divā svapna* – sleeping in the daytime; *purovātān* – eastern wind; *parityajet* – avoid

Translation

Avoid exposure to fog, *kṣāra*, eating to a full stomach, yogurt, sesame oil, marrow, sun, strong alcoholic beverages, sleeping in the daytime, and the eastern wind.

Commentary

An example of *kṣāra* is vinegar or betel leaf. *Kṣāra* is also prepared using many plants that have the qualities of being sharp, hot, light, and so on. Another example of *kṣāra* is cow urine which is commonly used in *Āyurvedic* treatments. We will learn more about *kṣāra* in the last chapter of the *Sūtra sthāna* of *Aṣṭāṅga Hṛdayam*.

Definition of *kṣāra*: *Kṣāra* is a substance that is cool, burning, ripening, bursting, pungent, penetrating, absorbing, liquefying, purifying, stopping, scarring, antiseptic, detoxifying, fat reducing, emasculating, and destroys *āma* and *kapha*. It can be prepared from plant ingredients (*Suśruta Samhita* Sū. 11.1–3).

It is to be understood that one of the characteristics of the autumn season is winds from the eastern direction.

The *guṇas* of *kṣāra* are similar to the *guṇas* of autumn seasons. Hence, it is advised not to use *kṣāra* during this season. Autumn season is a time of *pitta* predominance. This is because the fire of *pitta* that accumulated in the summer did not aggravate due to the cold during the rains, but with the end of the rainy season, it begins to manifest itself. The *agni* is of moderate strength. The *guṇa* of autumn season is *uṣṇa snigdha* (hot and unctuous).

During the autumn season, one is advised to avoid the following:

- Exposure to fog—increases kapha
- *Kṣāra* (sharp, penetrating)—increases *pitta*
- Eating to a full stomach—since *agni* is moderate
- Yogurt (*uṣṇa guṇa*)—increases *pitta*
- Sesame oil (heating)—increases *pitta*
- *Vasa* (animal fat)—since it is heavy to digest and *agni* is moderate at this time
- Exposure to sun—increases *pitta*
- Alcohol (sharp, hot, penetrating)—increases *pitta*
- Sleeping in daytime—vitiates *kapha* and reduces *agni*
- Eastern wind—vitiates all the three *doṣa*s

Thus end the recommendations of the regimen to be followed in the autumn season.

Vāgbhaṭa has completed the description of the regimen to the followed in each of the six *ṛtus* (seasons).

All the ṛtus are being experienced in the body each day (*Sarvāṅgasundara* Sū. 6.14). *Suśruta* describes that all the *ṛtus* can be seen as well as experienced in the body in each day as well:

During the forenoon the qualities of *vasanta ṛtu* (spring) should be expected in the body. During midday, those of *grīṣma ṛtu* (summer) are seen. During the afternoon, those of *prāvṛṭ* (early rainy season) are seen. During the evenings, the qualities of *varṣa ṛtu* (rainy season) are seen. During midnight we can experience the *śarad ṛtu* (autumn) and during the early mornings we experience *hemanta ṛtu* (winter season).

Thus we can conclude from the descriptions so far that the *ṛtus* can be appreciated on a daily, monthly as well as yearly basis.

If the seasons do not appear normally:

Suśruta Samhita explains what is to be done if the seasons do not appear as expected or their quality is vitiated. This is called *ṛtu vyāpat* (*Sarvāṅgasundara* Sū. 6.11, 19–20). The causes of *ṛtu* vyāpat (vitiation of the time, duration or qualities of the seasons) are as follows:

1. Curses
2. Unrighteous behavior of the people
3. Unfavorable movements of the planets
4. Smell of poisonous plants carried by the air
5. Qualities of house
6. Household equipments (*upakarana*)
7. Vehicles (*vahana*) and others...

Some of the remedial measures advised are as follows:

1. *Sthāna parityāga* (change of place of residence)
2. *Śānti karma* (pacificatory rites and rituals)
3. *Prāyaścitta* (atonement)
4. *Maṇḍala japa*, *homa* (auspicious rituals)
5. *Añjali namaskāra* (praying to deities with folded hands)
6. *Tapa* (performing penances)
7. *Niyama* (observing vows)
8. *Daya* (showing compassion)
9. *Dāna* (giving charity)
10. *Dīkṣa* (accepting initiation)
11. *Deva, brāhmaṇa, guru parair* (staying close to gods, brahmaṇas, and gurus)

In the next few verses, *Vāgbhaṭa* summarizes the dietary recommendations for different seasons given thus far.

AH Sū. 3.55b–56a

Tastes to be used in each of the seasons summarized

शीते वर्षासु चाद्यांस्त्रीन् वसन्तेऽन्त्यान् रसान्भजेत् ॥५५॥

स्वादुं निदाघे, शरदि स्वादुतिक्तकषायकान् ॥५६॥

śīte varṣāsu cādyāṁstrīn vasante 'ntyān rasān-bhajet //55//

svāduṁ nidāghe śaradi svādu tikta kaṣāyakān

śīte – in the winter; *varṣāsu* – in the rainy season; *ca* – and; *ādyāṁs* – the initial ; *trīn* – three; *vasante* – in the spring; *antyān* – the latter three; *rasān* – tastes; *bhajet* – should be used;

svāduṁ – sweet taste; *nidāghe* – in the summer; *śaradi* – in the autumn; *svādu* – sweet; *tikta* – bitter; *kaṣāyakān* – astringent

Translation

In early winter, late winter, and rainy season the first three tastes (sweet, sour, salty) are recommended. In the spring the last three tastes (pungent, bitter, astringent) are recommended. In the summer, sweet taste should be used and in the autumn season, sweet, bitter, and astringent tastes should be used.

Commentary

In the winter and rainy seasons—the first three tastes (sweet, sour, salty)

In spring season—the last three tastes (pungent, bitter, astringent)

In summer season—sweet taste

In autumn season—sweet, bitter, astringent tastes

This is a general principle wherein the first three tastes are good for *ādāna kāla*, as these tastes are more strengthening.

Vākyapradīpika: Though sweet and astringent tastes are *pitta* pacifying, bitter taste is specifically mentioned here, to be used in autumn. That is because of its *pitta-kapha*-reducing property, its natural ability to pacify the *jvara* that appears in *śarad* (autumn), ability to treat *agni* mandya (diminished digestive fire), *aruci* (loss of appetite), and *tṛṣṇa* (craving).

AH Sū. 3.56b–57a

Use of dry and unctuous foods in different seasons

शरद्वसन्तयो रूक्षं शीतं घर्मघनान्तयोः ॥५६॥

अन्नपानं समासेन विपरीतमतोऽन्यदा ॥५७॥

śarad vasantayo rūkṣaṁ śītaṁ gharma ghanāntayoḥ //56//

annapānaṁ samāsena viparītam ato'nyadā

śarad – autumn; *vasantayo* – in the spring; *rūkṣaṁ* – dry, dehydrating; *śītaṁ* – winter; *gharma* – summer; *ghana antayoḥ* – autumn (i.e. end of rainy season); *anna-pānaṁ* – food and drinks; *samāsena* – together; *viparītam* – opposite (opposite quality to dry is unctuous); *ataḥ* – therefore; *anyadā* – the others (the other four seasons – *śiśira, hemanta, grīṣma, varṣa*)

Translation

Food and drinks having drying quality are recommended in autumn and spring. Those that are unctuous can be used in the other four seasons.

Commentary

Season	Recommended	Recommended
Early winter	Sweet, sour, salty	*Snigdha, uṣṇa*
Extreme winter	Same	*Snigdha, uṣṇa*
Rainy season	Same	*Snigdha, uṣṇa*
Spring	Pungent, bitter,	*Rūkṣa, śīta*

Summer	Sweet	*Snigdha, śīta*
Autumn (*śarad*)	Sweet, bitter,	*Rūkṣa, śīta*

Of course this does not mean that only the recommended tastes are to be used in those seasons. Tastes undergo *vṛddhi* (increase) and *kṣaya* (decrease) similar to the *dhātu*s. Hence, one should analyze the strength or weakness of the *dhātu*s and use the tastes appropriately in the respective seasons.

AH Sū. 3.57b

नित्यं सर्वरसाभ्यासः स्वस्वाधिक्यमृतावृतौ ॥५७॥

nityaṁ sarva rasābhyāsaḥ sva svādhikyam-ṛtāvṛtau //57//

nityaṁ – regularly, always; *sarva* – all; *rasa* – tastes; *abhyāsaḥ* – use or practice; *sva-sva* – in each one's own; adhikyam – predominantly; *ṛtāvṛtau* (*ṛtau-ṛtau*) – particular season

Translation

All the tastes should be used regularly at all times. The specific tastes recommended for particular seasons should be used predominantly.

Commentary

This is the methodology of the *Vedic* teachings. There is a *sāmānya* (general rule) that is to be followed at all times, and there is also a *viśeṣa* (special rule), which should be applied in specific circumstances. It can be misunderstood that certain tastes are to be absolutely abandoned in certain seasons. But here it is emphasized and clarified that the tastes that are recommended to be avoided in a particular season, need not be absolutely abandoned in that season. All tastes should be used in all seasons, but the tastes that are not recommended should be used sparingly.

AH Sū. 3.58

Regimen to be followed at the junction of two seasons

ऋत्वोरन्त्यादि सप्ताहावृतुसन्धिरिति स्मृतः

तत्र पूर्वे विधिस्त्याज्यः सेवनीयोऽपरः क्रमात् ॥५८॥

ṛtvor-antyādi saptāhāv-ṛtu sandhir-iti smṛtaḥ

tatra pūrve vidhis-tyājyaḥ sevanīyo 'paraḥ kramāt //58//

ṛtvor – each of the two seasons; *anti* – end of; *ādi* – beginning of; *saptāhāu* – seven days; *ṛtu sandhir* – transition period of the season; *iti* – it is; smṛtaḥ – known as; *tatra* – therefore; *pūrve* – previous; *vidhis* – regimen; *tyājyaḥ* – give up; *sevanīyo* – practice that of; *aparaḥ* – the next; *kramāt* – gradually

Translation

Seven days at the beginning and end of each of the seasons are known as the junctions of the seasons. Therefore the practice of the previous seasonal regimen should be given up and next regimen adopted in a gradual manner.

Commentary

The transition period between two seasons is fourteen days—seven from the previous season and seven from the next. As much as the previous regimen is given up, the regimen of the next season must be adopted, and in fourteen days there should be a complete transition. This is also emphasized in AH Sū 4.25–26.

If we closely observe the timing of the outbreak of any major epidemic in the world, we will find that they invariably occur during the junction of the change from one season to the next. This is called *ṛtu sandhi* in *Āyurveda*.

Does that give a clue as to how we can prevent epidemics and save millions of lives in the future? The diet and lifestyle recommendations to be followed during the *ṛtu sandhis* form a major part of community medicine from the *Āyurvedic* perspective. The way to deal with epidemics is not to find out vaccines or medicines to attack the virus but to tune the body in such a way to discourage the virus from entering.

We cannot attribute these epidemics to any other factor since apart from the change in climate, nothing else really changes as far as regular activities in life are concerned in the mass population.

AH Sū. 3.59½

Do not immediately abandon any practice

असात्म्यजा हि रोगाः स्युः सहसा त्यागशीलनात् ॥५९ १/२॥

asātmyajā hi rogāḥ syuḥ sahasā tyāga-śīlanāt //59½ //

asātmyajā – arising from non-adaptation; *hi* – certainly; *rogāḥ* – diseases; *syuḥ* – will happen; *sahasā* – abruptly; *tyāga* – abandonment; *śīlanāt* – of the practice of

Translation

Abruptly abandoning any regimen or practices (which have been going on) will certainly cause diseases arising from inability (of the body and mind) to adapt to the new regimen.

Commentary

The importance of changing the seasonal regimen was explained in the previous verse. How to do it is explained here. Abruptly changing a life style that the body is accustomed to can be worse than not making any change at all. Accepting or rejecting any practice abruptly should be avoided. It should be a gradual and smooth transition.

At the end of the chapter, you should be able to recognize the characteristic features of the seasons, analyze the seasons and their changes in your region, and construct a seasonal regimen according to the *doṣa* and *guṇa* variations observed with respect to the change of seasons all year round. The *doṣa* variations during each of the seasons and change of seasons can also be understood by observing the flora, fauna and patterns of presentation of diseases in the general population during the course of the year. Look out for the time of the year when *kapha, pitta, or vāta* predominant diseases are more prevalent. This will give a clue. The understanding of *ṛtucaryā* can be utilized in physiological and pathological situations. This is the practical utility of studying this chapter called *ṛtucaryā*. This principle will be explained elaborately in AH. Sū Ch 7.48[7]

इति श्रीवैद्यपतिसिंहगुप्तसूनुश्रीमद्वाग्टविरचितायामष्टाङ्गहृदय संहितायां सूत्रस्थाने ऋतुचर्या नाम तृतीयोऽध्यायः ॥३॥

iti śrī-vaidyapati-simhaguptasūnu-vāgbhaṭa-viracitāyām-aṣṭāṅga-hṛdaya-samhitāyām sūtrasthāne ṛtucaryā nāma tṛtīyodhyāyaḥ

iti - this; śrī vaidyapati simhagupta sūnu - the son of Śrī vaidyapati Simhagupta; śrī Vāgbhaṭa viracitāyām - composed by Śrī Vāgbhaṭa; aṣṭāṅga-hṛdaya saṁhitāyāṁ - of the aṣṭāṅga hṛdaya samhita; sūtra-sthāne - of the sūtra sthāna; ṛtucaryā nāma - named ṛtucaryā; tṛtīyodhyāyaḥ - the third chapter

---

[7] pādenāpathyam abhyastham...

Translation

Thus ends the third chapter of the *Sūtra sthāna* of the *Aṣṭāṅga Hṛdaya samhita*, named *ṛtucaryā* composed by *Śrī Vāgbhaṭa*, the son of *Śrī Vaidyapati Simhagupta.*

---

1. *Rasāla* has several meanings—sugarcane, wheat, mango, grapes, yogurt with black pepper, sugar, and other spices or *śikhariṇi* (*lassi*).
2. It is a *pitta* stage of transformation.
3. Heat and wetness combine to produce this condition.
4. The word *enema* has been used to denote *vasti*, because there is no other suitable word available in English. In reality, *vasti* is much more than an enema, as its intention is to produce a systemic effect on the body rather than a local cleansing effect.

Topics in the Chapter

The division of the year into seasons—1

Uttarāyaṇa (ādānakāla)—2

Description of *ādāna kāla* (sun travels toward the north)—3, 4

Dakṣiṇāyana (visarga kāla) (sun travels to the south)—3.4b to 5a

Strength of moon and sun during *dakṣiṇāyana*—3.5b to 6

Bodily strength in the different seasons—3.7a

Hemanta beginning—3.7b to 8

Early mornings in early winter (*hemanta*)—3.9, 10

Removing the excess oil after oil massage—3.11

Diet for *hemanta* (early winter)—3.12, 13

Sleeping, sunbathing, and wearing footwear in winter—3.14

Utilization of body heat to keep warm—3.15

Tastes to be used in each of the seasons—3.55b to 56a

Use of dry and unctuous foods in different seasons—3.56b to 57a

Regimen to be followed during the transition of one season to the other—3.58

Do not immediately abandon any practice—3.59½

Chapter 4

रोगानुत्पादनीयम्

Rogānutpādanīyam *(roga-anutpādanīyam)*

Prevention of the Origin of Disease

Summary of the chapter

Chapters 2 and 3 describe the different activities required to be performed for the purpose of maintaining health. This chapter describes the items that should be avoided at all times for maintaining health. Though the previous chapters also describe prevention of disease, this chapter is a culmination of that description, and hence, is given this specific title.

There are voluntary and involuntary activities going on in the body. Many of the physiological activities going on within the body can be voluntarily blocked. These activities are essential for the maintenance of good health. Blocking[8] these physiological phenomena will result in manifestation of disease. Hence, the knowledge of these activities that can be blocked

[8] Blocking any process in the body, will result in vata aggravation. This could be the cause of side effects in case of some allopathic medicines which block certain biochemical reactions.

voluntarily is very essential. Conventionally they are fourteen in number and are commonly called the *vegas*.

This chapter describes some urges that should not be suppressed and other urges that should be controlled. Another reason why the chapter is given this name is because practically every disease in *Nidāna sthāna* has *vegodīraṇadhāraṇa* (forceful expression and suppression of the natural urges) as a cause. The items mentioned in this chapter play a key role in the manifestation of every endogenous and exogenous disease. This is the first time in *Aṣṭāṅga Hṛdayam,* that *Ācārya Vāgbhaṭa* begins to speak of diseases and their treatments. One may wonder why the diseases and their treatments (*cikitsa*) have been included in the section that discusses about health. This is because prevention of diseases is also a part of *cikitsa*.

Sections in the chapter

I. ***Nija rogas***
   A. List of *vegas* (Physical Urges)—1
   B. *Adho vāta* (*Apāna Vāta*)—2 to 7
   C. Hunger, thirst, and sleep—10 to 13, 21
   D. *Ūrdhva vāta*—13 to 20
   E. Mental urges—24
   F. Prophylactic cleansing—25 to 30

II. ***Āgantu rogas***—31

III. **Conclusion**—32 to 35

Key *Sanskṛt* words in this chapter

vega, vāta, viṭ, mūtra, kṣavathu, tṛṭ, kṣut, nidra, kāsa, śvāsa, jṛmbha, aśru, chardi, retas, piṇḍika udveṣṭanam, pratiśyāya, parikartika, aśmarī, meḍhra, vaṅgṣaṇa, avapīḍaka, udgāra, ādhmāna, hidhma, kampa, vibandha, śoṣa, bādhirya, aṅgamarda, gulma, hṛdroga, pīnasa, visarpa, kuṣṭha, pāṇḍu, jvara, śvayathu, rasāyana, vṛṣya, laṅghana, pācana, prajñāparādha, samīkṣyakārī

Title verse

अथातो रोगानुत्पादनीयाध्यायं व्याख्यास्यामः ।
इति ह स्माहुरात्रेयादयो महर्षयः ॥

athāto rogānutpādanīyādhyāyaṁ vyākhyāsyāmaḥ
iti ha smāhur ātreyādayo maharṣayaḥ

athāta – therefore; *rogānutpādanīyam* – prevention of the origin of diseases; *adhyāyaṁ* – chapter; *vyākhyāsyāmaḥ* – will describe; *iti* – this; *ha sma-āhur* – as spoken by; *ātreyādayo* – *Ātreya ṛṣi* and others; *maharṣayaḥ* – the sages

Translation

Therefore as spoken by the great hermit *Ātreya* and the group of sages, thus is described the chapter on the prevention of the origin of diseases.

Commentary

Āyurvedarasāyana: In the last chapter, the regimen to be followed when the seasons manifest in an orderly manner (*niyata kāla*) were described. Now the regimen to be observed at all times irrespective of day or season (*aniyata kāla*) will be described. Five items will be described in this chapter:

1. *Vegodīraṇam* (forceful expression of natural urges) and *Vegadhāraṇam* (suppression of natural urges)
2. *Mānasika vega nigrahaṇam* (suppression of mental urges)
3. *Śodhanam* at the appropriate times (cleansing)
4. *Bṛṁhaṇam* (nourishing), *rasāyanam* (increasing vitality), *vājīkaraṇam* (increasing virility)
5. *Bhūtādyasparśanam* (due to other living entities or spooked by spirits)

The first two are meant for prevention of diseases and the remaining three are for treatment.

Till the end of chapter 3, the regimens described were *niyata kala* (time specific) or those that come at a fixed time. In chapter 4 the author describes the *vegas*, which are *aniyata kala* (not specific to time), and these urges can manifest at any given time without any previous warning.

Two things are described in this chapter. One is *roga hetu* (cause of disease) and other is *ārogya hetu* (cause of health).

In order to prevent disease, one should understand both. The practices to prevent disease will include regular cleansing, which will be described later. The practices to promote or preserve health include the right way of addressing all the *vegas* (urges) in the body.

There are two ways in which disease can occur: *prāk abhāva* and *pradhvamsa abhāva*. The first one is a case where the disease is in the seed form. In this case, the person has never been affected by the disease, and the chances of contracting the disease are to be thwarted. The second one is the chance of getting the disease after it has been cured (a relapse). In this case the person has been affected by the disease once and cured. So he or she needs to be given practices suitable to prevent any kind of relapse. Both are included within the title *rogānutpādanīya* or "prevention of diseases."

One may ask the question, "There are people who follow a strict diet and lifestyle but still become diseased, but there are others who do not follow any of the rules and regulations but still remain healthy. Then what is the use of describing all these rules if sickness is not dependent on following or not following them?" The answer is that above all the things that we do to avoid disease, there is something higher called *daiva* (destiny), which plays a crucial role. We can see at times that one may have access to the best treatment and yet not survive, but another person has no access to any treatment and still survives. Someone may contract a severe illness and still get cured. On the contrary another person may develop a minor illness and eventually die from it. *Daiva* (destiny) is the reason these unexpected or unexplainable phenomena occur.

Note that a simple reflex like yawning has been associated with blindness, deafness and even a stroke. How important are these *vegas* which we do not take so seriously!

AH Sū. 4.1

Thirteen urges not to be suppressed

वेगान्न धारयेद्वातविण्मूत्रक्षवतृट्क्षुधाम् ॥१॥

निद्राकासश्रमश्वासजृम्भाश्रुच्छर्दिरेतसाम् ॥१॥

vegānna dhārayed vāta viṇ mūtra kṣava tṛṭ kṣudhām

nidrā kāsa śrama śvāsa jṛmbhā 'śru cchardi retasām //1//

vegan – the urges; *na* – not; *dhārayed* – to be suppressed; *vāta* – flatus and belching; *viṇ* - stool; *mūtra* - urine; *kṣava* - sneeze; *tṛṭ* - thirst; *kṣudhām* - hunger; *nidrā* - sleep; *kāsa* - cough; *śrama śvāsa* - breathing on exertion; *jṛmbha* - yawn; *aśru* - tears; *chardi* - vomiting; *retasām* - of semen

Translation

The urges which should not be suppressed/ blocked are flatus, belching, fecal urge, urine, sneezing, thirst, hunger, sleep, cough, heavy breathing after exertion, yawning, tears, vomiting, and seminal discharge.

Commentary

The natural urges or *vegas* are the means by which the body lets out the unwanted accumulated *doṣas* or *malas* present in the body. In one sense it is a *śodhana* (natural cleansing). Suppressing or restraining them will lead to accumulation inside the body and complications.

It is explained by the experts that the physical urges can be classified into:

- *Langhana* (depleting) – *śrama śvāsa, retasa* (making the *dhātus* to work more to burn)
- *Brmhana* (nourishing) - *kṣud, tṛṭ, nidra, jṛmbha*
- *Śodhana* (cleansing) - *vāta, viḍ, mūtra, kṣavathu, chardi, kāsa, aśru*

The *vegas* can also be classified according to the five types of *vāta* involved:

1. Flatus – *apāna*
2. Burping – *udāna*
3. Stool – *apāna*
4. Urine – *apāna*
5. Sneezing – *udāna*
6. Thirst – *samāna*
7. Hunger – *samāna*
8. Sleep – *prāṇa*
9. Cough – *prāṇa*

10. Exertional dyspnea – *prāṇa*
11. Yawning – *prāṇa*
12. Tears – *prāṇa*
13. Vomiting - *udāna*
14. Ejaculation - *apāna*

There are many urges like the urge to speak, fight, and so on, which are not included here because restraining them will not cause an increase in *vāta*, and it is recommended to control them. They are all mental urges that are expressed through the body. The ones mentioned here are the physical bodily urges, which if restrained will affect the mind adversely and also aggravate *vāta*. One should especially note that the vegas mentioned here are not *rogas*. *Vegas* are only natural urges. They are protective reflexes. Some of these *vegas* can also be found as symptoms of *rogas* and that is at times conceptually different from what is described here.

Āyurvedarasāyana: The word *vāta* includes *adhovāta* (flatus) and *ūrdhva vāta (belching)*. *Ūrdhva vāta* includes belching and hiccups. In a broader sense, *ūrdva vāta* includes all the activities of *vāta* in the upper part of the body. The word *aśru* includes happy tears, sad tears, and tearing of eyes.

AH Sū. 4.2

Disorders due to suppression of flatus

अधोवातस्य रोधेन गुल्मोदावर्तरुक्क्लमाः ॥२॥

वातमूत्रशकृत्सङ्गदृष्ट्यग्निवधहृद्गदाः ॥२॥

adhovātasya rodhena gulmodāvarta-ruk klamāḥ
vāta-mūtra-śakṛt-saṅga-dṛṣṭy-agnivadha-hṛd-gadāḥ //2//

adhovātasya - of the flatus; *rodhena* - by suppression; *gulma* – a space occupying lesion that feels or presents like a swelling in the abdomen; *udāvarta* – reverse movement of *vāta* (e.g., reverse peristalsis); *ruk* - pain; *klamāḥ* - fatigue in spite of rest; *vāta mūtra śakṛt-saṅga* - obstruction to passage of flatus, urine and feces; *dṛṣṭi-vadha* - destruction of vision; *agni-vadha* - destruction of digestive power; *hṛd-gadāḥ* - heart diseases

Translation

The suppression of the *vāta* that flows in the downward direction causes *gulma*, *udāvarta*, pain, fatigue, urinary obstruction, constipation, obstructed flatus, loss of vision, destruction of digestive fire, severe indigestion, and heart disorders.

Commentary

Notice that in this verse, *adho vāta* is mentioned separately from *vāta*. Why? The second vāta is mentioned to denote that the downward propulsion of flatus is no more present due to repeated obstruction of the reflex. It is called *ruddha vāta*.

***Sarvāṅgasundara*:** When the *ūrdhva-vāta* is vitiated by obstructing *udgāra*, the symptoms like loss of appetite that are caused can be easily cured. *Udāvarta* (pathological movement of *vāta* in the upward direction) is also related to the cause of *arśas* (haemorrhoids) and is described in *Nidāna sthāna*.

Āyurvedarasāyana: *Ruk* in this context refers to pain in the *koṣṭha* (gastrointestinal tract especially the lower part). The physiological movement of vāta is lost. *Dṛṣṭivadha* refers to *timira*. What is *timira*? A type of eye disease predominantly due to *vāta* aggravation, affecting the cornea in its initial stage, where it appears like a curtain over the eyes causing darkness and the object is blurred. The pathology gradually spreads inward and symptoms become more intensified.

In this verse, the distortion that happens to *agni* is described as "*agni vadha*". We have earlier studied three types of *doṣa* vitiations of *agni* in AH Sū 1.8 namely, *vaiṣamya* (distortion), *taikṣṇya* (intensification) and *māndya* (diminution). But this is an extreme vitiation. Before it reaches this condition, the *agni* can go through one or more of the other three stages as well. The word '*vadha'* means 'to completely destroy'. So here a total annihilation of *agni* is what is indicated. This is a serious and almost fatal condition.

Among all the five sense organs, the eyes are specifically connected to *agni*. The eyes are described as āgneya (fiery). So in this description, we can also understand that the agni of the eyes is destroyed. There can be other pathologies related to the eyes due to excess water or kapha. But here it is the fire element of the eye that is destroyed.

A client might come to you with a condition that apparently appears to be independent of any causative factor but when you look at it from the "*vegarodha*" point of view, you should be able to see the cause. A *cikitsa* (treatment) of any condition becomes complete only when the *nidāna* is identified and stopped. This approach helps you to find the *nidāna* in many situations.

You should also note that the sequence of symptoms described here are progressively moving upwards. This is a condition called *udāvarta* (upward spiralling). Beginning from the lower part of the body and moving upwards towards the head which can even result in *unmāda* (affliction of the mind).
Agnivadha indicates death of the body. So one can imagine the extreme consequences of blocking *adho vāta*.

Remember that the consequences of blocking the *vegas* (physiological movements of vāta) described here are not usually manifested due to a single incident of the same, rather they are caused due to a long term habitual suppression, though the possibility cannot be denied.

Note: *Gulma* is a pathology that can occur in any part of the body due to the obstruction of *vāta* though it is more often associated with the abdomen. It thus causes a space-occupying lesion at the site and a feeling of blockage.

AH Sū. 4.3–4a

Disorders due to the suppression of fecal urge

शकृतः पिण्डिकोद्वेष्टप्रतिश्यायशिरोरुजः ॥ ३ ॥

ऊर्ध्ववायुः परीकर्तो हृदयस्योपरोधनम् ॥ ३ ॥

मुखेन विट्प्रवृत्तिश्च पूर्वोक्ताश्चामयाः स्मृताः ॥४॥

śakṛtaḥ piṇḍikodveṣṭa pratiśyāya śiro rujaḥ
ūrdhva vāyuḥ parīkarto hṛdayasyoparodhanam //3//
mukhena viṭ-pravṛttiśca pūrvoktāścāmayāḥ smṛtāḥ

śakṛtaḥ – (suppression of) defecation; *piṇḍikaḥ udveṣṭa* – cramping of calf muscles; *pratiśyāya* - running nose; *śiro rujaḥ* - headaches; *ūrdhva vāyuḥ* - belching; *parīkarto* - fissure in ano, colicky pain; *hṛdayasya uparodhanam*[9] – spasmodic pain at the esophago -gastric junction, cardiac pain; *mukhena viṭpravṛttiḥ* - feces coming out of the mouth; *ca* - and; *pūrva-uktāḥ* – as mentioned before (in the previous verse); *ca* - and; *āmayāḥ* - disorders; *smṛtāḥ* - is known as

Translation

Suppression of the defecation urge causes cramping pain in the calf muscles, running nose, headache, belching, fissure in ano (severe pain while passing stools), feeling like an obstruction at the heart, expulsion of feces through the mouth, and the disorders mentioned in the previous verse (due to suppression of flatus).

Commentary

The calf muscles become stiff and painful especially in the evening. The obstruction to downward *vāta* also causes *ānāha*

[9] Uparodhanam – obstruction. It means that there is a feeling of some obstruction in the region of the heart causing pain.

(distention of abdomen). Cramping and constricting pain in the calf muscles can be a precursor to a disease like colon cancer or other pathologies of the colon causing incomplete obstruction of the bowels.

The obstruction of the downward *vāta* makes it *viguṇa* (lose its natural quality) in terms of the direction of flow. So the downward *vāta* changes the direction and moves upward (*ūrdhva gati)*. On the way it disturbs the digestive fire, heart, nose, and goes right up to the head. Fecal vomiting is commonly seen in palliative cancer patients with complete intestinal obstruction. This is a very advanced end stage of the disease and is *asādhya* (incurable). So we should understand that the symptoms due to obstruction of defecation (*śakṛd rodha*) can be due to voluntarily suppressing the reflex or due to obstruction caused by certain pathological conditions.

We can infer from this verse that in the case of some people with an intractable cold and running nose, the actual cause may be constipation. No matter how effectively we treat the cold on a local level, it will continue to relapse unless the constipation is addressed.

Since the fecal, urinary, flatus urges or reflexes are all due to the vitiation of the same *apāna vāta*, the symptoms produced as a result can overlap between them.

Note that obstruction of the fecal reflex can cause blockage of the heart (*hṛdayasya uparodhanam)* resulting in chest pain which can mimic a heart attack.

Āyurvedarasāyana: The description of fecal, urinary and flatus reflex is described prior to ūrdhva vāta rodha because the symptoms of the former three closely resemble those of adho vāta rodha.

AH Sū. 4.4b–5a

Disorders due to the suppression of urinary urge

अङ्गभङ्गाश्मरीवस्तिमेढ्रवंक्षणवेदनाः ॥४॥

मूत्रस्य रोधात्पूर्वे च प्रायो रोगास्तदौषधम् ॥५॥

aṅga-bhaṅgāśmarī-vasti-meḍhra-vaṁkṣaṇa vedanāḥ //4//

mūtrasya rodhāt-pūrve ca prāyo rogāḥ ....

aṅga-bhaṅga – cutting type of body pain; *aśmarī* - calculi; *vasti* – urinary bladder; *meḍhra* - penis; *vaṁkṣaṇa* - inguinal or pelvic region; *vedanāḥ* - pain; *mūtrasya rodhanāt* - due to obstruction of urinary reflex; *pūrve* - in the previous verses; *ca* - also; *prāyo* – almost all; *rogāḥ* - diseases;

Translation

Cutting type of pain in the body; calculi; pain along the urinary bladder, penis, and pelvic region; and almost all the disorders enumerated in the previous verses are caused due to suppression of the urinary urge.

Commentary

Initially *abhyaṅga* (oil massage) may be done all over the body and especially the perineal regions and area below the navel with warm oil. If there is insufficient relief, then *vasti* (therapeutic administration of medications through anus) will be necessary.

All the *vegas* have their own *udāvartas* as the *vata* when blocked will turn around producing a whirl and move along the path of least resistance producing associated symptoms along its path.

The word *'prāyo'* is significant. This means that there will be some symptoms which will be common in the case of the obstruction of fecal and flatus urges and there will be some symptoms which are exclusively specific to urinary obstruction. All the symptoms will not appear since the movement of *vata* in the case of obstruction of urinary reflex compared to the blockage of the other reflexes of fecal and flatus will be slightly different. So all the symptoms will not manifest but some of them will.

The *apāna vāta* disturbance extends into *vyāna vāta* causing a generalized bodyache. The function of *vyāna* – AH Sū 12.6 – is said to be *dehacārī* (moving all over the body) and thus its affliction causes generalized body ache. The other symptoms mentioned here are due to the affliction of the local actions of *apāna vāta*.

AH Sū. 4.5–6a

Treatment of diseases due to suppressing the urge of flatus, feces, and urine

....तदौषधम्

वर्त्यभ्यङ्गावगाहाश्च स्वेदनं वस्तिकर्म च ॥५॥

अन्नपानं च विड्भेदि विड्रोधोत्थेषु यक्ष्मसु ॥६॥

.. ...tad-auṣadham

varty-abhyaṅgāvagāhāśca svedanaṁ vasti-karma ca //5//

annapānaṁ ca viḍ-bhedi vid-rodhotthesu yakṣmasu

tad-auṣadham - the treatments, *varti* - herbal suppository; *abhyaṅga* - oil application over the body; *avagāhā* - immersion of the whole body in oil or medicated water; *ca* - and; *svedanaṁ* - sudation; *vasti karma* - medicated enema;[1] *ca* - and; *annapānaṁ* - food and drinks; *ca* - and; *viḍ-bhedi* - laxative (by disintegrating the feces) *viḍ rodhotthesụ* - caused due to stopping the defecation reflex (*utthesụ* – caused due to); *yakṣmasu* – diseases due to

Translation

The treatments recommended for these disorders are herbal suppository, oil application over the body, immersion in herbal water or oil bath, sudation, and medication through enema. Foods and drinks that help disintegrate the hardened feces should be used in diseases caused due to the suppression of fecal urge.

Commentary

First the general treatment principle for all the three types of obstructions is mentioned. Then the specific recommendations for each are given. Beginning with food and drinks, the specific protocol for constipation is given. Specifically the word *viḍ bhedi* is used. There are four types of laxatives used in *Āyurvedic* treatment—*bhedana* (breaking into pieces), *sramsana* (gentle laxative effect), *anulomana* (inducing normal physiological movement), and *virecana* (strong purgation). Here specifically the *bhedi* type of laxatives are recommended to break the hardened feces formed due to long-standing constipation. An example of a *bhedi* laxative is *Aloe vera*. Drinking coconut water is a good way to activate and cleanse the urinary bladder.

Sarvāṅgasundara: *Varti* (herbal suppository), which represents the *phala varti* that is made of the fruit of *madana phala* (*Randia dumetorum*), is introduced into the rectum.

Almost all the urges mentioned in the chapter are meant for the release of *vāta*. So when an urge is suppressed, the *vāta* that was supposed to be expelled out gets stuck in that position.

The principle of treating the symptoms caused by the suppression of the urges is to once again evoke the urge and release it. Once the blockage of *vāta* caused by the suppression has been removed, one can treat the complications caused due to the suppression. Since the suppression of the urge has blocked the movement of *vāta*, first it has to be released and then allowed to flow freely again. The *avagāha* (immersion in a tub) recommended here has to be done with *vāta* pacifying herbs to apply the medicines directly in the rectal area.

Sarvāṅgasundara/Āyurvedarasāyana: Some of the foodstuffs, which are *bhedi* (having the property of breaking) are *yāvaka* (barley), *mastu* (whey), and *vāstuka* (*Chenopodium alba*) (AH Sū. 6.72), which is a type of weed that grows all over the world and was consumed regularly as a vegetable in Europe and West Asia. It is commonly used in India and called *bathua* in Hindi. According to *Ṛg Veda, Atharva Veda, Caraka*, and *Suśruta* it is a laxative, cures piles, worms, and many other diseases and enhances digestive power, appetite, and memory. The word *ca* indicates all the general measures in previous verses like *varti*, *abhyaṅga*, and so on.

This system of analysis is followed all throughout the *Aṣṭāṅga Hṛdayam.* First the general principles are mentioned and then the specific variations. It is called *sāmānya* (general) and *viśeṣa* (specific). That is the methodology of *Vedic* teaching. The example given by *Hemādri* is that yoghurt is usually given in general to all *brāhmaṇas* but in specific cases (eg. *Kauṇdinya brāhmaṇas*) were given *takra* (buttermilk)

***Aruṇodaya** by Govindan vaidya*: Suppression of stool, urine, and flatus cause the *vaigunya* (distortion of the qualities) of *apāna vāta* resulting in the distortion of their activities. The treatments recommended to each of them are actions that bring about *anuloma* (restoration of the physiological movement) of *apana vāta*. Foods that are *vātānulomana* must be used in the obstruction of downward *vāta*. Especially in the case of urinary obstruction, the foods must be *mūtra virecanīya* (diuretic) as well. *Varti* (suppository) is especially recommended for constipation and *uttara vasti* is recommended for urinary obstruction.

Yakṣma represents a syndrome of symptoms. *Rājayakṣma* is the king of diseases because even the symptoms are different diseases of their own and it affects all the *dhātus* from top to bottom.

AH Sū. 4.6b–7

Treatment for the suppression of urination

मूत्रजेषु तु पाने च प्राग्भक्तं शस्यते घृतम् ॥६॥

जीर्णान्तिकं चोत्तमया मात्रया योजनाद्वयम् ॥७॥

अवपीडकमेतच्च संज्ञितं धारणात्पुनः ॥७॥

mūtrajeṣu tu pāne ca prāgbhaktaṁ śasyate ghṛtam //6//

jīrṇāntikaṁ cottamayā mātrayā yojanādvayam

avapīḍakam-etacca saṁñjitam dhāraṇāt-punaḥ //7//

mūtrajeṣu - due to micturition reflex; *tu* - but; *pāne* - having drunk; *ca* - and; *prāgbhaktaṁ* - taken before a meal; *śasyate* – approved procedure; *ghṛtam* - ghee; *jīrṇāntikaṁ* - after the digestion of; *ca* - and; *uttamayā* - the perfect; *mātrayā* - amount (*uttama mātra* is the amount that can be digested by the person in twenty-four hours); *yojanādvayam* - in two divided doses; *avapīdakam-etacca* - it is called *avapīḍaka*; *saṁñjitam* – known by the meaning of the word; *dhāraṇāt* - ingested; *punaḥ* – again

Translation

A process of intake of ghee called *avapīḍaka* is employed in the treatment of diseases due to suppression of the urinary urge (micturition reflex). In this process, *ghee* is ingested in *uttama mātra* (a quantity that takes twenty-four hours to be digested in the person) in two divided doses, before and after food.

Commentary

This is a special procedure called *avapīḍaka snehapāna*. In this process, the amount of ghee that can be digested by the person in twenty-four hours is estimated by trial. This amount is divided into two equal parts. One part is given before food and then moderate amount of food is consumed. The second part of the ghee is taken after the first part of the ghee and the food have been completely digested. This is the correct procedure.

Sesame oil, plain or medicated, can be used to pacify *vāta* in certain cases of *asātmya* or reduced urine output instead of ghee (AH Sū. 5.55).

Tailam has been explained earlier in *Aṣṭāṅga Hṛdayam* to be better than *ghṛta* for pacifying *vāta* (*pavana*). Then why is *taila* not used for *avapīḍaka snehapāna* to pacify *adhovāta*? This is because *tailam* causes constipation and reduced urinary output.

Hence it is not suitable. In chapter 5 the *sāmānya guṇa* of *tailam* is explained as *baddha viṭ* and in chapter 6 the *viśeṣa guṇa* of tila (sesame) is explained to be *alpa mūtrata*. Hence it is not advisable to use *tila tailam* for *avapīdaka snehapāna* though it pacifies *vāta*.

Sarvāṅgasundara: Since the food is caused to undergo *avapīḍana* (compression) from above and below, the procedure is called *avapīḍaka*. Due to the suppression of the urge, *vāta* aggravates. For such a *vāta* aggravation, sesame oil is best. But in this particular case, to show that ghee is best, the word *tu* has been used in the verse. Although *taila* (oil) is *vāta* pacifying, since it causes constipation and also concentrates the urine, in this circumstance it is not preferred according to *Aruṇadutta*.

Why are these treatments mentioned here in *hetu skanda* (section discussing cause of disease) rather in the *auṣadha skanda* (section discussing treatment of disease)? This is because when the disease is in an unmanifest potential stage avoiding the cause is also a treatment. When the disease is in a manifest stage, it is described in *auṣadha skanda*.

After describing the suppression of downward *vāta*, the *ācārya* describes symptoms due to the suppression of upward *vāta*.

AH Sū. 4.8

Suppression of belching and Treatment

उद्गारस्यारुचिः कम्पो विबन्धो हृदयोरसोः ॥८॥

आध्मानकासहिध्माश्च हिध्मावत्तत्र भेषजम् ॥८॥

udgārasyāruciḥ kampo vibandho hṛdayorasoḥ

ādhmāna-kāsa-hidhmāśca hidhmāvat-tatra bheṣajam //8//

udgārasya – due to (suppression of) belching; *aruciḥ* - loss of appetite, anorexia; *kampa* - tremors; *vibandho hṛdayo* - obstruction in the epigastric or cardiac region; *uras* - chest; *ādhmāna* - distension of abdomen; *kāsa* - cough; *hidhmāśca* - and hiccup; *hidhmāvat* - similar to belching; *tatra* - that of; *bheṣajam* - treatment is

Translation

Suppression of belching causes anorexia, tremors, a feeling of obstruction over the chest and cardiac region, distention of abdomen, and cough like pathology. The treatment for these conditions are the same as that for hiccup (AH Ci. Chapter. 4).

Commentary

The treatment is said to be similar to that of hiccup. When you refer the treatment of hiccup in *Aṣṭāṅga Hṛdayam Cikitsa sthāna*, you will find that it is the same as that of *kāsa* which is in chapter 3. This is how the text is arranged with cross connections between the various diagnoses and treatments. *Vibandha hrdayo* means a feeling like the heart is bound with a rope. Please note that many of the lakṣaṇas in the *Āyurvedic* texts are explained in the same words that a patient would express.

AH Sū. 4.9–10a

Suppression of sneezing and treatment

शिरोऽर्तीन्द्रियदौर्बल्यमन्यास्तम्भार्दितं क्षुतेः ॥९॥

तीक्ष्णधूमाञ्जनाघ्राणनावनार्कविलोकनैः ॥९॥
प्रवर्तयत्क्षुतिं सक्तां स्नेहस्वेदौ च शीलयेत् ॥१०॥

śiro'rtīndriya-daurbalya-manyāstambhārditaṁ kṣuteḥ
tīkṣṇa-dhūmāñjanā-ghrāṇa-nāvanārka-vilokanaiḥ //9//
pravartayat-kṣutiṁ saktāṁ sneha-svedau ca śīlayet

śiro 'rti - headache; *indriya-daurbalya* - weakness of the senses; *manyā-stambha* - neck rigidity; *arditaṁ* - facial palsy; *kṣuteḥ* – (due to suppression of) sneezing; *tīkṣṇa* - sharp; *dhūma* - therapeutic smoking; *añjnā* - collyrium application; *ghrāṇa* – inhalation of; *nāvana* (*nasya*) - errhines (nose drops); *arka-vilokanaiḥ* - looking at the sun; *pravartayat* – is provoked; *kṣutiṁ* - sneezing; *saktāṁ* – which has been obstructed or stuck; *snehasvedau* - oiling and sudation; *ca* - and; *śīlayet* - practiced

Translation

Suppression of the urge to sneeze causes headache, weakness of the senses, rigidity of the neck, and facial palsy. The sneezing reflex, which is stuck, is provoked by inhalation of herbal smoke, collyria (eye applications) and nose drops having sharp quality or by gazing at the sun. Oiling and sudation are also practiced.

Commentary

Weakness of the senses (*indriya-daurbalya*) means lack of strength to perceive the sense objects. Because *vāta kopa* (aggravation) is the principal result of every *vega rodha* (obstruction), oiling and sudation are mentioned as the principal treatments. Whenever a client presents with the above mentioned diseases or symptoms, we should remember to ask about the history of obstruction of sneezing reflex without fail. They may present to you with cervical issues (*manyāstambha*). Looking at the sun is advised in order to induce sneezing.

Suppression of the sneezing reflex results in vitiation of the *prāṇa vāta*. The route and functions of *prāṇa vāta* are explained in AH. Sū 12. 4. We can see that all the symptoms enumerated in the present verse are manifesting in structures along the route of *prāṇa vāta*. *Prāṇa vāta* moves towards the top of the head, hence headache, it moves along the neck (throat) and hence *manyāstambha*; the working of the senses is regulated by *prāṇa vāta* and hence they are also disturbed and so on.

Sarvāṅgasundara: Sneezing is caused due to an imbalance between the *prāṇa* and *udāna vāyus* in the head region. Examples of herbs that are used for *tīkṣṇa dhūmapāna* are *jyotiṣmati*, *niśā* (turmeric), *daśamūla*, *triphala*, *lākṣā* and so on. (Refer AH Sū 21.17)

Āyurvedarasāyana: For diseases caused due to the obstruction of *kṣavathu* (sneezing), it is advised to use *tīkṣṇa dhūma* (herbal smoke inhalation with substances having sharp penetrating quality, e.g., garlic) which will irritate the mucosa and *marma* in that region, inducing sneezing. It is also possible to induce sneezing by gazing directly at the sun. It should be followed by *sneha* and *sveda*. And then suitable foods that are *vāta* pacifying along with *ghee* are to be consumed.

AH Sū. 4.10b–11a
Suppression of thirst

शोषाङ्गसादबाधिर्यसम्मोहभ्रमहृद्गदाः ॥१०॥

तृष्णाया निग्रहात्तत्र शीतः सर्वो विधिर्हितः ॥११॥

śoṣāṅgasāda-bādhirya-sammoha-bhrama-hṛd-gadāḥ //10//

tṛṣṇāyā nigrahāt-tatra śītaḥ sarvo vidhir-hitaḥ

śoṣa - dehydration, drying up; *aṅga-sāda* - bodily fatigue; *bādhirya* - deafness; *sammoha* - unconsciousness; *bhrama* - giddiness; *hṛd gadāḥ* - epigastric distress; *tṛṣṇāyā* – of thirst; *nigrahāt* - by suppression; *tatra* – in that case; *śītaḥ* - cooling; *sarvo* - of all; *vidhir* - regulations (of food and regimen); *hitaḥ* – beneficial

Translation

Suppression of thirst causes drying up of the body, fatigue, deafness, loss of consciousness, giddiness, and epigastric distress. It is beneficial in these cases to use applications that are cooling.

Commentary

Here it is evident that these pathologies are due to excessive heat in the body. Thirst is produced when there is excess heat in the body, and the body wants to cool down. If this is not acknowledged and pacified, the heat goes on increasing and results in the listed complications.

Sometimes when we ask clients about the amount of water they drink, they often say that we drink teas or juices. It is to be understood that teas and juices have a different *guṇa* and will not fulfill the body's need for water. Similarly, the intake of ice-cold water is also not cooling. The ice water has to be brought to normal temperature for the body to digest it. The body has to first create heat in order to warm the water. This causes a resultant increase in body heat. Sodas cause the release of gas inside the stomach and irritate the gastric mucosa. This causes a type of agitation that results in *vāta-pitta* aggravation in most cases.

Drinking excessive amounts of water in spite of not feeling thirsty can be considered as an unnatural forceful expression of thirst.

Sarvāṅgasundara: All the *śīta* activities like *śīta snāna* (cool water bath), *śīta anna* (cooling foods) and *śīta pāna* (cooling drinks) are advised.

Āyurvedarasāyana: *Bhrama* is dizziness that is the feeling similar to riding on the giant wheel in an amusement park.

AH Sū. 4.11b–12a

Suppression of hunger and treatment

अङ्गभङ्गारुचिग्लानिकार्श्यशूलभ्रमाः क्षुधः ॥११॥

तत्र योज्यं लघु स्निग्धमुष्णमल्पं च भोजनम् ॥१२॥

aṅga-bhaṅgāruci-glāni-kārśya-śūla-bhramāḥ kṣudhaḥ //11//
tatra yojyaṁ laghu snigdham-uṣṇām-alpaṁ ca bhojanam

aṅga bhaṅga - bodyache; *aruci* - loss of appetite; *glāni* - weakness; *kārśya* - emaciation, weight loss; *śūla* - abdominal colic; *bhramāḥ* - giddiness; *kṣudhaḥ* - supression of hunger; *tatra* - here; *yojyaṁ* - connected to; *laghu* - light (to digest); *snigdham* - unctuous; *uṣṇām* - hot; *alpaṁ* - limited quantity; *ca* - and; *bhojanam* – food

Translation

Suppression of hunger causes body aches, anorexia, weakness, emaciation, abdominal colic, and giddiness. In this case, food that is light (easy to digest), unctuous, and hot should be given in limited quantity.

Commentary

Excessive fasting will result in starvation and depletion of the *dhātus*. But a moderate amount of fasting will help to stabilize the *agni* and digest *āma*. This has to be done judiciously. It is described here about how to identify when the fasting is becoming pathological. The basic principle is that one should not feel excessive weakness while fasting.

The suppression of this *vega* is seen in the background of many cases of hyperacidity in the modern world where people are too busy to have time to even have their food at regular times. Many busy people even consider eating and sleeping a waste of time and something to be quickly done with. This is wrong and one should show adequate respect to the needs of the body as well. The excessive indulgence in this *vega* results in obesity and associated complications. Detailed discussion of different eating disorders and their results will be detailed in the second volume of this series.

Sarvāṅgasundara: The six important symptoms of excessive suppression of hunger are enumerated. The term "*śūla*" indicates pain in the colon (*pakvāśaya*). Suppression of hunger results in *vāta* aggravation. *Pakvāśaya* (colon) is the seat of vāta and hence the pain is felt in that region.

AH Sū. 4.12a

Suppression of sleep

निद्राया मोहमूर्धाक्षिगौरवालस्यजृम्भिकाः ॥१२॥

आङ्गमर्दश्च, तत्रेष्टः स्वप्नः संवाहनानि च ॥१३॥

nidrāyā moha-mūrdhākṣi-gauravālasya-jṛmbhikāḥ //12//

aṅga-mardaśca tatreṣtaḥ svapnaḥ saṁvāhanāni ca

nidrāyā - of sleep; *moha* - confusion; *mūrdha* - top of head; *akṣi* - eyes; *gaurava* - heaviness; *ālasya* - laziness; *jṛmbhikāḥ* - yawning, and so on; *aṅga mardaḥ* - body pain; *ca* - and; *tatra* – in that case; *iṣtaḥ* - it is desirable, advisable; *svapnaḥ* – to sleep; *saṁvāhanāni* – caressing soft massage; *ca* - and

Translation

Suppression of sleep causes confusion, heaviness in the head and eyes, laziness, yawning, and a cutting type of body ache. In this case it is desirable to sleep and also receive a soft, caressing massage.

Commentary

Sleep is a basic need and one of the three pillars of health. Loss of sleep results in depletion of *ojas* and disturbance of *prāṇa vāta* which controls the mind and the senses. This is the reason for confusion and heaviness of head and eyes. *Prāṇa vāta* disturbs *vyāna* and results in generalized body ache. Detailed discussion of sleep is undertaken in the second volume of this series.

AH Sū. 4.13b–14a

Suppression of cough and treatment

कासस्य रोधात्तद्वृद्धिः श्वासारुचिहृदामयाः ॥१३॥

शोषे हिध्मा च, कार्योत्र कासहा सुतरां विधिः ॥१४॥

kāsasya rodhāt-tad-vṛddhiḥ śvāsāruci-hṛdāmayāḥ //13//

śoṣo hidhmā ca kāryo 'tra kāsahā sutarāṁ vidhiḥ

kāsasya - of cough; *rodhāt* - suppression; *tad* – of that; *vṛddhiḥ* – increases, aggravation; *śvāsa* - difficulty in breathing; *aruci* - loss of appetite; *hṛdāmayāḥ* - epigastric distress; *śoṣa* -

emaciation; *hidhmā* - hiccup; *ca* - and; *kāryo* – procedure, management; *atra* - in that case; *kāsahā* - termination of cough; *sutarāṁ* - primarily, definitely; *vidhiḥ* - things to be done

Translation

Suppression of cough causes aggravation of the same cough, breathlessness (dyspnea), loss of appetite, epigastric or cardiac distress, drying up, and hiccup. In that case, the procedure for the termination of cough is to be definitely adopted.

Commentary

The procedure for the management of *kāsa* can be found in AH Ni. Ch. 3. The term *śoṣa* indicates the pathology called *rājayakṣma* described in AH Ni. Ch. 5. Just as how *aṅgamarda* (body ache) is seen in many types of *vega-rodha*, another disease that is commonly seen due to *vega-rodha* is disease connected to *hṛdaya*[10]. In the present day when heart disease is one of the leading causes of death all over the world, it is only *Āyurveda* that can reveal *vegarodha* as the underlying cause for that increase.

Kāsa is a physiological reflex of the *prāṇavaha srotas.* Obstruction of this *srotas* will increase the pressure and aggravate the *kāsa* to make it pathological causing all the enumerated disorders. *Kāsa* naturally progresses to *śvāsa* as

---

[10] Hṛdaya has a wider connotation than just the physical heart including emotional and intellectual paradigms as well. This versatile term is used in āyurveda to indicate the mind and feelings of satisfaction etc.

the *vāta* disturbs the *kapha* in the chest region causing symptoms like epigastric distress.

When the *udāna vāta* is affected, it results in hiccups. If the *vāta* comes to the stomach region, it disturbs the *agni* resulting in loss of appetite. Due to long standing suppression, it can result in depletion of the *dhātus* called *śoṣa*. This is how habitual suppression of a simple cough reflex can snowball into a serious disease like *rājayakṣma* (a syndrome seen in severely depleting diseases like carcinoma) and become fatal.

AH Sū. 4.14b–15a

Suppression of heavy breathing (panting) and treatment

गुल्महृद्रोगसम्मोहाः श्रमश्वासाद्विधारितात् ॥१४॥
हितं विश्रमणं तत्र वातघ्नश्च क्रियाक्रमः ॥१५॥

gulma-hṛdroga-sammohāḥ śrama-śvāsād-vidhāritāt //14//
hitaṁ viśramaṇaṁ tatra vātaghnaśca kriyā-kramaḥ

gulma - trapped *vāta* in abdomen causing a space occupying lesion; *hṛdroga* - epigastric distress, cardiac ailments; *sammohāḥ* - complete confusion; *śrama-śvāsād* - of heavy breathing; *vidhāritāt* – upon the suppression of the urge; *hitaṁ* - beneficial; *viśramaṇaṁ* - proper rest; *tatra* - herein; *vātaghnaḥ* - pacify *vāta*; *ca* - and; *kriyā-kramaḥ* - the sequence of activities, measures

Treatment

Suppression of laboured breathing (panting) causes *gulma* (space-occupying lesion mostly in the abdomen), cardiac disorders, and confusion. Rest and *vāta*-pacifying measures are advised.

Commentary

Heavy panting can be a result of work or exercise. Some people have a habit of supressing or neglecting the exertional breath as part of their occupation. When one has this kind of breathing, he or she is suppose to rest till the breath comes back to normal. But in certain circumstances, there is no facility to rest and one has to keep on working. In this case the suppression means, suppressing the urge of the body to rest and to keep on working. The exertional breathing is an indication of over exercising or over work and that it is time to rest. This verse enumerates some of the diseases that can occur due to suppressing the exertional breath. One must look for a history of over exercising in clients who present with the list of disorders enumerated in this verse.

The heavy breathing is due to the acute *dhātu śoṣa* which occurs from the hard work. It can also be due to the constriction of the *prāṇavaha srotas*. The more we try to force ourselves, the more pressure *vāta* exerts on the *srotas* causing a vitiation. That can produce a vicious circle.

If we look across all the diseases caused due to suppression of urges, we find that cardiac disorders are the major group. This could be an important reason why cardiac disease is the major cause of death in the present time. It warrants a detailed study in this area by national and international health institutions to determine the fact of the matter.

We must remember that the list of diseases given here are only examples and many more diseases can result from the suppression of the urges.

AH Sū. 4.15b

Suppression of yawning

जृम्भायाः क्षववद्रोगाः, सर्वश्चानिलजिद्विधिः ॥१५॥

jṛmbhāyāḥ kṣavavad-rogāḥ sarvaścānilajid-vidhiḥ //15//

jṛmbhāyāḥ - (suppression) of yawning; *kṣavavad* - similar to sneezing; *rogāḥ* - diseases; *sarvaḥ* - all (measures); *ca* - which; *anilajit* - pacify *vāta*; *vidhiḥ* - procedures

Translation

Suppression of yawning causes disorders similar to that of the suppression of sneezing. The procedures for pacifying *vāta* are advised.

Commentary

The definition of yawning given in *Suśruta Samhita* Śā. 4.50, "*pītvaikam-anilotśvāsa*..." may be explained as "swallowing air through inspiration and expelling it out through the open mouth accompanied by flow of tears in the eyes is called *jhṛmbhā*."

Refer to the verse on sneezing (AH Sū 4.9-10a) for the disorders caused due to suppression of yawning. This is a very common urge that is suppressed when we feel sleepy in a public place or meeting due to embarrassment. All clients should be advised to never do it.

AH Sū. 4.16

Suppression of tears

पीनसाक्षिशिरोहृद्रुङ्मन्यास्तम्भारुचिभ्रमाः ॥१६॥

सगुल्मा बाष्पतस्तत्र स्वप्नो मद्यं प्रियाः कथाः ॥१६॥

pīnasākṣi śiro-hṛdruṅg-manyāstambhāruci-bhramāḥ

sagulmā bāṣpatas-tatra svapno madyaṁ priyāḥ kathāḥ //16//

pīnasa - running nose; *akṣi roga* – eye disorders; *śiro roga* – diseases of the head*; hṛd roga* – cardiac disorders; manyā stambha - neck rigidity; *aruci* - loss of appetite; *bhramāḥ* - giddiness; *sagulmā* – accompanied by a space occupying lesion; *bāṣpatas* - (suppression) of tears; *tatra* - therein; *svapno* - sleep; *madyaṁ* - alcoholic beverages; *priyāḥ kathāḥ* - (listening to) pleasant talks

Translation

Suppression of crying causes running nose, eye disorders, diseases of the head, cardiac disorders, rigidity of neck, loss of appetite, giddiness, and *gulma*. In that case, sleep, alcoholic beverages, and listening to pleasant talks are recommended.

Commentary

Could the same symptoms result if the lacrimation reflex is suppressed due to injury to the lachrymal nerve where the gland is unable to express the tears? If the tears are not being produced at all, it will not cause any of the problems enumerated above. But if tears are being produced by the gland, and the release is being blocked, it will cause symptoms.

In certain communities it is a custom to invite professional wailers to cry at the funeral of a loved one. The reason is that people often suppress their sorrow and tears thus resulting in complications later. The wailers bring the relatives in front of the dead body and cry so much that the relatives also burst out crying. This is good for physical and mental well-being.

In certain societies, men are expected to maintain a macho image and it is considered a sign of weakness to cry. This results in the suppression of tears as well as emotion by the men and thus resulting in various illnesses.
It actually means to hold back one's emotions. For example, when someone dies, the male members of the family hold back their tears due to social reasons or sometimes due to the shock of an event a person is unable to cry.

Pīnasa is the mildest manifestation wherein the fluids find an alternative pathway to exit out of the body. The complications can go upto affecting the heart (*hṛdaya*) and even the head (*bhrama*). *Bhrama – rajaḥ pittānilāt bhrama* (caused by *rajas guṇa*, *pitta* and *vāta* aggravation in the head)

Suppression of crying has a very intense effect on the neck muscles. Many causes of cervical spondylosis and other types of neck strain can present being resistant to all treatment. One must consider this cause.

Aruci can be caused due to two factors – 1. *Hṛdaya* (emotional factor) 2. *Jihva* (the taste factor)
Here the *gulma* presents in the region of the body on the level of heart and above.
Priya katha – when someone has suppressed emotions, the person needs counselling done with affection. This is *priya katha*.
Madyam – it is *srotosodana* (clearing the channels) and gives a pleasant feeling to the mind. It should be a *vāta pacifying* type of alcoholic beverage.

Note: If take a look at all the diseases occurring due to *vegāvarodha*, you will notice that *hṛd roga* (cardiac disease) is the most commonly occurring disease. This is a very significant observation with respect to present times since cardiac disorders occupy the position as the most common cause of death.

AH Sū. 4.17–19a

Suppression of vomiting urge and its treatment

विसर्पकोठकुष्ठाक्षिकण्डूपाण्ड्वामयज्वराः ॥१७॥

सकासश्वासहृल्लासव्यङ्गश्वयथवो वमेः ॥१७॥

गण्डूषधूमानाहारा रूक्षं भुक्त्वा तदुद्वमः ॥१८॥

व्यायामः स्रुतिरस्रस्य शस्तं चात्र विरेचनम् ॥१८॥

सक्षारलवणं तैलमभ्यङ्गार्थं च शस्यते ॥१९॥

Diseases caused

visarpa-koṭha-kuṣṭhākṣi-kaṇdū-pāṇdvāmaya-jvarāḥ

sakāsa-śvāsa-hṛllāsa-vyaṅga-śvayathavo-vameḥ //17//

Treatment

gaṇḍūṣa-dhūmānāhārā rūkṣaṁ bhuktvā tadudvamaḥ

vyāyāmaḥ srutir-asrasya śastaṁ cātra virecanam //18//

sakṣāra-lavaṇaṁ tailam-abhyaṅgārthaṁ ca śasyate

visarpa - cellulitis (an inflammatory skin lesion that spreads rapidly); *koṭha* – urticaria (a region that is reddish and hard to touch); *kuṣṭha* - skin diseases; *akṣi* - eyes; *kaṇdu* - itching; *pāṇdu* - causing pallor; *āmaya* - diseases; *jvarāḥ* - inflammation; *sakāsa* - cough; *śvāsa* - dyspnea; *hṛllāsa* – acidity, palpitations; *vyaṅga* - hyperpigmentation of face; *śvayathu* - edema; *vameḥ* - vomiting;

gaṇḍūṣa - gargle; *dhūma* - therapeutic smoking; *anāhārā* - fasting; *rūkṣa bhuktvā* - eat dry foods; *tad-udvamaḥ* - followed by vomiting; *vyāyāmaḥ* - exercise; *srutir-asrasya* - blood-letting;

śastaṁ - recommended, approved; *ca* - and; *atra* - here; *virecanam* - purgation; *sakṣāra* - with alkalis; *lavaṇaṁ* - salt; *tailam* - sesame oil; *abhyaṅgārthaṁ* - in order to massage; *ca* - and; *śasyate* - recommended

Translation

Suppression of the vomiting urge causes fast-spreading inflammation of skin, *urticaria*, *kuṣṭha*, diseases of the eyes, itching, *pāṇḍu*, *jvara*, *kāsa* (pathology resembling cough), *śvāsa* (dyspnea), *hṛllāsa*,[2] *vyaṅga* (hypopigmentation), and edema. Gargling, inhalation of herbal smoke, fasting or consumption of dry foods followed by vomiting, exercises, blood-letting, and purgation are advised in this condition. Massaging the body with sesame oil mixed with alkali (*kṣāra*[3]) and salt is also desirable.

Commentary

What are the types of physical exercises recommended in this condition? Yoga postures that promote the normalization of *udāna vāta* can be adopted.

How do we understand *chardi*? Whatever the cause may be, *chardi* is a mechanism by which the body expels the *utkliṣṭa kapha (kapha* that has been separated from the *dhātus* and freely accumulated in the body) that has accumulated inside.

Antiemetics should not be used indiscriminately. It should not be administered in the case of *kapha utkleśa* in *āmāśaya.* This will cause the *doṣa* to go into *rakta* (from *koṣṭha* to *śākha*) and become *kleda* in *rakta* causing *visarpa*. Another example is when all the *doṣās* have not been eliminated completely after *vamana* (*ayoga* or *hīnayoga* of *vamana*). In the *ayoga lakṣaṇa* of *vamana* you will see symptoms similar to the suppression of vomiting reflex. Not making the person vomit when there is *utkleśa avastha* in *jvara*. When the toxins are not eliminated in case of food poisoning is another such instance.

Vyaṅga is due to *rakta duṣṭi (kleda in rakta)*.
Āma in the *koṣṭha (GIT – in this context)* = *śopha* in the *parva (joints)* = *kleda* in the *rakta (blood)* = *abhiṣyanda* in the *netra (eye)*. All these similar conditions are caused due to *kapha utkleśa*. Suppression of vomiting reflex causes *kapha utkleśa*. Blood letting, *vamana* and *virecana* are a part of *visarpa cikitsa*. The *vamana* and *virecana* should be conducted using *rūkṣa* (drying) substances.

Sarvāṅgasundara: The exercises recommended here are those that gently help the *prāṇa vāyu* move in the proper physiological direction once again. This means that *prāṇavaha srotas* is the one that is most affected by the suppression of vomiting reflex.

Āyurvedarasāyana: The words *koṭha* and *vyaṅga* used here indicate a group of disorders called *kṣudra rogas* in *Āyurveda*. This is a list of disorders that cannot be grouped under any specific classification, and hence, such conditions are given a unique category. There are several disorders under this category and beyond the scope of the present book. Commonly they refer to a list of skin disorders since many diseases described under this name are connected to the skin. The word *kṣudra* means "less," because the *nidāna* for these diseases are described very briefly in the books.

AH Sū. 4.19b–21a

Suppression of seminal urge

शुक्रात्तत्स्रवणं गुह्यवेदनाश्वयथुज्वराः ॥१९॥

हृद्व्यथामूत्रसङ्गाङ्गभङ्गवृद्ध्यश्मषण्ढताः ॥२०॥

ताम्रचूडसुराशालिवस्त्यभ्यङ्गावगाहनम् ॥२०॥

वस्तिशुद्धिकरैः सिद्धम् भजेत्क्षीरं प्रियाः स्त्रियः ॥२१॥

śukrāt-tat-sravaṇaṁ guhya-vedanā-śvayathu-jvarāḥ //19//

hṛdvyathā-mūtrasaṅgāṅga-bhaṅga-vṛddhy-aśma-ṣaṇḍatāḥ

Treatment

tāmra-cūda-surāśāli-vasty-abhyaṅgāvagāhanam //20//

vasti-śuddhikaraiḥ siddhaṁ bhajet kṣīraṁ priyāḥ striyaḥ

śukrāt – the semen; *tat* - that; *sravaṇaṁ* - the exudation; *guhya-vedanāḥ* - pain in perineal region; - *śvayathu* - testicular edema; *jvaraḥ* - inflammation; *hṛdvyathā* - epigastric distress; *mūtrasaṅga* - obstruction of urine flow; *aṅgabhaṅga* - body pain (of cutting type); *vṛddhi* - increase in size (hydrocele); *aśma* - (seminal) calculi; *ṣaṇḍatāḥ* – impotency, not strong enough to perform intercourse (premature ejaculation);

tāmra cūda – chicken; *surā* - beer; *śāli* - a variety of rice reddish in color that grows in sixty days; *vasti* - medicated enema; *abhyaṅga* - oil application on the body; *avagāhanam* - immersion of body or part in medicated oil or herbal water; *vasti śuddhikaraiḥ* - cleansing the urinary bladder; *siddhaṁ* – (herbs) having the potency; *bhajet* - to partake; *kṣīraṁ* - milk; *priyāḥ* – affectionate; *striyaḥ* – intercourse with females

Translation

Suppression of the ejaculation of semen causes exudation of semen, pain along the perineal region or sexual organs, edema (of the penis, testes and other parts of reproductive apparatus), *jvara*, epigastric or cardiac distress, urinary obstruction, cutting pain over the body, increase in size of scrotum (eg. hydrocele, hernia), seminal calculi, and impotency.

Consumption of chicken, beer, *śālī* (a variety of rice), administration of *vasti*, oil application all over the body, immersion of the body in a tub of oil or herbal water, milk decoction of herbs that helps to cleanse the urinary bladder, and affectionate sexual intercourse are recommended in this situation.

Commentary

How does this translate in females? It is known that the females also secrete a small quantity of semen during sexual intercourse. But the secretion in females does not have the same function as in males. The *vegarodha* described here is referring to the suppression of orgasm and holding it back at a point when it is just about to be released. This is applicable in

females too as it will block the *apana vāta*. All complications related to imbalance and misdirected flow of *apana vāta* can occur.
There may be other *vegas* which was not part of the lifestyle in those days. One example very common in the present times is the withholding of menstruation using hormonal drugs. This suppression of the *ārtava pravṛtti (*menstrual flow) also is found to result in many complications in due course of time.

Srāva of semen is involuntary exudation or release of seminal fluid (involuntary ejaculation at night?). *śvayathu* could indicate testicular edema which is also indicated by the term *vṛddhi*.
Substances which purify the bladder should be used – for example *kūṣmāṇda kṣīra* (milk decoction of white pumpkin) can be used for clearing the bladder. Drinking coconut water will also be a good choice in this case.

Some of these symptoms are those that can be experienced immediately; some after a while; and some after years. So a client may have engaged in suppression of a certain urge sometime in the past, but the manifestation may come about many years later. Due to this reason, the *vaidya* will have to carefully inspect any such habits of suppression in the past, through discussions with the client to find the culprit.

Diseases caused due to suppression of the *dhāraṇīya vegas* (urges which should be suppressed) are revised in the table.

Adhovāta (flatus)	*Gulma, udāvarta, ruk, klama, flatus obstruction, mūtra rodha, śakṛd rodha, dṛṣṭi vadha, agni vadha, hṛdgada*
Śakṛd / Viṭ	*Piṇḍikodveṣṭa, pratiśyāya, śiro rujaḥ, belching, parikartika, hṛdayasya uparodhanam, mukhena viḍ pravṛtti & all the symptoms in No. 1*
Mūtra	*Aṅga bhaṅga, aśmarī, vasti meḍhra vaṁkṣaṇa vedana and all the symptoms of No 1 & 2*
Udgāra	*Aruci, kampa, vibandha hṛdayo, vibandha uras, ādhmāna, kāsa, hidhma*
Kṣavathu	*Śiro arti, indriya daurbalyam, manyāstambha, ardita*
Tṛṣṇa/tṛṭ	*Śoṣa, aṅgasāda, bādhirya, sammoha, bhrama, hṛdgadāḥ*
Kṣud	*Aṅga bhaṅga, aruci, glāni, kārśya, śūla, bhrama*
Nidrā	*Moha, mūrdha gaurava, akṣi gaurava, ālasya, jṛmbhika, aṅga marda*
Kāsa	*Vṛddhi, śvāsa, aruci, hṛdāmaya, śoṣa, hidhma*
Śvāsa	*Gulma, hṛdroga, sammoha*
Jṛṁbha	*All diseases similar to kṣavathu*
Aśru	*Pīnasa, akṣi roga, śiro roga, hṛd roga, manyā stambha, aruci, bhrama, sagulma*
Chardi	*Visarpa, koṭha, kuṣṭha, akṣi, kaṇḍu, pāṇḍu, jvara, kāsa, śvāsa, hṛllāsa, vyaṅga, śvayathu*
Retasā	*Guhya vedana, śvayathu, jvaraḥ, hṛdvyathā, mūtrasaṅga, aṅga bhaṅga, vṛddhi, aśma, ṣaṇḍataḥ*

AH Sū. 4.–21b

When to reject curative options

तृट्शूलार्तं त्यजेत् क्षीणं विड्वमं वेगरोधिनम् ॥२१॥

tṛṭśulārtaṁ tyajet kṣīṇaṁ viḍvamaṁ vegarodhinam //21//

tṛṭ - intense thirst; *śūla* - severe pain; *ārtaṁ* - the diseased who has; *tyajet* - is to be given up; *kṣīṇaṁ* - emaciated; *vid-vamaṁ* – fecal vomiting; *vegarodhinam* - one who is suppressing the urges

Translation

A client who shows up with intense thirst, severe pain in the body, emaciated, and vomiting fecal matter with a history of suppressing the urges is to be rejected.

Commentary

This is to indicate that this is an incurable situation. The word *tyajet* is used here in the sense as to indicate that the option for a cure should be given up. It does not mean that the patient should not be given any care. It means that the preparation for a peaceful departure should be initiated. These symptoms are called *ariṣṭa lakṣaṇa* in *Āyurveda* and herald impending death. They are described in more detail at the end of *Śārīra sthāna*.

AH Sū. 4.22–23

Vāta aggravation is the result of all suppression of urges

रोगाः सर्वेऽपि जायन्ते वेगोदीरणधारणैः ॥२२॥

निर्दिष्टं साधनं तत्र भूयिष्ठं ये तु तान् प्रति ॥२२॥

ततश्चानेकधा प्रायः पवनो यत्प्रकुप्यति ॥२३॥

अन्नपानौषधं तस्य युञ्जीतातोऽनुलोमनम् ॥२३॥

rogāḥ sarve 'pi jāyante vego-dīraṇa-dhāraṇaiḥ
nirdiṣtaṁ sādhanaṁ tatra bhūyiṣṭham ye tu tān prati //22//
tataś-cānekadhā prāyaḥ pavano-yat-prakupyati
annapān-auṣadhaṁ tasya-yuñjītāto 'nulomanam //23//

rogāḥ - diseases; *sarve* - all; *api* - certainly; *jāyante* - is caused by; *vegaḥ* - urges; *dīraṇa* - forceful expression; *dhāraṇaiḥ* - suppression;
nirdiṣtaṁ - indicated; *sādhanaṁ* - (with) management; *tatra* - there; *bhūyiṣṭham* - for the most part; *ye* - these; *tu* - but; *tān* - in; *prati* - each and every (case)
tataḥ - therefore; *ca* - and; *anekadhā* - in various ways; *prāyaḥ* - almost all of them; *pavano* - of *vāta*; *yat* - which; *prakupyati* – aggravates; *annapāna* - foods; *auṣadhaṁ* - medicines; *tasya* - for that purpose; *yuñjītāto* - is therefore applied; *anulomanam* – to cause movement in the physiological direction

Translation

All the diseases can be caused by forceful expression and suppression of the natural urges. Most of the diseases have been described here along with their management. Almost all of them are due to the aggravation of *vāta* in various ways, and therefore, all the foods and medicines are also applied for facilitating the physiological movement of *vāta*.

Commentary

Ācārya Vāgbhaṭa is boldly stating here that the root cause of almost *all* diseases is in one way or another related to suppression or forceful expression of the urges. One who does not suppress or force the expression of urges will almost never fall sick. A *vaidya* must take special care to take detailed history of any suppression or forceful unnatural expression of urges in all clients irrespective of what their disease is and include the remedy in the management protocol.

If we carefully examine the list of all the pathologies enumerated in this chapter, it will practically include all the diseases that are described ahead in the *Aṣṭāṅga Hṛdayam*. .

Sarvāṅgasundara: All these diseases are caused usually due to chronic and habitual suppression of these physiological reflexes.

***Aruṇodaya by Govindan vaidya*:** All diseases can be caused by obstruction or forced expression of the urges because *vāta prakopa* is involved. A strong *vāta* aggravation can also agitate and aggravate *pitta, kapha, malas*, and *dhātus.* That includes all the diseases. The diseases that are predominantly associated with each *vegarodha* (suppression of urges) have been enumerated along with some of their treatments. But one should not misunderstand that these are the only diseases than can be caused or these are the only treatments that can be done. Hence, all *vāta anulomana* treatments can be used suitably in all disease conditions. In the case of the suppression of *tṛṣṇa* (thirst) and *chardi (vomiting), pitta* and *kapha*, which get aggravated, need to be treated as well. We should remember that *vāta* aggravation is also present here and *vāta*-pacifying treatments are not contraindicated in these conditions.

AH Sū. 4.23b–24a

Urges to be controlled

धारयेत्तु सदा वेगान् हितैषी प्रेत्य चेह च ॥२४॥

लोभेर्ष्याद्वेषमात्सर्यरागादीनां जितेन्द्रियः ॥२४॥

dhārayet-tu sadā vegān hitaiṣī pretya ceha ca

lobherṣyā-dveṣa-mātsarya-rāgādīnāṁ jitendriyaḥ //24//

dhārayet - to be controlled; *tu* - in any case; *sadā* - always; *vegān* - urges; *hitaiṣi* – one desirous of beneficial results; *pretya* – hereafter (the next world); *ca* - and; *iha* - in this world; *ca* - and; *lobha* – greed, *īrṣya* – jealousy, *dveṣa* – hatred, *mātsarya* – envy; *rāgādināṁ* – attachments, longings; *jitendriyaḥ* - those who have conquered their senses and mind

Translation

One who desires beneficial results in this life and the next should at all times control the urges of greed, jealousy, hatred, envy, and the various longings and attachments by conquering the mind and senses.

Commentary

Kāma and *krodha* are not mentioned here. They are included in the word *ādi.* In chapter 1, the word *ādi* is already explained in such a way that *rāgādi* includes *kāma*, *krodha*, and others.

The urges mentioned here are called *manovegas* or urges of the mind. Some of the prominent *manovegas* (urges of the mind) are mentioned here and the others are included in the word *ādi.*

It should be noted that the use of the word "suppressed" in the context of dealing with the mental urges does not mean that they should be forcefully retained inside. Forceful suppression will lead to many chronic diseases. What is meant is that one should be able to prevent the mind from coming under the influence of these urges. It is possible to create such an atmosphere in the mind by which the negative urges will not manifest. This atmosphere is called *sattva*. This is the reason why a healthy mind is also referred to as *sattva* in the texts. The unhealthy mind cannot be referred to as *sattva*.

In the first chapter it was described that *rajas* and *tamas* are the two *doṣas* which cause vitiation of the mind. The mental urges described here are the outcome of *rajas* and *tamas*. Once we slip down into *rajas* or *tamas*, it starts a vicious cycle and it is very difficult to stop these urges from evolving in the mind. The only way is to attain and maintain a predominant atmosphere of *sattva* in the mind which will automatically prevent these urges from taking birth. Trying to forcefully suppress anger or any other mental urges while remaining in a *rajasik* or *tamasik* atmosphere will be futile and detrimental.

Aruṇodaya by Govindan vaidya: The urges are of two types: of the body and of the mind. Those described thus far are bodily urges that should not be suppressed. But the urges mentioned here (*lobha, īṛsya*, etc.) should be sublimated, because it is this transformation of the mind that is the solution from all suffering. They are also natural for the conditioned mind and not easy to suppress. If the mind is positively engaged or fixed on a positive object, it is possible to control these mental urges.

In the *Bhagavad Gīta* 2.59, it is explained that one cannot suppress the mind by denial. But by giving the mind a higher positive engagement, it is possible to overcome the lower negative urges. When the mind gets a higher taste, it automatically gives up the lower taste.

When *Arjuna* told Lord *Krishna* that the mind is too flickering, strong, obstinate, turbulent, and difficult to control, Lord *Kṛṣṇa* replied that it is possible to control the mind by practice and detachment. As explained above, detachment does not mean forceful separation. It is the transfer of the attachment to higher, more meaningful, and joyful engagements and emotions.

The mind is a neutral entity. When it is controlled, it can work wonders and be our best friend, but when it is uncontrolled, it can wreak havoc and be our worst enemy. Controlling the mind is not a one-time process. It is a continuous exercise that goes on from moment to moment—a spontaneous byproduct of understanding the self.

Why are the bodily urges to be expressed and mental urges to be suppressed? This is because the more we try to satisfy the mental urges, the more they increase. And the more we satisfy the bodily urges, the more they decrease. Suppression does not mean a forceful exercise. The way to control envy has already been described in AH Sū 2.25. In the same way, all the other mental urges should also be redirected in a positive way. That is the method of controlling the mind.

AH Sū. 4.25–26

Importance of seasonal cleansing

यतेत च यथाकालं मलानां शोधनं प्रति ॥२५॥

अत्यर्थसञ्चितास्ते हि क्रुद्धाः स्युर्जीवितच्छिदः ॥२५॥

दोषाः कदाचित्कुप्यन्ति जिता लङ्घनपाचनैः ॥२६॥

ये तु संशोधनैः शुद्धा न तेषां पुनरुद्भवः ॥२६॥

yateta ca yathā kālaṁ malānāṁ śodhanaṁ prati
atyartha sañcitāste hy kruddhāḥ syur-jīvitacchidaḥ //25//
doṣāḥ kadācit-kupyanti jitā langhana pācanaiḥ
ye tu samśodhanaiḥ śuddhā na teṣāṁ punar-udbhavaḥ //26//

yateta – endeavor to; *ca* – and; *yathā kālaṁ* – at the appropriate time; *malānāṁ* – vitiated *doṣas*; *śodhanaṁ* – eliminate; *prati* - every; *atyartha* – due to excessive; *sañcitāste* – having accumulated; hi – certainly; *kruddhāḥ* – aggravate; *syuḥ* – happening; *jīvitat* – of; *chidaḥ* – cutting off

doṣāḥ – the *doṣas*; *kadācit* – possibly; *kupyanti* – will aggravate (again); *jitā* – having been conquered by; *langhana* – depleting therapies; *pācanaiḥ* – digesting therapies; *ye* – these; *tu* – but; *samśodhanaiḥ* – cleansing (cathartic, eliminative) procedures; *śuddhā* – purified; *teṣāṁ* – of them; *na punar-udbhavaḥ* – will not recur again

Translation

One should endeavor to eliminate the aggravated *doṣas* at the appropriate time (season), since they can accumulate and cause loss of life. *Doṣas* pacified by depleting (reducing) and digesting therapies can aggravate again later, but those that are eliminated by cleansing therapies will not recur again.

Commentary

Here the superiority of *śodhana* over *śamana* is also explained in terms of recurrence of symptoms. *Śodhana* involves the removal of the accumulated or aggravated *doṣas* from the body. *Śamana* does not remove the *doṣas*. They are still in the body but pacified. Whenever there is a provocation of the *doṣas*, they will come up and cause the same problems again. But if a *śodhana* is done, they are gone for good, and a fresh accumulation of *doṣas* will have to occur for the disease to manifest again. The words *langhana pācanaiḥ* denote *śamana cikitsa*.

This verse is often quoted by those who want to establish the effectiveness of *śodhana* over *śamana* in all cases. There is another perspective. This verse has to be understood in the context of the *doṣā caya* and *kopa* due to the influence of *kāla*. It means that if one tries to employ *śāmana* upon the *doṣās* that have accumulated due to the influence of *kāla*, there is a possibility that they will aggravate. This is because, by the time we accomplish *langhana* and *pācana*, the *ṛtu* has already changed to the next. Since the time available is very limited (seven days before and after the *ṛtu sandhi*), in this scenario *śodhana* may be better than *śamana*.

In the light of *cikitsa* in general, *śodhana* is also dependent on *śamana* to be done at the end of *śodhana* for achieving non-relapse of *doṣa* aggravation and disease. In the case of low *rogi bala* (strength of client), though all other factors indicate a *śodhana*, it is contraindicated. On the other hand, there is never an instance where a *śamana cikitsa* is contraindicated.

The conclusive fact is that no *cikitsa* is superior over any other *cikitsa*. It all depends on the circumstance, which one is more warranted and becomes effective.

Āyurvedarasāyana: *śodhana* is given more importance than *śamana*. *laṅghana* can be done by fasting alone. For *pācana*, other methods have to be adopted.

Aruṇodaya: Regular cleansing is necessary to remove the accumulated *doṣas* from time to time though they do not cause any symptoms. If we allow them to accumulate, they can aggravate and cause diseases. Hence prophylactic cleansing is recommended. There are two kinds of *svastha* (healthy persons). One has *sañcita doṣa (*accumulated *doṣas*) and the other does not have *sañcita doṣā*. The cleansing is being recommended for the first type of healthy person. The second type of person does not need it.

AH Sū. 4.27

Rejuvenation and strengthening after cleansing

यथाक्रमं यथायोगमत ऊर्ध्वं प्रयोजयेत् ॥२७॥

रसायनानि सिद्धानि वृष्ययोगांश्च कालवित् ॥२७॥

yathā-kramam yathā-yogam ata-ūrdhvaṁ prayojayet

rasāyanāni siddhāni vṛṣya-yogāmśca kālavīt //27//

yathā-kramam – in that order; *yathā-yogama* – suitable formulations; *ataḥ ūrdhvaṁ* – the above (mentioned procedures); *prayojayet* – after completing; *rasāyanāni* – rejuvenative medicines; *siddhāni* – proven, potent; *vṛṣya* – aphrodisiacs; *yogāmśca* – and formulations; *kālavīt* – the physician (who acts in a timely manner)

Translation

After completing the above-mentioned procedures (of cleansing), in the same order, suitable, proven, and potent formulations for rejuvenation and aphrodisiacs are administered by the physician, who knows the right time to administer them.

Commentary

Sarvāṅgasundara: *Kālavit* refers to a physician who knows the influence of time. Which time? The time that is most favourable and appropriate for the administration of a medicine or performing a procedure.

Ataḥ indicates that only after cleansing should the *rasāyanas* be used. The word *kāla* includes *deśa* (place), *bala* (strength), *śarīra* (body), *āhāra* (diet), *sātmya* (habits), *sattva* (mind), and *prakṛti* (constitution).

Some of the popular *rasāyanas* as given in AH Ut. 39.11 are *harītakī, āmalaki, saindhava, nāgara,* and *vacā.*

Here the time of administration of the *rasāyanas* and *vājīkaraṇa* medicines is stressed. If the timing is not correct, one will not obtain the desired result. This is why the physician is also known as *kālavit.* The place *(deśa)* and age *(vayas)* should also be considered. In this context the *rasāyana* mentioned is not *kuṭi prāveśika* (a type of intense *rasāyana* procedure). It is more *vṛṣya* (increasing *śukra dhātu*) and suitable for each *doṣa* type, since it is being mentioned in the context of *svastha vṛtta.* In AH Ut 40.7, a *rasāyana vasti* is mentioned: *"atha snigdha visuddhanam..."*

Āyurvedarasāyana: It is *bṛmhaṇa* (nourishing therapy). The methods used are *rasāyana*, *vājīkaraṇa*, *āhāra* and so on. One who has undergone purification is eligible for *rasāyana* and *vājīkaraṇa* in that order. *Siddhāni* means many people have obtained the results from this process. The word *kālavit* indicates one who know the *avastha* of the disease. After completing *rasāyana*, the process of *vājīkaraṇa* can be done.

Aruṇodaya: When *śodhana* is performed and *doṣas* are expelled, some of the healthy *dhātu* is also stripped away, along with the vitiated *doṣas*. This causes *dhātu kṣaya* and weakens the body. In order to replenish the lost *dhātus* and strengthen them again, *rasāyana* and *vājīkaraṇa* therapies are employed by the *vaidya*.
Rasāyanas should not be administered without cleansing if *āma* is present. Otherwise they will not give any result and might even produce a negative result.

Āyurvedarasāyana: Here *bheṣaja* refers to *śodhana* (purificatory) treatments. After purificatory treatments, a nourishing therapy is always essential because the purification results in depletion of *dhātus* and aggravation of *vāta*. *Bheṣajena* means the purification that is done in accordance with the *prakṛti*. For those who are emaciated due to *śodhana*, the *bṛmhaṇa* has to be done using *rasāyana*. *Kramāt* indicates that the nourishment has to be done in a particular order taking into account the *bala* (strength of the person) and *anala* (digestive fire).

The next verse elaborates the benefits of performing these procedures described above.

AH Sū. 4.28–29

The sequence of purification, nourishment, and rejuvenation

भेषजक्षपिते पथ्यमाहारैर्बृंहणं क्रमात् ॥२८॥

शालिषष्टिकगोधूममुद्गमांसघृतादिभिः ॥२८॥

हृद्यदीपनभैषज्यसंयोगाद्रुचिपक्तिदैः ॥२९॥

साभ्यङ्गोद्वर्तनस्नाननिरूहस्नेह वस्तिभिः ॥२९॥

bheṣaja-kṣapite pathyam-āhārai-bṛmhaṇaṁ kramāt
śāli-ṣaṣṭika-godhūma-mudga māmsa-ghṛtādibhiḥ //28//
hṛdya-dīpana bhaiṣajya saṁyogād-rucipaktidaiḥ
sābhyaṅgodvartana snāna nirūha-sneha-vastibhiḥ //29//

bheṣaja – treatments; *kṣapite* – after having completed, exhausted; *pathyam* – desirable, according to the prescription of the diet to be taken after the treatment; *āhārai* – foods; *bṛmhaṇaṁ* – nourishing; *kramāt* – gradually, in a particular order; *śāliṣaṣṭika* – two varieties of rice; *godhūma* – wheat; *mudga* – green gram; *māmsa* – meat; *ghṛta* – ghee; *ādibhiḥ* – etc; *hṛdya* – pleasing; *dīpana* – digestive; *bhaiṣajya* – treatments; *saṁyogād* – in conjunction with; *ruci-paktidaiḥ* – tastily prepared; *sa* – along with; *abhyaṅga* – oil massage;

udvartana – powder massage; *snāna* – bath; *nirūha-sneha-vastibhiḥ* – decoction and oil enemas;

Translation

After having completed the various treatments, one should resort to nourishment of the body in a certain specified order by consuming *śāli* rice, wheat, green gram, meat, *ghee*, and so on, prepared with pleasing-to-eat and digestive ingredients. This can be done in conjunction with oil application on the body, powder massages, bath, decoction enemas, and oil enemas.

Commentary

Sarvāṅgasundara: The type of food that is given should be *hṛdyāni* (pleasing), *dīpanāni* (igniting digestion), and *bhaiṣajyāni* (medicinal)—containing herbs like ginger, *pippali, ārdraka, tvak, elā*, and so on. The word *samyoga* indicates that the food should be pleasing, digestive, and medicinal, as mentioned above. The art of dietetics according to *Āyurveda* is to be able to optimally bring together the three components to make it pleasing (taste factor), easily digestible (nutrition factor), and medicinal (healing factor).

Āyurvedarasāyana: Here *bheṣaja* refers to *śodhana* (purificatory) treatments. After purificatory treatments, a nourishing therapy is always essential because the purification results in depletion of *dhātus* and aggravation of *vāta*. *Bheṣajena* means the purification that is done in accordance with the *prakṛti*. For those who are emaciated due to *śodhana*, the *bṛmhaṇa* has to be done using *rasāyana*. *Kramāt* indicates that the nourishment has to be done in a particular order taking into account the *bala* (strength of the person) and *anala* (digestive fire).

The next verse elaborates the benefits of performing these procedures described above.

AH. Sū. 4.30

Benefits of performing the purification and nourishment

तथा स लभते शर्म सर्वपावकपाटवम् ॥३०॥

धीवर्णेन्द्रियवैमल्यं वृषतां दैर्घ्यमायुषः ॥३०॥

tathā sa labhate śarma sarva-pāvaka-pāṭavam

dhī-varṇendriya-vaimalyaṁ vṛṣatāṁ dairghyam-āyuṣaḥ //30//

tathā – thus; *sa* – the patient; *labhate* – obtains; *śarma* – comfort; *sarva-pāvaka* – all the *agnis* at various levels; *pāṭavam* – sharpness, dexterous; *dhī* – intellect; *varṇa* – complexion; *indriya-vaimalyaṁ* – clarity of the senses; *vṛṣatāṁ* – virility; *dairghyam-āyuṣaḥ* – long life

Translation

Thus the patient obtains comfort, ignited digestion at all levels, sharpness of intellect, clear complexion, clarity of the senses, virility, and a long life.

Commentary

The word *tathā* indicates 'thus having undergone *śodhana*, *bṛmhaṇa* and *rasāyana'*. The word *'sa'* in this verse indicates the person who has undergone all these procedures. The word *'sarva pāvaka'* indicates that there are many fires situated at various locations in the human body. These fires are explained in AH Śā 3.59 (*bhaumāpya...*)

Pañcamahābhūta agni, sapta dhātu agni, trayodaśa jaṭharāgni are the different agnis in the body. *Vṛṣatā* is explained as *'strī gamana sāmarthya'* meaning 'expertise in dealing with women'. From this expression we can understand that it is not just about the physical act but it also denotes the sex appeal.

AH Sū. 4.31

Āgantu rogaḥ: Diseases due to external causes

ये भूतविषवाय्वग्निक्षतभङ्गादिसम्भवाः ॥३१॥

रागद्वेषभयाद्याश्च ते स्युरागन्तवो गदाः ॥३१॥

ye bhūta-viṣavāyvagni-kṣata-bhaṅgādi-sambhavāḥ
raga dveṣa[4]*-bhayādyāśca te syur-āgantavo gadāḥ //31//*

ye – those which; *bhūta* – (due to) other living entities; *viṣa* – toxins, poisons; *vāyu* – (polluted) air; *agni* – fire; *kṣata* – trauma; *bhaṅgādi* – fracture, and so on; *sambhavāḥ* – caused by; *kāma* – lust; *krodha* – anger; (*rāga* – attachment; *dveṣa* – aversion); *bhaya* – fear; *ādyāśca* – and others; *te* – they; *syur*

– are; *āgantavo* – caused due to external factors; *gadāḥ* – *diseases*

Translation

The diseases that arise due to other living entities, toxic substances, polluted air, fire, traumatic injury, fracture, and emotions such as such as lust, anger, attachments, hatred, fear, and so forth are called known as *āgantu roga*s.

Commentary

Till the previous verse, the diseases described were *nija* (endogenous). In this verse, examples of *āgantu* (exogenous) diseases are given.

Sarvāṅgasundara: There are two types of causes for *āgantu rogas*. One is due to living entities, and another is due to nonliving entities.

AH Sū. 4.32

To prevent endogenous and exogenous diseases

त्यागः प्रज्ञापराधानामिन्द्रियोपशमः स्मृतिः ॥३२॥

देशकालात्मविज्ञानं सद्वृत्तस्यानुवर्तनम् ॥३२॥

tyāgaḥ prajñāparādhānām-indriyopaśamaḥ smṛtiḥ

deśa-kālātma-vijñānaṁ sadvṛttasyānuvartanam //32//

tyāgaḥ - avoiding; *prajñāparādhānām* - the insult of the intelligence (in other words, heeding to the voice of intellect); *indriya* - senses; *upaśamaḥ* - having control over; *smṛtiḥ* -

(retrospective) cognizance; *deśa* - place; *kāla* - time; *ātma* - of the self; *vijñānaṁ* – being aware of; *sadvṛttasya* - having good conduct; *anuvartanam* – undertaking, executing

Translation

Giving up the tendency to ignore our own intelligence (conscience); controlling the senses; being aware of past experiences; being aware of place, time, and body constitution one should perform all activities according to principles of *sadvṛtta* (good conduct).

Commentary

After explaining *nija* (endogenous) and *āgantu* (exogenous) *rogas*, the author tells us how to prevent them.

It is from the *smṛti* (memory) that we develop *dhī* (intelligence). Our intelligence depends upon past memory retrieval to discriminate and make the right decisions. *Prajñāparādha* is the result of vitiation (*bhramśā*) of the *dhī*, *dhṛti* and *smṛti*. The only way to avoid *prajñāparādha* is to prevent the vitiation of intellect, patience and memory. This is possible only by controlling the senses (*indriyopaśamaḥ*). The spiral of how the loss of *dhī, dhṛti and smṛti* result in prajñāparādha is most beautifully and simply is described in *Bhagavad Gīta* 2.62 (*dhyāyato viṣayān puṁsaḥ…)*. It is not true that a person deliberately ignores his or her intelligence. When one sparks off this spiral as a result of which the intelligence is destroyed, one is helplessly dragged away by the uncontrolled senses and mind towards performing wrong actions. This is the truth.

Contemplates on the objects of the senses

↓

Develops attachment to the sense objects

↓

Attachment turns into an intense craving

↓

The intense craving turns into frustration or anger

↓

Anger causes delusion

↓

Delusion causes confusion of memory

↓

Confusion of the memory causes destruction of intelligence

↓

Destruction of intelligence (prajñāparādha) causes wrong actions

↓

Wrong actions cause disease

Aṣṭāṅga ṣaṅgraha also adds *atharva vihitā śāntiḥ pratikūla grahārcanam, bhūtādyaspraśanopāyo nirdiṣṭaśca pṛthak pṛthak*

meaning that one can also perform the required rituals, prayers to the deities of the planets who are not favorable and perform the other activities to prevent being affected by other living entities.

Sarvāṅgasundara: *Deśa* refers to *jānghala* (dry), *ānūpa* (wet) or *sādhāraṇa* (moderate) places. *Kāla* refers to the seasons; *ātma* refers to our *prakṛti.*

AH Sū. 4.33

Nontouch therapies

अथर्वविहिता शान्तिः प्रतिकूलग्रहार्चनम् ॥३३॥

भूताद्यस्पर्शनोपायो निर्दिष्टश्च पृथक् पृथक् ॥३३॥

atharva-vihitā śāntiḥ pratikūla grahārcanam

bhūtādya sparśanopāyo nirdiṣṭaśca pṛthak pṛthak //33//

atharva – the *atharva veda*; *vihitā* – devoid of; *śāntiḥ* – peace, relief; *pratikūla* – as opposed to, in contrast; *graha-arcanam* – prayers to the planets; *bhūtādi* – other living beings etc; *asparśana* – devoid of touch; *upāyaḥ* – methods; *nirdiṣṭaśca* – and specified; *pṛthak pṛthak* – many different

Translation

In contrast (to *Āyurvedic* therapies that use touch), the *Atharva Veda* specifies many different methods for obtaining relief by offering prayers to planets, other living beings, and so on by methods that are devoid of touch.

Commentary

The *Atharva Veda* is replete with different recommendations of incantations and rituals (*pujas*). There are different texts named *Sāyaṇīya, Vīrasimhāvalokanam, Hārita samhita* and others that explain the specific sinful activity that cause specific diseases. They also explains the atonement and rituals that are to be performed to cure diseases. These are a part of the *Atharva Veda* and are called *daiva vyapāśraya cikitsa*—one of the three types of treatments in *Āyurveda*. The other two types are *yukti vyapāśraya* and *sattvavajaya*.

AH Sū. 4.34

Pacifying both manifested and unmanifested diseases

अनुत्पत्त्यै समासेन विधिरेषः प्रदर्शितः ॥३४॥
निजागन्तुविकाराणामुत्पन्नानां च शान्तये ॥३४॥

anutpatyai samāsena vidhireṣa pradarśitaḥ
nijāgantu-vikārāṇām-utpannānāṁ ca śāntaye //34//

anutpatyai – to prevent from manifesting; *samāsena* – in brief; *vidhiḥ-eṣa* – these instructions; *pradarśitaḥ* – has been explained; *nijāgantu* – endogenous and exogenous; *vikārāṇām* – diseases; *utpannānāṁ* – and those already manifested; *ca* – and; *śantaye* – will pacify

Translation

These instructions that have been briefly explained prevent endogenous as well as exogenous diseases from manifesting. They will also pacify the diseases that have already manifested.

Commentary

If you follow the instructions mentioned here, it will even significantly alter the course of diseases that appear due to the influence of *kāla* (time)—that is, geriatric diseases. This is the treatment for both *nija* (endogenous) and *āgantu vikāras* (exogenous diseases) if they have already manifested. *Sāmānya cikitsā kramam* (general treatment method) is the method to be adopted in case one has not understood the exact *nidāna* (cause) and *samprāpti* (pathogenesis), and one does not know whether it is *nija* (endogenous) or *āgantu (exogenous)*.

Sarvāṅgasundara: The word *vidhireṣa* means to give up *prajñāparādha* and so forth (the three causes of diseases) and follow the principles of *sadvṛtta* (as explained in chapter 2). The rules and regulations are not only meant for preventing unmanifested diseases but also for treating manifested diseases.

AH Sū. 4.35

Cleanse on time to avoid diseases originating due to season changes

शीतोद्भवं दोषचयं वसन्ते विशोधनं ग्रीष्मजमभ्रकाले ॥३५॥

घनात्यये वार्षिकमाशु सम्यक् प्राप्नोति रोगानृतुजान्न जातु ॥३५॥

śītodbhavaṁ doṣa-cayaṁ vasante
viśodhayan grīṣmajam-abhrakāle
ghanātyaye vārṣikam-āśu samyak
prāpnoti rogān-ṛtujān-na jātu //35//

śītodbhavaṁ - that which originates in the cold season; *doṣa-cayaṁ* - accumulation of the *doṣās*; *vasante* - in the spring; *viśodhayan* - is evacuated; *grīṣmajam* - in the summer; *abhrakāle* - rainy season (*abhra* - clouds); *ghana* - autumn (autumn is called *ghana vyapāya*); *atyaye* - terminated in, removed in; *vārṣikam* - the increase is; *āśu* - quickly; *samyak* - completely; *prāpnoti* - be affected by; *rogan* - diseases; *ṛtujān* - originating from the seasonal changes; *na jātu* - will never at any time

Translation

The *doṣas* that accumulate in *hemanta* and *śiśira ṛtus* (cold seasons) are cleansed in *vasanta ṛtu* (spring season). Those that accumulate in *grīṣma ṛtu* (summer) are cleansed in the *abhraka ṛtu* (rainy season); and those that accumulate in *abhraka ṛtu* (rainy season) are cleansed in *śarad ṛtu* (autumn). The cleansing should be done quickly (before the next season begins), and thus one will never be affected by diseases originating due to the changing of seasons.

Commentary

The term *āśu* (quickly) used here indicates that the cleansing should be done quickly, before the *ṛtu sandhi* (transition period between two seasons) is over, and should avoid entering into the next *ṛtu* (season).

The words *na jātu* are very emphatic. This means that if the accumulated *doṣas* are regularly evacuated, one will never become sick in life. In this case it is during the changing of the seasons. But the same principle can be applied to other causes of accumulation of the *doṣas* as well. Thus *śodhana* is the best form of treatment if all the factors are favourable for its performance.

Sarvāṅgasundara: The word *śīta* includes both *hemanta* and *śiśira*. If the seasons go according to the schedule of two months each, *śrāvaṇa, kārtika*, and *caitra* are the times for cleansing the *doṣās, vāta, pitta*, and *kapha* accumulating in the summer, rainy, and winter seasons, respectively. The cleansing in *vasanta ṛtu* has to be done at the beginning of the season.

Āyurvedarasāyana: The same principle has been explained in AH Sū 13.33 in terms of the names of the months which is here explained in terms of the names of seasons. As explained in the beginning of the chapter, the seasons can be calculated according to calendar months, planetary movements or *guṇa* changes in the atmosphere.

AH Sū. 4.36

Formula for freedom from all diseases

नित्यं हिताहारविहारसेवी समीक्ष्यकारी विषयेष्वसक्तः ॥३६॥

दाता समः सत्यपरः क्षमावानाप्तोपसेवी च भवत्यरोगः ॥३६॥

nityam hitāhāra-vihāra-sevī

samīkṣyakārī viṣayeṣv-asaktaḥ

dātā samaḥ satyaparaḥ kṣamāvān

āptopasevī ca bhavaty-arogaḥ //36//

nityam - always; *hitāhāra* - eats beneficial food; *vihāra* - (beneficial) regimen; *sevī* - adopts; *samīkṣyakārī* - is objective, closely observing everything and mindful of what one is doing; *viṣayeṣu-asaktaḥ* - free from attachment to the sense objects; *dātā* - munificent; *samaḥ* - equal to all (just); *satya-paraḥ* - honest (taken shelter of the truth); *kṣamāvān* - patient; *āptopasevī* - one who values traditional wisdom from the great authorities; ca - and; *bhavati* - becomes; *arogaḥ* - free from diseases

Translation

One who always eats only what is beneficial, performs only those activities that are beneficial, is closely observant and mindful of everything, is free from any attachment to sense objects, is munificent, is equally disposed to all, is honest, is patient, and accepts the words of the authorities will be free from all diseases.

Commentary

The last point is significant. It may not be always possible to understand why an instruction is being given, but we need to have faith in the words of the *āpta* (definition of *āpta* is given below) based on the fact that what they have said earlier has proved to be true and beneficial.

The definition of an *āpta* is given in *Caraka Samhita* Sū. 11.18, "*yeṣāṁ trikālam amalaṁ....*" One should be cautious in performing every activity. One is said to be *kṣamāvān* when one has the power to inflict a punishment but still forgives and lets the offender go free.

Meaning of *āpta* (authority)

The *āptas* are those who have sharpened their faculties, comprehension, and thinking with discipline and penance. They are endowed with *pratibha* (intuition) and can visualize solutions during their meditative state. Their words can be relied upon, because they are impartial, sincere, and without any prejudice. However, the intuitive solutions have to be verified by actual experience.

The special features of an *āpta* (authoritative person) include

1. sharp faculties;
2. discipline;
3. penance;

4. intuition;
5. impartiality;
6. lack of prejudice;
7. lack of impulsivity;
8. constantly thinking towards bettering the science; and
9. purity in thought, word, and deed.

इति श्रीवैद्यपतिसिंहगुप्तसूनुश्रीमद्वाग्टविरचितायामष्टाङ्गहृदय संहितायां सूत्रस्थाने रोगानुत्पादनीयोनाम चतुर्थोध्यायः ॥४॥

iti śrī vaidyapati simhagupta sūnu śrī vāgbhaṭa viracitāyām-aṣṭāṅga-hṛdaya saṁhitāyāṁ sutra-sthāne rogānutpādanīyo-nāma caturthodhyāyaḥ

iti - this; śrī vaidyapati simhagupta sūnu - the son of Śrī vaidyapati Simhagupta; śrī Vāgbhaṭa viracitāyām - composed by Śrī Vāgbhaṭa; aṣṭāṅga-hṛdaya saṁhitāyāṁ - of the aṣṭāṅga hṛdaya samhita; sūtra-sthāne - of the Sūtra sthāna; rogānutpādanīyo-nāma - named rogānutpādanīyam; caturthodhyāyaḥ - the fourth chapter

Translation

This is the fourth chapter of the *Sūtra sthāna* of the *Aṣṭāṅga Hrdaya Samhita*, named "Prevention of Diseases," composed by *Śrī* Vāgbhaṭa, the son of *Śrī vaidyapati Simhagupta*.

1. *Vasti* cannot be literally called enema, since the effects are different. Enema intends only a local cleansing effect, but *vasti* has an effect on the entire system.
2. This is a condition where there is vomiting/regurgitation of salty, watery liquid (*Āyurvedarasāyana* commentary).
3. Alkaline-soluble residue made from ash of burned herbs.
4. *Kāma-krodha bhyādyāśca...*—this is another variation of this verse [end of review]

Topics in the Chapter

Thirteen urges not to be suppressed—4.1

Disorders due to suppression of flatus—4.2

Disorders due to the suppression of fecal urge—4.3 to 4a

Disorders due to the suppression of urinary (micturition) urge—4.4b to 5a

Treatment of diseases due to suppressing the urge of flatus, feces, and urine—4.5 to 6a

Treatment of the suppression of urination—4.6b to 7

Suppression of belching and treatment—4.8

Suppression of sneezing and treatment—4.9 to 10a

Suppression of thirst—4.10b to 11a

Suppression of hunger and treatment—4.11b to 12a

Suppression of sleep—4.12a

Suppression of cough and treatment—4.13b to 14a

Suppression of heaving (panting) and treatment—4.14b to 15a

Suppression of yawning—4.15b

Suppression of tears—4.16

Suppression of vomiting urge and treatment—4.17 to 19a

Suppression of seminal urge—4.19b to 21a

When to reject curative options—4.21b

Vāta aggravation is the result of all suppression of urges—4.22, 23

Urges to be controlled—4.23b to 24a

Importance of seasonal cleansing—4.25, 26

Rejuvenation and strengthening after cleansing—4.27

The sequence of purification, nourishment, and rejuvenation—4. 28 to 30

Āgantu rogaḥ: diseases due to external causes—4.31

To prevent endogenous and exogenous diseases—4.32

Nontouch therapies—4.33

Pacifying both manifested and unmanifested diseases—4.34

Cleanse on time to avoid diseases originating due to season changes—4.35

Formula for freedom from all diseases—4.36

Notes

Notes

Notes

Notes

Author contact information:

Dr Sanjay Pisharodi welcomes your valuable feedback, comments, and suggestions about this book. Please feel free to write to him at contact@purnarogya.com
He also has a facebook group - "Acharya Vagbhata's Ashtanga Hridayam" - where you can ask doubts related to this book and also discuss some interesting case studies
Facebook page: Purnarogya Holistic Health Care
Website: www.purnarogya.com
He is the founder and director of Purnarogya Holistic Health Care and Research Pvt Ltd, which is an academy for advanced studies in Āyurveda and a Holistic healing center for different kinds of ailments. He is also involved in teaching Online classes on Ashtanga Hridayam to students around the world.

Appendix 1

Sanskrit Verse Index

Appendix 2

For daily śloka recitation

Chapter 1

Invocation of auspiciousness

रागादिरोगान् सततानुषक्तानशेषकायप्रसृतानशेषान्
औत्सुक्यमोहारतिदान् जघान योऽपूर्ववैद्याय नमोस्तुतस्मैः ॥१॥
rāgādi-rogān satatānuṣaktān-
aśeṣa-kāya-prasṛtān-aśeṣān
autsukya-mohāratidān jaghāna
yo'pūrva-vaidyāya namo'stu-tasmai //1//

Name of chapter & Blessings of the sages

अथात आयुष्कामीयमध्यायं व्याख्यास्यामः
इति ह स्माहुरात्रेयादयो महर्षयः ॥ *गद्य सूत्रम्* १॥
athāta āyuṣkāmīyam-adhyāyaṁ vyākhyāsyāmaḥ
iti ha smāhur-ātreyādayo maharṣayaḥ // prose 1//

Purpose of *āyurveda*

आयुःकामायमानेन धर्मार्थसुखसाधनम् ।
आयुर्वेदोपदेशेषु विधेयः परमादरः॥२॥
āyuḥ-kāmayamānena dharmārtha-sukha-sādhanam
āyurvedopadeśeṣu vidheyaḥ paramādaraḥ //2//

Āyurvedāgamanam - Advent of *āyurveda*

ब्रह्मा स्मृत्वायुषोवेदं प्रजापतिमजिग्रहत् ।
सोऽश्विनौ तौ सहस्राक्षं सोऽत्रिपुत्रादिकान्मुनीन् ॥३॥
तेऽग्निवेशादिकांस्ते तु पृथक् तन्त्राणि तेनिरे ।

brahmā smṛtvāyuṣo-vedaṁ prajāpatim-ajigrahat
so'śvinau tau sahasrākṣaṁ so'tri-putrādikān-munīn //3//
te'gniveśādikāṁste tu pṛthak tantrāṇi tenire //4a//

Why was the *aṣṭāṅga hṛdayam* written

तेभ्योऽतिविप्रकीर्णेभ्यः प्रायः सारतरोच्चयः॥४॥
क्रियतेऽष्टाङ्गहृदयं नातिसंक्षेपविस्तरम् ।

tebhyo'ti-viprakīrṇebhyaḥ prāyaḥ sārataroccayaḥ //4//
kriyate'ṣṭāṅga-hṛdayam nāti-saṅkṣepa-vistaram

Eight branches of *āyurveda*

कायबालग्रहोर्ध्वाङ्गशल्यदंष्ट्राजरावृषान् ॥५॥
अष्टावङ्गानि तस्याहुश्चिकित्सा येषु संश्रिताः ।

kāya-bāla-grahordhvānga-śalya-daṁṣṭrā-jarā-vṛṣāṅ //5//
aṣṭāvaṅgāni tasyāhuś-cikitsā yeṣu saṁśritāḥ

Three *doṣas* maintain and destroy the body

वायुः पित्तं कफश्चेति त्रयो दोषाः समासतः॥६॥
विकृताऽविकृता देहं घ्नन्ति ते वर्तयन्ति च ।

vāyu pittaṁ kaphaśceti trayo doṣāḥ samāsataḥ //6//
vikṛtā 'vikṛtāḥ dehaṁ ghnanti te vartayanti ca

The predominant locations of three *doṣas* in body / Predominant *doṣa* periods related to age, day, night & digestion

ते व्यापिनोऽपि हृन्नाभ्योरधोमध्योर्ध्वसंश्रयाः॥७॥
वयोऽहोरात्रिभुक्तानां तेऽन्तमध्यादिगाः क्रमात् ।

te vyāpino 'pi hṛnnābhyor-adho-madhyordhva-saṁśrayāḥ //7//
vayo'ho-rātri-bhuktānāṁ te'nta-madhyādigāḥ kramāt

4 types of fires (*agni)*

तैर्भवेद्विषमस्तीक्ष्णो मन्दश्चाग्निः समैः समः॥८॥

tair-bhaved-viṣamas-tīkṣṇo mandaś-cāgniḥ samai samaḥ //8//

Three types of channels - *koṣthas)*

कोष्ठः क्रूरो मृदुर्मध्यो मध्यः स्यात्तैः समैरपि ॥९॥

koṣṭhaḥ krūro mṛdur-madhyo madhyaḥ syāttaiḥ samair-api

prakṛtiḥ (Individual body constitution)

शुक्रार्तवस्थैर्जन्मादौ विषेणेव विषक्रिमेः॥९॥

तैश्च तिस्रः प्रकृतयो हीनमध्योत्तमाः पृथक् ।

समधातुः समस्तासु श्रेष्ठा निन्द्या द्विदोषजाः॥१०॥

śukrārtava-sthair-janmādau viṣeṇeva viṣakrimeḥ //9//
taiśca tisraḥ prakṛtayo hīna-madhyottamāḥ pṛthak
samadhātuḥ samastāsu śreṣṭhā nindyā dvidoṣajāḥ //10//

Qualities of three *doṣas* 11-12

Qualities of *vāta*

तत्र रूक्षो लघुः शीतः खरः सूक्ष्मचलोऽनिलः॥११॥

tatra rūkṣo laghu śītaḥ kharaḥ sūkṣmaś-calo 'nilaḥ

Qualities of *pitta*

पित्तं सस्नेहतीक्ष्णोष्णं लघु विस्रं सरं द्रवम् ॥११॥

pittaṁ sasneha tīkṣṇoṣṇaṁ laghu visraṁ saraṁ dravaṁ //11//

Qualities of *kapha*

स्निग्धः शीतो गुरुर्मन्दः श्लक्ष्णो मृत्स्नः स्थिरः कफः॥१२॥

snigdhaḥ śīto gurur mandaḥ ślakṣṇo mṛtsnaḥ sthiraḥ kaphaḥ

Types of imbalances

संसर्गः सन्निपातश्च तद्द्वित्रिक्षयकोपतः॥१२॥

samsargaḥ sannipātaśca tad-dvi-tri-kṣaya-kopataḥ //12//

Seven *dhātūs* (also known as *dūṣyas*)

रसासृङ्मांसमेदोऽस्थिमज्जशुक्राणि धातवः॥ १ ३॥

rasāsṛṇg-māṁsa-medo-'sthi majja-śukrāni dhātavaḥ

Three *malās*

सप्त दूष्याः मला मूत्रशकृत्स्वेदादयोऽपि च ॥ १ ३॥

sapta dūṣyāḥ malāḥ mūtra śakṛt svedādayo 'pi ca //13//

Increase and decrease of *doṣa*

वृद्धिः समानैः सर्वेषां विपरीतैर्विपर्ययः॥ १ ४।

vṛddhiḥ samānaiḥ sarveṣāṁ viparītair-viparyayaḥ

Six tastes enumerated

रसाःस्वाद्वम्ललवणतिक्तोषणकषायकाः॥ १ ४॥

षड् द्रव्यमाश्रितास्ते च यथापूर्वंबलावहाः॥ १ ५॥

rasāḥ svādvamla-lavaṇa-tiktoṣaṇa-kaṣāyakāḥ //14//

ṣaḍ dravyam- āśritāste ca yathā-pūrvaṁ-balāvahāḥ

How the six tastes affect the *doṣās*

तत्राद्या मारुतं घ्नन्ति त्रयस्तिक्तादयः कफम् ॥ १ ५॥

कषायतिक्तमधुराः पित्तमन्ये तु कुर्वते ॥ १ ६॥

tatrādyā mārutaṁ ghnanti trayas tiktādayaḥ kaphaṁ //15//

kaṣāya-tikta madhurāḥ pitta-manye tu kurvate

Three kinds of substances *(dravya)*

शमनं कोपनं स्वस्थहितं द्रव्यमिति त्रिधा ॥ १ ६॥

śamanaṁ kopanaṁ svastha hitaṁ dravyamiti tridhā //16//

Two types of potencies *(vīrya)*

उष्णशीतगुणोत्कर्षात्तत्र वीर्यं द्विधा स्मृतम् ॥ १ ७॥

uṣṇa śīta guṇotkarṣāt tatra vīryaṁ dvidhā smṛtaṁ

Three kinds of post digestive effects *(vipākaḥ)*

त्रिधा विपाको द्रव्यस्य स्वाद्वम्लकटुकात्मकः॥१७॥

tridhā vipāko dravyasya svādvamla katukātmakaḥ //17//

Twenty basic qualities (*guṇāḥ*)

गुरुमन्दहिमस्निग्धश्लक्ष्णसान्द्रमृदुस्थिराः॥१८॥

गुणाः ससूक्ष्मविशदा विंशतिः सविपर्ययाः॥१८॥

guru-manda-hima-snigdha-ślakṣṇa-sāndra-mṛdu-sthirāḥ
guṇāḥ sa-sūkṣma-viśadā viṁśatiḥ sa-viparyayāḥ //18//

Three causes of disease and health

कालार्थकर्मणां योगो हीनमिथ्यातिमात्रकः॥१९॥

सम्यग्योगश्च विज्ञेयो रोगारोग्यैककारणम्॥१९।

kālārtha-karmaṇāṁ yogo hīna-mithyāti-mātrakaḥ
samyag-yogaś-ca vijñeyo rogārogyaika-kāraṇaṁ //19//

Definition of disease and health

Two types of diseases - based on origin

रोगास्तु दोषवैषम्यं, दोषसाम्यमरोगता॥२०॥

निजागन्तुविभागेन तत्र रोगा द्विधा स्मृताः॥२०॥

rogastu doṣa vaiṣamyaṁ doṣa-sāmyam-arogatā
nijāgantu vibhāgena tatra rogā dvidhā smṛtāḥ //20//

Foundation of disease *(rogāḍhiṣṭhānam)*

तेषां कायमनोभेदादधिष्ठानमपि द्विधा॥२१

teṣām kāya-mano-bhedād-adhiṣthānam-api dvidhā

Two kinds of *doṣas* of the mind *(mānasika doṣa)*

रजस्तमश्च मनसो द्वौ च दोषावुदाहृतौ॥२१॥

rajas-tamas-ca manaso dvau ca doṣāvudāhṛtau //21//

Examination of patient (*rogi parīkṣā*)

दर्शनस्पर्शनप्रश्नैः परीक्षेत च रोगिणम्॥२२॥

darśana-sparśana-praśnaiḥ parīkṣeta ca rogiṇaṁ

Examination of disease (*roga parīkṣā*) - *nidāna pañcakam*

रोगं निदानप्राग्रूपलक्षणोपशयाप्तिभिः॥२२॥

rogaṁ nidāna-prāgrūpa-lakṣaṇopaśayāptibhiḥ //22//

Three kinds of lands or countries *(deśa)*

भूमिदेहप्रभेदेन देशमाहुरिह द्विधा॥२३॥

जाङ्गलं वातभूयिष्ठमानूपं तु कफोल्बणम्॥२३॥

साधारणं सममलं त्रिधा भूदेशमादिशेत्॥२४॥

bhūmi-deha-prabhedena deśamāhur iha dvidhā

jāṇgalaṁ vāta-bhūyiṣṭhaṁ-ānūpaṁ tu kapholbaṇaṁ //23//

sādhāraṇaṁ sama-malaṁ tridhā bhūdeśam-ādiśet

Determining the right timing for therapies and medicines

क्षणादिर्व्याध्यवस्था च कालो भेषजयोगकृत्॥२४॥

kṣaṇādir-vyādhy-avasthā ca kālo bheṣaja-yoga-kṛt //24//

Two kinds of treatments

शोधनं शमनं चेति समासादौषधं द्विधा॥२५॥

śodhanaṁ śamanaṁ ceti samāsād-auṣadhaṁ dvidhā

Three kinds of therapies for *doṣās* in the body

शरीरजानां दोषाणां क्रमेण परमौषधम्॥२५॥

वस्तिर्विरेको वमनं तथा तैलं घृतं मधु॥२६॥

śarīrajānāṁ doṣāṇāṁ krameṇa param-auṣadhaṁ

vastir-vireko vamanaṁ tathā tailaṁ ghṛtaṁ madhu

Three therapies for the *doṣas* of the mind

धीधैर्यात्मादिविज्ञानं मनोदोषौषधं परम्॥ २६॥

dhī-dhairyātmādi-vijñānaṁ mano-doṣauṣadhaṁ paraṁ

Four limbs of treatment

भिषक् द्रव्याण्युपस्थाता रोगी पादचतुष्टयम्॥ २७॥

चिकित्सितस्य निर्दिष्टं, प्रत्येकं तच्चतुर्गुणम्॥ २७॥

bhiṣak dravyāṇyupasthātā rogī pāda-catuṣṭayam
cikitsitasya nirdiṣṭaṁ pratyekaṁ taccatur-guṇam //27//

Qualities of physician and other limbs of treatment

दक्षस्तीर्थात्तशास्त्रार्थो दृष्टकर्मा शुचिर्भिषक्॥ २८॥

बहुकल्पं बहुगुणं सम्पन्नं योग्यमौषधम्॥ २८॥

dakṣas-tīrthātta-śāstrārthe dṛṣṭa-karmā śucir-bhiṣak
bahukalpaṁ bahuguṇaṁ sampannaṁ yogyam-auṣadhaṁ //28/

Four qualities of a nurse

अनुरक्तः शुचिर्दक्षो बुद्धिमान् परिचारकः॥ २९।

anuraktaḥ śucir-dakṣo buddhimān paricārakaḥ

Four qualities of patient

आढ्यो रोगी भिषग्वश्यो ज्ञापकः सत्त्ववानपि॥ २९॥

āḍhyo rogī bhiṣag-vaśyo jñāpakaḥ sattvavān-api //29//

Prognosis of diseases

साध्योऽसाध्य इति व्याधिर्द्विधा, तौ तु पुनर्द्विधा॥

सुसाध्यः कृच्छ्रसाध्यश्च, याप्यो यश्चानुपक्रमः॥

sādhyo'sādhya iti vyādhir-dvidhā tau tu punar-dvidhā
susādhyaḥ kṛcchra-sādhyaśca yāpyo-yaścānupakramaḥ

Features of curability and incurability:

Factors suggesting good prognosis

सर्वौषधक्षमे देहे यूनः पुंसो जितात्मनः॥ ३०॥

अमर्मगोऽल्पहेत्वग्ररूपरूपोऽनुपद्रवः॥ ३०॥

sarvauṣadha-kṣame dehe-yūnaḥ puṁso jitātmanaḥ

amarmago'lpa-hetvagra-rūpa-rūpo'nupadravaḥ //30//

Factors suggesting good prognosis (contd...)

अतुल्यदूष्यदेशर्तुप्रकृतिः पादसम्पदि॥ ३१॥

ग्रहेष्वनुगुणेष्वेकदोषमार्गो नवः सुखः॥ ३१॥

atulya-dūṣya-deśa-ṛtu-prakṛtiḥ pāda-sampadi

graheṣv-anuguṇeṣv-eka-doṣa-mārgo navaḥ sukhaḥ //31//

Difficult prognosis:

Curable with difficulty & Incurable but manageable diseases

(*kṛcchra sādhya & yāpya*)

शस्त्रादिसाधनः कृच्छ्रः सङ्करे च ततो गदः॥ ३२॥

शेषत्वादायुषो याप्यः पथ्याभ्यासाद्विपर्यये॥ ३२॥

śastrādi-sādhanaḥ kṛcchraḥ saṅkare ca tato gadaḥ

śeṣatvād-āyuṣo-yāpyaḥ pathyābhyāsād-viparyaye //32//

Incurable & fatal diseases (*anupakrama*)

अनुपक्रम एव स्यात्स्थितोऽत्यन्तविपर्यये॥ ३३॥

औत्सुक्यमोहारतिकृद् दृष्टरिष्टोऽक्षनाशनः॥ ३३॥

anupakrama eva syāt-sthito'tyanta-viparyaye

autsukya-mohārati-kṛd dṛṣṭariṣṭo'kṣa-nāśanaḥ //33//

Situations when patients may be avoided

त्यजेदार्तं भिषग्भूपैर्द्विष्टं तेषां द्विषं द्विषम्॥ ३४॥

हीनोपकरणं व्यग्रमविधेयं गतायुषम्॥ ३४॥

चण्डं शोकातुरं भीरुं कृतघ्नं वैद्यमानिनम्॥ ३५॥

tyajedārta bhiṣag-bhūpair-dviṣṭaṁ teṣāṁ dviṣaṁ dviṣaṁ

hīnopakaraṇaṁ vyagram-avidheyaṁ gatāyuṣaṁ //34//
caṇḍaṁ śokāturaṁ bhīruṁ kṛtaghnaṁ vaidyamāninaṁ

Index of the 120 chapters of *Aṣṭāṅga Hṛdayaṁ*

तन्त्रस्यास्य परं चातो वक्ष्यते'ध्यायसङ्ग्रहः॥ ३५॥
tantrasyāsya param cāto vakṣyate'dhyāya-sangrahaḥ //35//

Section 1: sūtrasthānam: 36 to 39

आयुष्कामदिनर्त्वीहारोगानुत्पादनद्रवाः॥ ३६॥
अन्नज्ञानान्नसंरक्षामात्राद्रव्यरसाश्रयाः॥ ३६॥
āyuṣkāma-dina-rtvīhā rogānutpādana-dravāḥ
annajñānānnarasaṁ-rakṣā mātrā-dravya-rasāśrayāḥ //36//
दोषादिज्ञानतद्भेदतच्चिकित्साद्युपक्रमाः॥ ३७॥
शुद्ध्यादिस्नेहनस्वेदरेकास्थापननावनम्॥ ३७॥
doṣādi-jñāna-tad-bheda-tac-chikitsā-dvyupakramāḥ
śudhyādi-snehana-sveda-rekāsthāpana-nāvanaṁ //37//
धूमगण्डूषदृक्सेकतृप्तियन्त्रकशस्त्रकम्॥ ३८॥
सिराविधिः शल्यविधिः शस्त्रक्षाराग्निकर्मिकौ॥ ३८॥
dhūma-gaṇḍūṣa-dṛk-seka tṛpti-yantraka-śastrakaṁ
sirā-vidhi-śalya-vidhi śastra-kṣārāgni-karmikau //38//
सूत्रस्थानमिमेऽध्यायास् त्रिम्शत् ....
sūtrasthānam-ime'dhyāyās-trimśat ....

Section 2: śārīra sthānam

......................................शारीरमुच्यते॥ ३९॥
गर्भावक्रान्तितद्व्यापदङ्गमर्मविभागिकम्॥ ३९
विक्रितर् दूतजम् षष्टम् ....
.... śārīram-ucyate
garbhāvakrānti-tad-vyāpad-aṅga-marma-vibhāgikaṁ //39//
vikṛtir-dūtajaṁ ṣaṣṭham ....

Section 3: nidāna sthānam

................................निदानं सार्वरोगिकम्॥४०॥

ज्वरासृक्श्वासयक्ष्मादिमदाद्यर्शोतिसारिणाम्॥४०॥

मूत्राघातप्रमेहाणां विद्रध्याद्युदरस्य च॥४१॥

पाण्डुकुष्ठानिलार्तानां वातास्रस्य च षोडश्च॥४१॥

... nidānaṁ sārvarogikaṁ

jvarā-sṛk-śvāsa-yakṣmādi-madādy-arśo-'tisāriṇāṁ //40//

mūtrāghāta-pramehāṇāṁ vidradhyādy-udarasya ca

pāṇḍu-kuṣṭhānilārtānāṁ vātāsrasya ca ṣoḍaśa //41//

Section 4: cikitsā sthānam. 42 & 43

चिकित्सितं ज्वरे रक्ते कासे श्वासे च यक्ष्मणि॥४२॥

वमौ मदात्ययेऽर्शःसु विशि द्वौ द्वौ च मूत्रिते॥४२॥

विद्रधौ गुल्मजठरपाण्डुशोफविसर्पिषु॥४३॥

कुष्ठश्वित्रानिलव्याधिवातास्रेषु चिकित्सितम्॥४३॥

द्वाविंशतिरिमेऽध्यायाः ....

cikitsitaṁ jvare rakte kāse śvāse ca yakṣmaṇi

vamau madātyaye-'rśaḥsu viśi dvau dvau ca mūtrite //42//

vidradhau gulma-jaṭhara-pāṇḍu-śopha-visarpiṣu

kuṣṭha-śvitrānila-vyādhi- vātāsreṣu-cikitsitaṁ //43//

dvāvimśatir-ime-'dhyāyāḥ ....

Section 5: kalpa siddhi sthāna

.... कल्पसिद्धिरतः परम् ॥४४॥

कल्पो वमेर्विरेकस्य तत्सिद्धिर्वस्तिकल्पना॥४४॥

सिद्धिर्वस्त्यापदां षष्ठो द्रव्यकल्पोऽत उत्तरम्॥४५॥

.... kalpasiddhir-ataḥ paraṁ

kalpo vamor-virekasya tat-siddhir-vasti-kalpanā //44//

siddhir-vastyāpadāṁ ṣaṣṭho dravya-kalpo'ta uttaraṁ

Section 6*: uttara sthāna:* 45 to 48

बालोपचारे तद्व्याधौ तद्ग्रहे, द्वौ च भूतगे॥४५॥

जन्मादेऽथ स्मृतिभ्रंशे द्वौ द्वौ वर्त्मसु सन्धिषु॥४६॥

दृक्तमोलिङ्गनाशेषु त्रयो द्वौ द्वौ च सर्वगे॥४६॥

bālopacāre tad-vyādhau tad-grahe dvau ca bhūtage //45//
unmāde'tha smṛti-bhraṁśe dvau dvau vartmasu sandhiṣu
dṛk-tamo-liṅganāśeṣu trayo ....

कर्णनासामुखशिरोव्रणे भङ्गे भगन्दरे॥४७॥

ग्रन्थ्यादौ क्षुद्ररोगेषु च गुह्यरोगे पृथग्द्वयम्॥४७॥

..dvau dvau ca sarvage //46//
karṇa-nāsā-mukha-śiro-vraṇe bhaṅge-bhagandare
granthyādau kṣudra-rogeṣu ca guhyaroge pṛthak-dvayaṁ //47//

विषे भुजङ्गे कीटेषु च मूषकेषु रसायने॥४८॥

चत्वारिंशोऽनपत्यानामध्यायो बीजपोषणः॥४८॥

viṣe bhujaṅge kīṭeṣu ca mūṣakeṣu rasāyane
catvāriṁśo'napatyānām-adhyāyo bīja-poṣaṇaḥ //48//

इत्यध्यायशतं विंशं षड्भिः स्थानैरुदीरितम् ॥४८ १/२॥

ityadhyāya-śataṁ viṁśaṁ ṣadbhiḥ sthānair-udīritam //48 ½ //

Chapter 2

अथातो दिनचर्याध्यायं व्याख्यास्यामः ।

इति ह स्माहुरात्रेयादयो महर्षयः ॥

athāto dinacaryādhyāyam vyākhyāsyāmaḥ
iti ha smāhur-ātreyādayo maharṣayaḥ

Time of waking up from sleep

ब्राह्मे मुहूर्त उत्तिष्ठेत्स्वस्थो रक्षार्थमायुषः ॥१॥

brāhme muhūrte uttiṣṭhet svastho rakṣārtham āyuṣaḥ

What to do immediately upon rising

शरीरचिन्तां निर्वर्त्य कृतशौचविधिस्ततः ॥१॥
śarīra cintāṁ nirvartya kṛta śauca vidhis-tataḥ //1//

Herbs used for cleansing oral cavity

अर्कन्यग्रोधखदिरकरञ्जककुभादिजम् ॥२॥
प्रातर्भुक्त्वा च मृद्वग्रं कषायकटुतिक्तकम् ॥२॥
arka nyagrodha khadira karañja kakubhādijam
prātar-bhuktvā ca mṛdvagraṁ kaṣāya kaṭu tiktakam //2//

Size of the brush twig and method of brushing

कनीन्यग्रसमस्थौल्यं प्रगुणं द्वादशाङ्गुलम् ॥३॥
भक्षयेद्दन्तपवनं दन्तमांसान्यबाधयन् ॥३॥
kanīny-agra-sama sthaūlyaṁ praguṇaṁ dvādaśāṅgulam
bhakṣayed-danta-pavanaṁ danta-māmsāny-abādhayan //3//

Contraindications for brushing teeth

नाद्यादजीर्णवमथुश्वासकासज्वरार्दिती ॥४॥
तृष्णास्यपाकहृन्नेत्रशिरःकर्णामयी च तत् ॥४॥
nādyād-ajīrṇa-vamathu śvāsa-kāsa jvarārditī /
tṛṣṇāsya-pāka-hṛn-netra-śiraḥ karṇāmayī ca tat //4//

Eye care

सौवीरमञ्जनं नित्यं हितमक्ष्णोस्ततो भजेत् ॥५॥
लोचने तेन भवतः सुस्निग्ध घनपक्ष्मणी ॥५॥
व्यक्त त्रिवर्णे विमले मनोज्ञे सूक्ष्म दर्शने
sauvīram-añjanaṁ nityaṁ hitam-akṣṇos-tato bhajet
locane tena bhavātaḥ susnigdha-ghanapakṣmaṇī //5//
vyakta-trivarṇe vimale manojñe sūkṣma-darśane

Protecting the eyes from excess *kapha*

चक्षुस्तेजोमयं तस्य विशेषात् श्लेष्मतो भयम् ॥६॥
योजयेत्सप्तरात्रेस्मात्स्रावणार्थं रसाञ्जनम्
cakṣus-tejomayaṁ tasya viśeṣāt śleṣmato bhayam //6//
yojayet sapta-rātre 'smāt srāvaṇārtham rasāñjanam
ततो नावनगण्डूषधूमताम्बूलभाग्भवेत् ॥७॥
tato nāvana-gaṇḍūṣa-dhūma-tāmbūla-bhāg-bhavet //6//

Contraindications for chewing betel leaf

ताम्बूलं क्षतपित्तास्ररूक्षोत्कुपितचक्षुषाम् ॥८॥
विषमूर्च्छामदार्तानामपथ्यं शोषिणामपि ॥८॥
tāmbūlaṁ kṣata pittāsra rūkṣotkupita cakṣuṣām
viṣa mūrcchā madārtānām apathyaṁ śoṣiṇām api //7//

Benefits of body massage - with oil

अभ्यङ्गमाचरेन्नित्यं, स जराश्रमवातहा ॥९॥
दृष्टिप्रसादपुष्ट्यायुःस्वप्नसुत्वक्त्वदार्ढ्यकृत् ॥९॥
abhyañgam ācaren-nityaṁ sa jarā-śrama-vātahā
dṛṣti-prasāda-puṣtyāyuḥ-svapna-sutvaktva dārḍhya kṛt //8//

Where to massage?

शिरःश्रवणपादेषु तं विशेषेण शीलयेत् ॥१०॥
śiraḥ śravaṇa pādeṣu taṁ viśeṣeṇa śīlayet

Contraindications for massage

वर्ज्योभ्यङ्गः कफग्रस्तकृतसंशुद्ध्यजीर्णिभिः ॥१०॥
varjyo 'bhyaṅgaḥ kapha-grasta kṛta saṁśuddhy-ajīrṇibhiḥ //9//

Benefits of Exercise

लाघवं कर्मसामर्थ्यं दीप्तोग्निर्मेदसः क्षयः ॥११॥
विभक्तघनगात्रत्वं व्यायामादुपजायते ॥११॥
lāghavaṁ karma-sāmarthyaṁ dīpto 'gnir-medasaḥ kṣayaḥ
vibhakta-ghana-gātratvaṁ vyāyāmād-upajāyate //10//

Those who should avoid exercise

वातपित्तामयी बालो वृद्धोजीर्णी च तं त्यजेत् ॥१२॥

vāta pittāmayī bālo vṛddho'jīrṇī ca taṁ tyajet

How much, who should exercise and when

अर्धशक्त्या निषेव्यस्तु बलिभिः स्निग्धभोजिभिः ॥१२॥

शीतकाले वसन्ते च, मन्दमेव ततोन्यदा ॥१३॥

aṛdha-śaktyā niṣevyastu balibhiḥ snigdha-bhojibhiḥ
śīta-kāle vasante ca, mandam-eva tato'nyadā //11//

What to do after exercise

तं कृत्वानुसुखं देहं मर्दयेच्च समन्ततः ॥१३॥

taṁ kṛtvā 'nusukhaṁ dehaṁ mardayecca samantataḥ //12//

Consequences of too much exercise

तृष्णा क्षयः प्रतमको रक्तपित्तं श्रमः क्लमः ॥१४॥

अतिव्यायामतः कासो ज्वरच्छर्दिश्च जायते ॥१४॥

tṛṣṇā kṣayaḥ pratamako rakta pittaṁ śramaḥ klamaḥ
ativyāyāmataḥ kāso jvara cchardiśca jāyate //13//

Causes of untimely death

व्यायामजागराध्वस्त्रीहास्यभाष्यादि साहसम् ॥१५॥

गजं सिंह इवाकर्षन् भजन्नति विनश्यति ॥१५॥

vyāyāma jāgarādhva-strī hāsya bhāṣyādi sāhasaṁ
gajaṁ siṁha ivākarṣan bhajannati vinaśyati //14//

udvartanam (dry powder massage)

उद्वर्तनं कफहरं मेदसः प्रविलायनम् ॥१६॥

स्थिरीकरणमङ्गानां त्वक्प्रसादकरं परम् ॥१६॥

udvartanaṁ kaphaharaṁ medasaḥ pravilāyanaṁ
sthirīkaraṇam aṅgānāṁ tvak prasāda-karaṁ param //15//

snānaṁ (benefits of bathing)

दीपनं वृष्यमायुष्यं स्नानमूर्जाबलप्रदम् ॥१७॥
कण्डूमलश्रमस्वेदतन्द्रातृड्दाहपाप्मजित् ॥१७॥
dīpanaṁ vṛṣyam-āyuṣyaṁ snānam-ūrjā-balapradam
kaṇḍū-mala-śrama-sveda-tandrā-tṛṅg-dāha pāpmajit //16//

Usage of hot water for bathing

उष्णाम्बुनाऽधःकायस्य परिषेको बलावहः ॥१८॥
तेनैव तूत्तमाङ्गस्य बलहृत्केशचक्षुषाम् ॥१८॥
uṣṇāmbunā 'dhaḥ kāyasya pariṣeko balāvahaḥ
tenaiva-tūttamāṅgasya bala hṛt-keśa cakṣuṣām //17//

Those who should not bathe: contraindications

स्नानमर्दितनेत्रास्यकर्णरोगातिसारिषु ॥१९॥
आध्मानपीनसाजीर्णभुक्तवत्सु च गर्हितम् ॥१९॥
snānam-ardita netrāsya karṇa rogātisāriṣu
ādhmāna pīnasājīrṇa bhukta-vatsu ca garhitam //18//

Good eating and bowel habit

जीर्णो हितं मितं चाद्यान्नवेगानीरयेद्बलात् ॥२०॥
न वेगितोऽन्यकार्यः स्यान्नाजित्वा साध्यमामयम् ॥२०॥
jīrṇe hitaṁ mitaṁ cādyānnavegān-īrayed-balāt
na vegito 'nya-kāryaḥ syāt nājitvā sādhyam-āmayam //19//

Occupation, friends, others

सुखार्थाः सर्वभूतानां मताः सर्वाः प्रवृत्तयः ॥२१॥
सुखं च न विना धर्मात्तस्माद्धर्मपरो भवेत् ॥२१॥
भक्त्या कल्याणमित्राणि सेवेतेतरदूरगः ॥२२॥
sukhārthāḥ sarva bhūtānāṁ matāḥ sarvāḥ pravṛttayaḥ
sukhaṁ ca na vinā dharmāt tasmād dharma-paro bhavet //20//
bhaktyā kalyāṇa mitrāṇi sevet-etara dūragaḥ

10 sins to strictly avoid:

हिंसास्तेयान्यथाकामं पैशुन्यं परुषानृते ॥२२॥
सम्भिन्नालापं व्यापादमभिध्यां दृग्विपर्ययम् ॥२३॥
पापं कर्मेति दशधा कायवाङ्मानसैस्त्यजेत् ॥२३॥

hiṁsā-steyānyathā kāmaṁ paiśunyaṁ paruṣānṛte //21//
saṁbhinnālāpaṁ vyāpādam abhidhyā dṛk viparyayaṁ
pāpaṁ karmeti daśadhā kāya vāk mānasais tyajet //22//

People who must be helped

अवृत्तिव्याधिशोकार्तानिनुवर्तेतशक्तितः ॥२४॥
आत्मवत्सततं पश्येदपि कीटपिपीलिकम् ॥२४॥

āvṛtti vyādhi-śokārtān-anuvartet-aśaktitaḥ
ātmavat-satataṁ paśyed-api kīta-pipīlikam //23//

7 kinds of persons to be worshipped

अर्चयेद्देवगोविप्रवृद्धवैद्यनृपातिथीन् ॥२५॥
विमुखान्नार्थिनः कुर्यान्नावमन्येत नाक्षिपेत् ॥२५॥

arcayed-deva-go-vipra-vṛddha-vaidya-nṛpātithīṅ
vimukhān-nārthīnaḥ kuryāt-nāvamanyeta nākṣipet //24//

Helpfulness and envy

उपकारप्रधानः स्यादपकारपरेप्यरौ ॥२६॥
सम्पद्विपत्स्वेकमना, हेतावीर्ष्येत्फले न तु ॥२६॥

upakāra pradhānaḥ syād apakārapare 'pyarau
sampad vipatsv-ekamanā hetāv-īrṣyet-phale na tu //25//

The art of speaking

काले हितं मितं ब्रूयादविसंवादि पेशलम् ॥२७॥
पूर्वाभिभाषी, सुमुखः सुशीलः करुणामृदुः ॥२७॥

नैकः सुखी, न सर्वत्र विश्रब्धो, न च शङ्कितः ॥२८॥

kāle hitaṁ mitaṁ brūyād avisaṁvādi peśalam
pūrvābhibhāṣī sumukhaḥ suśīla karuṇā mṛduḥ
naikaḥ sukhī na sarvatra viśrabdho na ca śaṅkitaḥ //26//

Four things that should be concealed

न कञ्चिदात्मनः शत्रुं नात्मानं कस्यचिद्रिपुम् ॥२८॥
प्रकाशयेन्नापमानं न च निःस्नेहतां प्रभोः ॥२९॥

na kañcid-ātmanaḥ śatruṁ nātmānaṁ kasyacid ripuṁ
prakāśayen-nāpamānaṁ na ca niḥ-snehatāṁ prabhoḥ //27//

How to deal with people in general: to please them

जनस्याशयमालक्ष्य यो यथा परितुष्यति ॥२९॥
तं तथैवानुवर्तेत पराराधनपण्डितः ॥३०॥

janasyāśayam ālakṣya yo yathā parituṣyati
taṁ tathaivānuvarteta parārādhana paṇḍitaḥ //28//

The Golden Mean

न पीडयेदिन्द्रियाणि न चैतान्यतिलालयेत् ॥३०॥
त्रिवर्गशून्यं नारम्भं भजेत्तं चाविरोधयन् ॥३१॥
अनुयायात्प्रतिपदं सर्वधर्मेषु मध्यमाम् ॥३१॥

na pīḍayed-indriyāṇī na-caitāny-atilālayet //29//
trivarga śūnyaṁ nārambhaṁ bhajettaṁ cāvirodhayan
anuyāyāt pratipadaṁ sarva dharmeṣu madhyamām //30//

Norms of personal appearance: hygiene

नीचरोमनखश्मश्रुर्निर्मलाङ्घ्रिमलायनः ॥३२॥
स्नानशीलः सुसुरभिः सुवेषोऽनुल्बणोज्ज्वलः ॥३२॥
धारयेत्सततं रत्नसिद्धमन्त्रमहौषधीः ॥३३॥

nīca roma nakha śmaśru nirmalānghri malāyanaḥ
snāna-śīla susurabhiḥ suveṣo 'nulbaṇojjvalaḥ //31//
dhārayet satataṁ ratna siddha-mantra mahauṣadhīḥ

Rules to be followed before going out at night:

सातपत्रपदत्राणो विचरेद्युगमात्रदृक् ॥३३॥
निशि चात्ययिके कार्ये दण्डी मौली सहायवान् ॥३४॥
sātapatra padatrāṇo vicared-yugamātra-dṛk //32//
niśi cātyayike kārye daṇḍī maulī sahāyavān

11 items to avoid:

चैत्यपूज्यध्वजाशस्तच्छायाभस्मतुषाशुचीन् ॥३४॥
नाक्रामेच्छर्करालोष्टबलिस्नानभुवो न च ॥३५॥
caitya pūjya dhvajāśastac-chāyā bhasma tuṣāśucīn //33//
nā krāmec-charkarā-loṣta bali snāna bhuvo na ca

5 more items to avoid:

नदीं तरेन्न बाहुभ्यां, नाग्निस्कन्धमभिव्रजेत् ॥३५॥
सन्दिग्धनावं वृक्षं च नारोहेद्दुष्टयानवत् ॥३६॥
nadīṁ tarenna bāhubhyāṁ nāgni-skandham-abhivrajet //34//
sandigdha-nāvaṁ vṛkṣaṁ ca nārohed-duṣṭayānavat

7 more items to avoid

नासंवृतमुखः कुर्यात्क्षुतिहास्यविजृम्भणम् ॥३६॥
नासिकां न विकुष्णीयान्नाकस्माद्विलिखेद्भुवम् ॥३७॥
नाङ्गैश्चेष्टेत विगुणं, नासीतोत्कुटकश्चिरम् ॥३७॥
nāsaṁvṛta-mukhaḥ kuryāt-kṣuti-hāsya-vijṛmbhaṇam //35//
nāsikāṁ na vikuṣṇīyān-nākasmād-vilikhed-bhuvam
naṅgaiś-ceṣṭeta viguṇaṁ nāsītotkuṭakaś-ciram //36//

When to stop activities, prolonged squatting, place to avoid for night stay

देहवाक्चेतसां चेष्टाः प्राक् श्रमाद्विनिवर्तयेत् ॥३८॥
नोर्ध्वजानुश्चिरं तिष्ठेत् नक्तं सेवेत न द्रुमम् ॥३८॥
deha-vāk-cetasāṁ ceṣṭāḥ prāk śramād-vinivartayet
nordhva-jānuś-ciram tiṣṭhet naktaṁ seveta na drumam //37//

More places to be avoided in the day as well as night

तथा चत्वरचैत्यान्तश्चतुष्पथसुरालयान् ॥३९॥
सूनाटवीशून्यगृहश्मशानानि दिवापि न ॥३९॥
tathā catvara caityāntaś catuṣpatha surālayān
sūnāṭavī śūnya gṛha śmaśānāni divāpi na //38//

Looking at the sun, carrying weight, protecting eyes

सर्वथेक्षेत नादित्यं, न भारं शिरसा वहेत् ॥४०॥
नेक्षेत प्रततं सूक्ष्मं दीप्तामेध्याप्रियाणि च ॥४०॥
sarvathekṣeta nādityaṁ na bhāraṁ śirasā vahet
nekṣeta pratataṁ sūkṣmaṁ dīpt-āmedhy-āpriyāṇi ca //39//

dealing with alcohol, exposure to natural forces

मद्यविक्रयसन्धानदानपानानि नाचरेत् ॥४१॥
पुरोवातातपरजस्तुषारपरुषानिलान् ॥४१॥
madya vikraya sandhāna dāna-pānāni nācaret
purovāt-ātapa-rajas-tuṣāra paruṣānilān //40//

Avoid awkward body positions & 5 more things to avoid

अनृजुः क्षवथूद्गारकासस्वप्नान्नमैथुनम् ॥४२॥
कूलच्छायां नृपद्विष्टं व्यालदंष्ट्रिविषाणिनः ॥४२॥
anṛjuḥ kṣavathūdgāra kāsa svapnānna maithunam
kūlacchāyāṁ nṛpa dviṣṭam vyāla daṁṣtri viṣāṇinaḥ //41//

Association with different types of people, 5 activities to avoid during sandhya

हीनानार्यातिनिपुणसेवां विग्रहमुत्तमैः ॥४३॥
सन्ध्यास्वभ्यवहारस्त्रीस्वप्नाध्ययनचिन्तनम् ॥४३॥
hīnānāryātinipuṇa-sevāṁ vigraham-uttamaiḥ
sandhyāsv-abhyavahāra-strī-svapnādhyayana-cintanam //42//

Where not to accept food from, avoid making sounds using body parts

शत्रुसत्रगणाकीर्णगणिकापणिकाशनम् ॥४४॥
गात्रवक्त्रनखैर्वाद्यं हस्तकेशावधूननम् ॥४४॥
śatru-satra-gaṇākīrṇa-gaṇikā-paṇikāśanam
gātra-vaktra-nakhair-vādyaṁ hasta-keśāvadhūnanam //43//

6 items to avoid

तोयाग्निपूज्यमध्येन यानं धूमं शवाश्रयम् ॥४५॥
मद्यातिसक्तिं विश्रम्भस्वातन्त्र्ये स्त्रीषु च त्यजेत् ॥४५॥
toyāgni-pūjya-madhyena-yānaṁ dhūmaṁ śavāśrayam
madyātisaktiṁ viśrambha-svātantrye strīṣu ca tyajet //44//
आचार्यः सर्वचेष्टासु लोक एव हि धीमतः ॥४६॥
अनुकुर्यात्तमेवातो लौकिकेर्थे परीक्षकः ॥४६॥
ācāryaḥ sarva-ceṣṭāsu lokaeva hi dhīmataḥ
anukuryāt-tam-evāto laukike'rthe parīkṣakaḥ //45//

Definition of *sadvṛtta*

आर्द्रसन्तानता त्यागः कायवाक्चेतसां दमः ॥४७॥
स्वार्थबुद्धिः परार्थेषु पर्याप्तमिति सद्व्रतम् ॥४७॥
ārdra-santānatā tyāgaḥ kāya-vāk-cetasāṁ damaḥ
svārtha-buddhiḥ parārtheṣu paryāptam-iti sad-vratam //46//

Benediction to one who follows the rules of dinacarya

नक्तंदिनानि मे यान्ति कथम्भूतस्य सम्प्रति ॥४८॥
दुःखभाङ्नभवत्येवं नित्यं सन्निहितस्मृतिः ॥४८॥
naktaṁ dināni me yānti katham-bhūtasya samprati
duḥkha-bhāṅg-na-bhavaty-evaṁ nityaṁ sannihita-smṛtiḥ //47//

इत्याचारः समासेन, यं प्राप्नोति समाचरन् ॥४९॥
आयुरारोग्यमैश्वर्यं यशो लोकांश्च शाश्वतान् ॥४९॥
ityācāraḥ samāsena yaṁ prāpnoti samācaran
āyur-ārogyaṁ-aiśvaryaṁ-yaśo lokāṁśca śāśvatān //48//

इति श्रीवैद्यपतिसिंहगुप्तसूनु श्रीमद्वाग्भटविरचितायामष्टाङ्गहृदयसंहितायां सूत्रस्थाने दिनचर्या नाम द्वितीयोध्यायः ॥
iti śrī vaidyapati siṁhagupta sūnū vāgbhaṭa viracitāyām aṣṭāṅga hṛḍaya samhitāyām sutra sthāne dinacaryā nāma dvitīyodhyāyaḥ

Chapter 3

अथात ऋतुचर्याध्यायं व्याख्यास्यामः
इति ह स्माहुरात्रेयादयो महर्षयः
athāta ṛtucaryādhyāyām vyākhyāsyāmaḥ
iti ha smāhur ātreyādayo maharṣayaḥ

The division of the year into seasons

मासैर्द्विसंख्यैर्माघाद्यैः क्रमात् षड्ऋतवः स्मृताः ॥१॥
शिशिरोथ वसन्तश्च ग्रीष्मो वर्षाशरद्धिमाः ॥१॥
māsair-dvisankhyair-māghādyaiḥ kramāt ṣaḍ ṛtavaḥ smṛtāḥ
śiśiro'tha vasantaśca grīṣma-varṣā-śaraddhimāḥ //1//

uttarāyaṇa (*ādānakāla*) – verses 2 to 4

शिशिराद्यास्त्रिभिस्तैस्तु विद्यादयनमुत्तरम् ॥२॥
आदानं च, तदादत्ते नृणां प्रतिदिनं बलम् ॥२॥

śiśirādyais-tribhis-taistu vidyād-ayanam-uttaram
ādānaṁ ca tad-ādatte nṛṇāṁ pratidinaṁ balam //2//

uttarāyaṇa (*ādāna kāla)* - sun moves in north

तस्मिन् ह्यत्यर्थतीक्ष्णोष्णरूक्षा मार्गस्वभावतः ॥३॥
आदित्यपवनाः सौम्यान् क्षपयन्ति गुणान् भुवः ॥३॥
तिक्तः कषायः कटुको बलिनोत्र रसाः क्रमात् ॥४॥
तस्मादादानमाग्नेयम् ....॥४॥

tasmin-hy-atyartha-tīkṣṇoṣṇa-rūkṣā mārga-svabhāvataḥ
āditya-pavanāḥ saumyān kṣapayanti guṇān bhuvaḥ //3//
tiktaḥ kaṣāyaḥ kaṭuko balino'tra rasāḥ kramāt
tasmād-ādānam-āgneyaṁ ....

dakṣiṇāyana (visarga kāla) – sun moves in south

.... ऋतवो दक्षिणायनम् ॥४॥
वर्षादयो विसर्गश्च यद्बलं विसृजत्ययम् ॥५॥

.... *ṛtavo dakṣiṇāyanam //4//*
varṣādayo visargaśca yad-balaṁ visṛjatyayam

सौम्यत्वादत्र सोमो हि बलवान् हीयते रविः ॥५॥
मेघवृष्ट्यनिलैः शीतैः शान्ततापे महीतले ॥६॥
स्निग्धाश्चेहाम्ललवणमधुरा बलिनो रसाः ॥६॥

saumyatvād-atra somo hy balavān hīyate raviḥ //5//
megha-vṛṣṭy-anilaiḥ śītaiḥ śāntatāpe mahītale
snigdhāścehāmla-lavaṇa-madhurā balino rasāḥ //6//

Bodily strength in the different seasons

शीतेऽग्र्यं वृष्टिघर्मेऽल्पं बलं मध्यं तु शेषयोः ॥७॥

śīte'gryaṁ vṛṣṭi-gharme'lpaṁ balaṁ madhyam tu śeṣayoḥ

hemanta ṛtu (Early Winter)

बलिनः शीतसंरोधाद्धेमन्ते प्रबलोनलः ॥७॥

भवत्यल्पेन्धनो धातून् स पचेद्वायुनेरितः ॥८॥

अतो हिमेस्मिन्सेवेत स्वाद्वम्ललवणान् रसान् ॥८॥

balinaḥ śīta-saṁrodhād hemante prabalo'nalaḥ //7//

bhavaty-alpendhano dhātūn sa paced-vāyuneritaḥ

ato hime'smin seveta svādvamla lavaṇān rasān //8//

Early mornings in early winter (*hemanta*)

दैर्घ्यान्निशानामेतर्हि प्रातरेव बुभुक्षितः ॥९॥

अवश्यकार्यं सम्भाव्य यथोक्तं शीलयेदनु ॥९॥

वातघ्नतैलैरभ्यङ्गं मूर्ध्नि तैलं विमर्दनम् ॥१०॥

नियुद्धं कुशलैः सार्धं पादाघातं च युक्तितः ॥१०॥

dairghyān-niśānām-etarhi prātareva bubhukṣitaḥ

avaśyakāryaṁ saṁbhāvya yathoktaṁ śīlayedanu //9//

vātaghna-tailair-abhyaṅgam mūrdha-tailam vimardanam

niyuddhaṁ kuśalaiḥ sārdhaṁ pādāghātaṁ ca yuktitaḥ //10//

Removing the excess oil after oil massage

कषायापहृतस्नेहस्ततः स्नातो यथाविधि ॥११॥

कुङ्कुमेन सदर्पेण प्रदिग्धोगुरुधूपितः ॥११॥

kaṣāyāpahṛta-snehas-tataḥ snāto yathāvidhi

kuṅkumena sadarpeṇa pradigdho'garu-dhūpitaḥ //11//

Diet for early winter *(hemanta)*

रसान् स्निग्धान् पलं पुष्टं गौडमच्छसुरां सुराम् ॥१२॥
गोधूमपिष्टमाषेक्षुक्षीरोत्थविकृतीः शुभाः ॥१२॥
rasān snigdhān palaṁ puṣṭaṁ gauḍamacchasurāṁ surām
godhūma-piṣṭamāṣ-ekṣu-kṣīrottha-vikṛtīḥ śubhāḥ //12//

Diet, Cleansing & Clothing during winter

नवमन्नं वसां तैलं, शौचकार्ये सुखोदकम् ॥१३॥
प्रावाराजिनकौशेयप्रवेणीकौचवास्तृतम् ॥१३॥
navam-annaṁ vasāṁ tailaṁ śaucakārye sukhodakam
prāvārājina-kauśeya-praveṇī-kauthapāstṛtam //13//

Sleeping, sudation and footwear in winter

उष्णस्वभावैर्लघुभिः प्रावृतः शयनं भजेत् ॥१४॥
युक्त्यार्ककिरणान् स्वेदं पादत्राणं च सर्वदा ॥१४॥
uṣṇa-svabhāvair-laghubhiḥ prāvṛta-śayanaṁ bhajet
yuktyārka-kiraṇān svedaṁ pādatrāṇaṁ ca sarvadā //14//

Utilization of body heat to keep warm

पीवरोरुस्तनश्रोण्यः समदाः प्रमदाः प्रियाः ॥१५॥
हरन्ति शीतमुष्णाङ्ग्यो धूपकुङ्कुमयौवनैः ॥१५॥
pīvaroru-stana-śroṇyaḥ samadāḥ pramadāḥ priyāḥ
haranti śītam-uṣṇāṅgyo dhūpa-kumkuma-yauvanaiḥ //15//

Underground residence regulates temperature

अङ्गारतापसन्तप्तगर्भभूवेश्मचारिणः ॥१६॥
शीतपारुष्यजनितो न दोषो जातु जायते ॥१६॥
aṅgāra-tāpa-santapta-garbha-bhūveśma-cāriṇaḥ
śīta-pāruṣya-janito na doṣo jātu jāyate //16//

śiśira ṛtu (Late winter)

अयमेव विधिः कार्यः शिशिरेपि विशेषतः ॥१७॥
तदा हि शीतमधिकं रौक्ष्यं चादानकालजम् ॥१७॥
ayameva vidhiḥ kāryaḥ śiśire'pi viśeṣataḥ
tadā hi śītam-adhikamraukṣyam cādāna-kālajam //17//

vasanta ṛtu (spring)

कफश्चितो हि शिशिरे वसन्तेर्कांशुतापितः ॥१८॥
हत्वाग्निं कुरुते रोगानतस्तं त्वरया जयेत् ॥१८॥
kaphaścito hi śiśire vasante'rkāṁśu-tāpitaḥ
hatvā'gniṁ kurute rogānantastaṁ tvarayā jayet //18//

Nasal drops, massage, bath, diet, and drinks in spring

तीक्ष्णैर्वमननस्याद्यैर्लघुरूक्षैश्च भोजनैः ॥१९॥
व्यायामोद्वर्तनाघातैर्जित्वा श्लेष्माणमुल्बणम् ॥१९॥
स्नातोनुलिप्तः कर्पूरचन्दनागुरुकुङ्कुमैः ॥२०॥
पुराणयवगोधूमक्षौद्रजाङ्गलशूल्यभुक् ॥२०॥
सहकाररसोन्मिश्रानास्वाद्य प्रिययार्पितान् ॥२१॥
प्रियास्यसङ्गसुरभीन् प्रियानेत्रोत्पलाङ्कितान् ॥२१॥
सौमनस्यकृतो हृद्यान्वयस्यैः सहितः पिबेत् ॥२२॥
निर्गदानासवारिष्टसीधुमार्द्वीकमाधवान् ॥२२॥
शृङ्गबेराम्बु साराम्बु मध्वम्बु जलदाम्बु च ॥२३॥
tīkṣṇair-vamana-nasyādyair-laghu-rūkṣaiśca bhojanaiḥ
vyāyām-odvartan-āghātair-jitvā śleṣmāṇam-ulbaṇam //19//
snāto'nuliptaḥ karpūra-candanāgaru-kuṅkumaiḥ
purāṇa-yava-godhūma-kṣaudra-jāṅgala-śūlya-bhuk //20//
sahakāra-rasonmiśrān-āsvādya priyayā'rpitān
priyāsya-saṅga-surabhīn priyā-netrotpalā'ṅkitān //21//
saunasya-kṛto hṛdyān vayasyaiḥ sahitaḥ pibet

nigadān-āsavāriṣṭa-sīdhu-mārdvīka-mādhavān //22//
śṛṅga-verāmbu sārāṁbu madhvambu jaladāṁbu vā

Dwelling, activities, diet (the "ṣu" śloka)

दक्षिणानिलशीतेषु परितो जलवाहिषु ॥२३॥
अदृष्टनष्टसूर्येषु मणिकुट्टिमकान्तिषु ॥२४॥
परपुष्टविघुष्टेषु कामकर्मान्तभूमिषु ॥२४॥
विचित्रपुष्पवृक्षेषु काननेषु सुगन्धिषु ॥२५॥
गोष्ठीकथाभिश्चित्राभिर्मध्याह्नं गमयेत्सुखी ॥२५॥
dakṣiṇā'nila-śīteṣu parito jalavāhiṣu //23//
adṛṣṭa-naṣṭa-sūryeṣu maṇikuttima-kāntiṣu
parapuṣṭavighuṣṭeṣu kāmakarmānta-bhūmiṣu //24//
vicitra-puṣpa-vṛkṣeṣu kānaneṣu sugandhiṣu
goṣṭī-kathābhiś-citrābhir-madhyāhnam gamayet sukhī //25//

Activities to be avoided

गुरुशीतदिवास्वप्नस्निग्धाम्लमधुरांस्त्यजेत् ॥२६॥
guru-śīta-divāsvapna-snigdhāmla-madhurāms-tyajet

grīṣma ṛtu (summer)

Weakening effect of summer

तीक्ष्णांशुरतितीक्ष्णांशुर्ग्रीष्मे संक्षिपतीव यत् ॥२६॥
प्रत्यहं क्षीयते श्लेष्मा तेन वायुश्च वर्धते ॥२७॥
tīkṣṇāṁśur-atitīkṣṇāṁśu grīṣme saṁkṣipatīva yat //26//
pratyahaṁ kṣīyate śleṣmā tena vāyuśca vardhate

अतोऽस्मिन्पटुकट्वम्लव्यायामार्ककरांस्त्यजेत् ॥२७॥
ato'smin paṭu kaṭvamla vyāyāmārka karāṁs tyajet //27//

Qualities of foods consumed in summer

भजेन्मधुरमेवान्नं लघु स्निग्धं हिमं द्रवम् ॥२८॥
सुशीततोयसिक्ताङ्गो लिह्यात्सक्तून् सशर्करान् ॥२८॥
bhajen-madhuram-evānnaṁ laghu snigdhaṁ himaṁ dravam
suśīta-toya-siktāṅgo lihyāt-saktūn saśarkarān //28//

Consumption of alcohol in summer

मद्यं न पेयं, पेयं वा स्वल्पं, सुबहुवारि वा ॥२९॥
अन्यथाशोषशैथिल्यदाहमोहान् करोति तत् ॥२९॥
madyaṁ na peyaṁ peyaṁ vā svalpaṁ subahuvāri vā
anyathā śopha śaithilya dāha mohān karoti tat //29//

Different foods consumed in summer

कुन्देन्दुधवलं शालिमश्नीयाज्जाङ्गलैः पलैः ॥३०॥
पिबेद्रसं नातिघनं रसालां रागखाण्डवौ ॥३०॥
kundendu-dhavalaṁ śālim-aśnīyājjāṅgalaiḥ palaiḥ
pibed-rasaṁ nātighnaṁ rasālāṁ rāga-khāṇḍavau //30//

Different beverages used during summer

पानकं पञ्चसारं वा नवमृद्भाजने स्थितम् ॥३१॥
मोचचोचदलैर्युक्तं साम्लं मृन्मयशुक्तिभिः ॥३१॥
पाटलावासितं चाम्भः सकर्पूरं सुशीतलम् ॥३२॥
pānakaṁ pañcasāraṁ vā nava mṛdbhājana sthitam
moca-coca dalairyuktaṁ sāmlaṁ mṛnmaya-śuktibhiḥ //31//
pāṭalā-vāsitaṁ cāmbhaḥ sakarpūraṁ suśītalam

Summer nights - diet

शशाङ्ककिरणान् भक्ष्यान् रजन्यां भक्षयन् पिबेत् ॥३२॥

ससितं माहिषं क्षीरं चन्द्रनक्षत्रशीतलम् ॥३३॥

śaśāṇka-kiraṇān bhakṣyān rajanyāṁ bhakṣayan pibet //32//

sasitaṁ māhiṣaṁ kṣīraṁ candra nakṣatra śītalam

Recommendations for dwellings during the summer

अभ्रङ्कषमहाशालतालरुद्धोष्णरश्मिषु ॥३३॥

वनेषु माधवीश्लिष्टद्राक्षास्तबकशालिषु ॥३४॥

सुगन्धिहिमपानीयसिच्यमानपटालिके ॥३४॥

कायमाने चिते चूतप्रवालफललुम्बिभिः ॥३५॥

कदलीदलकह्लारमृणालकमलोत्पलैः ॥३५॥

कोमलैः कल्पिते तल्पे हसत्कुसुमपल्लवे ॥३६॥

मध्यंदिनेऽर्कतापार्तः स्वप्याद्धारागृहेऽथवा ॥३६॥

पुस्तस्त्रीस्तनहस्तास्यप्रवृत्तोशीरवारिणि ॥३७॥

abhraṅkaṣa-mahā-śāla-tāla-rūddhoṣṇa-raśmiṣu //33//

vaneṣu mādhavī-śliṣṭa-drākṣā-stabaka-śāliṣu

sugandhi-hima-pānīya-sicyamāna-paṭālike //34//

kāyamāne cite cūta-pravāla-phala-lumbibhiḥ

kadalīdala-kahlāra-mṛṇāla-kamalotpalaiḥ //35//

komalaiḥ kalpite talpe hasat-kusuma-pallave

madhyaṁ-dine'rka-tāpārtaḥ svapyād-dhārā-gṛhe'thavā //36//

pusta-strīstana-hastāsya-pravṛttośīra-vāriṇī

Moon bathing during summer nights

निशाकरकराकीर्णे सौधपृष्ठे निशासु च ॥३७॥

आसना स्वस्थचित्तस्य चन्दनार्द्रस्य मालिनः ॥३८॥

निवृत्तकामतन्त्रस्य सुसूक्ष्मतनुवाससः ॥३८॥

niśākara-karākīrṇe saudha-pṛṣṭhe niśāsu ca //37//

āsanā svastha-cittasya candanārdrasya mālinaḥ

nivṛtta-kāma-tantrasya susūkṣma-tanu-vāsasaḥ //38//

More recommendations for the summer

जलार्द्रास्तालवृन्तानि विस्तृताः पद्मिनीपुटाः ॥३९॥
उत्क्षेपाश्च मृदूत्क्षेपा जलवर्षिहिमानिलाः ॥३९॥
कर्पूरमल्लिकामाला हाराः सहरिचन्दनाः ॥४०॥
मनोहरकलालापाः शिशवः सारिकाः शुकाः ॥४०॥
मृणालवलयाः कान्ताः प्रोत्फुल्लकमलोज्ज्वलाः ॥४१॥
जङ्गमा इव पद्मिन्यो हरन्ति दयिताः क्लमम् ॥४१॥

jalārdrāstālavṛntāni vistṛtāḥ padminī-puṭāḥ
utkṣepāśca mṛdūtkṣepā jalavarṣi himānilāḥ //39//
karpūra-mallikā mālā hārāḥ saharicandanāḥ
manohara kalālāpāḥ śiśavaḥ sārikāḥ śukāḥ //40//
mṛṇāla valayāḥ kāntāḥ protphulla kamalojjvalāḥ
jaṅgamā iva padminyo haranti dayitāḥ klamam //41//

varṣa ṛtu (rains)

Vitiated water, *agni*, *doṣas* and dūṣyas

आदानग्लानवपुषामग्निः सन्नोऽपि सीदति ॥४२॥
वर्षासु दोषैर्दुष्यन्ति तेऽम्बुलम्बाम्बुदेऽम्बरे ॥४२॥
सतुषारेण मरुता सहसा शीतलेन च ॥४३॥
भूबाष्पेणाम्लपाकेन मलिनेन च वारिणा ॥४३॥
वह्निनैव च मन्देन, तेष्वित्यन्योन्यदूषिषु ॥४४॥
भजेत्साधारणं सर्वमूष्मणस्तेजनं च यत् ॥४४॥

ādāna-glāna-vapuṣām-agni sanno'pi sīdati
varṣāsu doṣair-duṣyanti te'mbulambāmbude'mbare //42//
satuṣāreṇa marutā sahasā śītalena ca
bhūbāṣpeṇāmlapākena malinena ca vāriṇā //43//
vahninaiva ca mandena teṣvity-anyonya dūṣiṣu
bhajet sādhāraṇaṁ sarvam-ūṣmaṇas-tejanaṁ ca yat //44//

Recommendations for rainy season

आस्थापनं शुद्धतनुर्जीर्णं धान्यं रसान् कृतान् ॥४५॥
जाङ्गलं पिशितं यूषान् मध्वरिष्टं चिरन्तनम् ॥४५॥
मस्तु सौवर्चलाढ्यं वा पञ्चकोलावचूर्णितम् ॥४६॥
दिव्यं कौपं शृतं चाम्भो भोजनं त्वतिदुर्दिने ॥४६॥
व्यक्ताम्ललवणस्नेहं संशुष्कं क्षौद्रवल्लघु ॥४७॥

āsthāpanaṁ śuddhatanu-jīrṇaṁ dhānyaṁ rasān kṛtān
jāṅgalaṁ piśitaṁ-yūṣān madhvariṣṭaṁ cirantanam //45//
mastu sauvarcalāḍhyaṁ vā pañcakolāva-cūrṇitam
divya kaupaṁ śṛtaṁ cāmbho bhojanaṁ tvatidurdine //46//
vyaktāmlalavaṇasnehaṁ saṁśukaṁ kṣaudravallaghu

More recommendations for rainy season

अपादचारी सुरभिः सततं धूपिताम्बरः ॥४७॥
हर्म्यपृष्ठे वसेद्बाष्पशीतशीकरवर्जिते ॥४८॥
नदीजलोदमन्थाहःस्वप्नायासातपांस्त्यजेत् ॥४८॥

apādacārī surabhiḥ satataṁ dhūpitāmbaraḥ //47//
harmya pṛṣṭhe vased-bāṣpa-śīta-śīkara-varjite
nadījaloda-manthāhaḥ svapnāyāsā tapāṁs-tyajet //48//

śarad ṛtu (autumn)

How *pitta* aggravates in autumn

वर्षाशीतोचिताङ्गानां सहसैवार्करश्मिभिः ॥४९॥
तप्तानां सञ्चितं वृष्टौ पित्तं शरदि कुप्यति ॥४९॥

varṣā śīto citāṅgānāṁ sahasaivārka raśmibhiḥ
taptānāṁ sañcitaṁ vṛṣṭau pittaṁ śaradi kupyati //49//

Treatment for aggravated *pitta* in autumn

तज्जयाय घृतं तिक्तं विरेको रक्तमोक्षणम् ॥५०॥
तिक्तं स्वादु कषायं च क्षुधितोऽन्नं भजेल्लघु ॥५०॥
शालिमुद्गसिताधात्रीपटोलमधुजाङ्गलम् ॥५१॥

tajjayāya ghṛtaṁ tiktaṁ vireko raktamokṣaṇam
tiktam svādu kaṣāyaṁ ca kṣudhito 'nnaṁ bhajellaghu //50//
śāli-mudga-sitā-dhātrī-paṭola-madhu-jāṅgalam

haṁsodakam – an elixir that pacifies all *doṣas*

तप्तं तप्तांशुकिरणैः शीतं शीतांशुरश्मिभिः ॥५१॥
समन्तादप्यहोरात्रमगस्त्योदयनिर्विषम् ॥५२॥
शुचि हंसोदकं नाम निर्मलं मलजिज्जलम् ॥५२॥
नाभिष्यन्ति न वा रूक्षं पानादिष्वमृतोपमम् ॥५३॥

taptaṁ taptāṁśu kiranaiḥ śītaṁ śītāṁśu-raśmibhiḥ //51//
samantādapy-ahorātram agastyodaya nirviṣam
śuci haṁsodakaṁ nāma nirmalaṁ malajijjalam //52//
nābhiṣyandi na vārūkṣaṁ pānādiṣv-amṛtopamam

Herbs and lifestyle for autumn nights

चन्दनोशीरकर्पूरमुक्तास्रग्वसनोज्ज्वलः ॥५३॥
सौधेषु सौधधवलां चन्द्रिकां रजनीमुखे ॥५४॥

candanośīra-karpūra muktā-srag-vasanojjvalaḥ //53//
saudheṣu saudha dhavalāṁ candrikāṁ rajanī-mukhe

Some things to avoid in the autumn

तुषारक्षारसौहित्यदधितैलवसाऽऽतपान् ॥५४॥
तीक्ष्णमद्यदिवास्वप्नपुरोवातान् परित्यजेत् ॥५५॥

tuṣāra kṣāra sauhitya dadhi taila vasā "tapān //54//
tīkṣṇa madya divā svapna purovātān parityajet

Tastes to be used in each of the seasons

शीते वर्षासु चाद्यांस्त्रीन् वसन्तेऽन्त्यान् रसान्भजेत् ॥५५॥
स्वादुं निदाघे, शरदि स्वादुतिक्तकषायकान् ॥५६॥

śīte varṣāsu cādyāṁstrīn vasante 'ntyān rasān-bhajet //55//
svāduṁ nidāghe śaradi svādu tikta kaṣāyakān

Use of dry and unctuous foods in different seasons

शरद्वसन्तयो रूक्षं शीतं घर्मघनान्तयोः ॥५६॥
अन्नपानं समासेन विपरीतमतोऽन्यदा ॥५७॥

śarad vasantayo rūkṣaṁ śītaṁ gharma ghanāntayoḥ //56//

annapānaṁ samāsena viparītam ato'nyadā

नित्यं सर्वरसाभ्यासः स्वस्वाधिक्यमृतावृतौ ॥५७॥

nityaṁ sarva rasābhyāsaḥ sva svādhikyam-ṛtāvṛtau //57//

Regimen to be followed at the junction of two seasons

ऋत्वोरन्त्यादि सप्ताहावृतुसन्धिरिति स्मृतः
तत्र पूर्वे विधिस्त्याज्यः सेवनीयोऽपरः क्रमात् ॥५८॥

ṛtvor-antyādi saptāhāv-ṛtu sandhir-iti smṛtaḥ
tatra pūrve vidhis-tyājyaḥ sevanīyo 'paraḥ kramāt //58//

Do not immediately abandon any practice

असात्म्यजा हि रोगाः स्युः सहसा त्यागशीलनात् ॥५९ १/२॥

asātmyajā hi rogāḥ syuḥ sahasā tyāga-śīlanāt //59 ½ //

इति श्रीवैद्यपतिसिंहगुप्तसूनुश्रीमद्वाग्टविरचितायामष्टाङ्गहृदयसंहितायां
सूत्रस्थाने ऋतुचर्या नाम तृतीयोध्यायः ॥३॥

iti śrī-vaidyapati-simhaguptasūnu-vāgbhaṭa-viracitāyām aṣṭāṅga-hṛdaya-samhitāyām sūtrasthāne ṛtucaryā nāma tṛtīyodhyāyaḥ

Chapter 4

अथातो रोगानुत्पादनीयाध्यायं व्याख्यास्यामः |

इति ह स्माहुरात्रेयादयो महर्षयः ||

athāto rogānutpādanīyādhyāyaṁ vyākhyāsyāmaḥ
iti ha smāhur ātreyādayo maharṣayaḥ

13 urges not to be suppressed

वेगान्न धारयेद्वातविण्मूत्रक्षवतृट्क्षुधाम् ॥१॥

निद्राकासश्रमश्वासजृम्भाश्रुच्छर्दिरेतसाम् ॥१॥

vegānna dhārayed vāta viṇ mūtra kṣava tṛt kṣudhām
nidrā kāsa śrama śvāsa jṛmbhā 'śru cchardi retasām //1//

Disorders due to suppression of flatus

अधोवातस्य रोधेन गुल्मोदावर्तरुक्क्लमाः ॥२॥

वातमूत्रशकृत्सङ्गदृष्ट्यग्निवधहृद्गदाः ॥२॥

adhovātasya rodhena gulmodāvarta-ruk klamāḥ
vāta-mūtra-śakṛt-saṅga-dṛṣṭy-agnivadha-hṛd-gadāḥ //2//

Disorders due to the suppression of fecal urge

शकृतः पिण्डिकोद्वेष्टप्रतिश्यायशिरोरुजः ॥३॥

ऊर्ध्ववायुः परीकर्तो हृदयस्योपरोधनम् ॥३॥

मुखेन विट्प्रवृत्तिश्च पूर्वोक्ताश्चामयाः स्मृताः ॥४॥

śakṛtaḥ piṇḍikodveṣṭa pratiśyāya śiro rujaḥ
ūrdhva vāyuḥ parīkarto hṛdayasyoparodhanam //3//
mukhena viṭ-pravṛttiśca pūrvoktāścāmayāḥ smṛtāḥ

Disorders due to the suppression of urinary urge

अङ्गभङ्गाश्मरीवस्तिमेढ्रवंक्षणवेदनाः ॥४॥

मूत्रस्य रोधात्पूर्वे च प्रायो रोगास्तदौषधम् ॥५॥

aṅga-bhaṅgāśmarī-vasti-medhra-vaṁkṣaṇa vedanāḥ //4//

mūtrasya rodhāt-pūrve ca prāyo rogās ....

Treatment of diseases due to suppressing the urge of flatus, feces & urine

.... तदौषधम्

वर्त्यभ्यङ्गावगाहाश्च स्वेदनं वस्तिकर्म च ॥५॥

अन्नपानं च विड्भेदि विड्रोधोत्थेषु यक्ष्मसु ॥६॥

.... tad-auṣadham

varty-abhyaṅgāvagāhāśca svedanaṁ vasti-karma ca //5//

annapānaṁ ca viḍ-bhedi vid-rodhottheṣu yakṣmasu

Treatment of the suppression of urination

मूत्रजेषु तु पाने च प्राग्भक्तं शस्यते घृतम् ॥६॥

जीर्णान्तिकं चोत्तमया मात्रया योजनाद्वयम् ॥७॥

अवपीडकमेतच्च संज्ञितं धारणात्पुनः ॥७॥

mūtrajeṣu tu pāne ca prāgbhaktaṁ śasyate ghṛtam //6//

jīrṇāntikaṁ cottamayā mātrayā yojanādvayam

avapīḍakam-etacca saṁñjitam dhāraṇāt-punaḥ //7//

Suppression of belching & Treatment

उद्गारस्यारुचिः कम्पो विबन्धो हृदयोरसोः ॥८॥

आध्मानकासहिद्धमाश्च हिद्धमावत्तत्र भेषजम् ॥८॥

udgārasyāruciḥ kampo vibandho hṛdayorasoḥ

ādhmāna-kāsa-hidhmāśca hidhmāvat-tatra bheṣajam //8//

Suppression of sneezing & treatment

शिरोऽर्तीन्द्रियदौर्बल्यमन्यास्तम्भार्दितं क्षुतेः ॥९॥

तीक्ष्णधूमाञ्जनाघ्राणनावनार्कविलोकनैः ॥९॥

प्रवर्तयेत्क्षुतिं सक्तां स्नेहस्वेदौ च शीलयेत् ॥१०॥

śiro'rtīndriya-daurbalya-manyāstambhārditaṁ kṣuteḥ
tīkṣṇa-dhūmāñjanā-ghrāṇa-nāvanārka-vilokanaiḥ //9//
pravartayet-kṣutiṁ saktāṁ sneha-svedau ca śīlayet

Suppression of thirst

शोषाङ्गसादबाधिर्यसम्मोहभ्रमहृद्दाः ॥१०॥

तृष्णाया निग्रहात्तत्र शीतः सर्वो विधिर्हितः ॥११॥

śoṣāṅgasāda-bādhirya-sammoha-bhrama-hṛd-gadāḥ //10//
tṛṣṇāyā nigrahāt-tatra śītaḥ sarvo vidhir-hitaḥ

Suppression of hunger & treatment

अङ्गभङ्गारुचिग्लानिकार्श्यशूलभ्रमाः क्षुधः ॥११॥

तत्र योज्यं लघु स्निग्धमुष्णमल्पं च भोजनम् ॥१२॥

aṅga-bhaṅgāruci-glāni-kārśya-śūla-bhramāḥ kṣudhaḥ //11//
tatra yojyaṁ laghu snigdham-uṣṇām-alpaṁ ca bhojanam

Suppression of sleep

निद्राया मोहमूर्धाक्षिगौरवालस्यजृम्भिकाः ॥१२॥

आङ्गमर्दश्च, तत्रेष्टः स्वप्नः संवाहनानि च ॥१३॥

nidrāyā moha-mūrdhākṣi-gauravālasya-jṛmbhikāḥ //12//
aṅga-mardaśca tatreṣṭaḥ svapnaḥ saṁvāhanāni ca

Suppression of cough & treatment

कासस्य रोधात्तद्वृद्धिः श्वासारुचिहृदामयाः ॥१३॥
शोषो हिध्मा च कार्योत्र कासहा सुतरां विधिः ॥१४॥

kāsasya rodhāt-tad vṛddhiḥ śvāsāruci hṛdāmayāḥ //13//
śoṣo hidhmā ca kāryo 'tra kāsahā sutarāṁ vidhiḥ

Suppression of heaving (panting) & treatment

गुल्महृद्रोगसम्मोहाः श्रमश्वासाद्विधारितात् ॥१४॥
हितं विश्रमणं तत्र वातघ्नश्च क्रियाक्रमः ॥१५॥

gulma-hṛdroga-sammohāḥ śrama-śvāsād-vidhāritāt //14//
hitaṁ viśramaṇaṁ tatra vātaghnaśca kriyā-kramaḥ

Suppression of yawning

जृम्भायाः क्षववद्रोगाः सर्वश्चानिलजिद्विधिः ॥१५॥

jṛmbhāyāḥ kṣavavad-rogāḥ sarvaścānilajid-vidhiḥ //15//

Suppression of tears

पीनसाक्षिशिरोहृद्रुङ्मन्यास्तम्भारुचिभ्रमाः ॥१६॥
सगुल्मा बाष्पतस्तत्र स्वप्नो मद्यं प्रियाः कथाः ॥१६॥

pīnasākṣi śiro-hṛdruṅ-manyāstambhāruci-bhramāḥ
sagulmā bāṣpatas-tatra svapno madyaṁ priyāḥ kathāḥ //16//

Suppression of vomiting urge & treatment

विसर्पकोठकुष्ठाक्षिकण्डूपाण्ड्वामयज्वराः ॥१७॥
सकासश्वासहृल्लासव्यङ्गश्वयथवो वमेः ॥१७॥
गण्डूषधूमानाहारा रूक्षं भुक्त्वा तदुद्भ्रमः ॥१८॥
व्यायामः स्तुतिरस्रस्य शस्तं चात्र विरेचनम् ॥१८॥

सक्षारलवणं तैलमभ्यङ्गार्थं च शस्यते ॥१९॥

visarpa-koṭha-kuṣṭhākṣi-kaṇdū-pāṇdvāmaya-jvarāḥ
sakāsa-śvāsa-hṛllāsa-vyaṅga-śvayathavo-vameḥ //17//
gaṇḍūṣa-dhūmānāhārā rūkṣaṁ bhuktvā tadudvamaḥ
vyāyāmaḥ srutir-asrasya śastaṁ cātra virecanam //18//
sakṣāra-lavaṇaṁ tailam-abhyaṅgārthaṁ ca śasyate

Suppression of seminal urge

शुक्रात्तत्स्रवणं गुह्यवेदनाश्वयथुज्वराः ॥१९॥
हृद्व्यथामूत्रसङ्गाङ्गभङ्गवृद्ध्यश्मषण्ढताः ॥२०॥
ताम्रचूडसुराशालिवस्त्यभ्यङ्गावगाहनम् ॥२०॥
वस्तिशुद्धिकरैः सिद्धम् भजेत्क्षीरं प्रियाः स्त्रियः ॥२१॥

śukrāt-tat-sravaṇaṁ guhya-vedanā-śvayathu-jvarāḥ //19//
hṛdvyathā-mūtrasaṅgāṅga-bhaṅga-vṛddhy-aśma-ṣaṇḍatāḥ
tāmra-cūda-surāśāli-vasty-abhyaṅgāvagāhanam //20//
vasti-śuddhikaraiḥ siddhaṁ bhajet kṣīraṁ priyāḥ striyaḥ

When to reject curative options

तृट्शूलार्तं त्यजेत् क्षीणं विड्वमं वेगरोधिनम् ॥२१॥

tṛṭśulārtaṁ tyajet kṣīṇaṁ vidvamaṁ vegarodhinam //21//

रोगाः सर्वेपि जायन्ते वेगोदीरणधारणैः ॥२२॥
निर्दिष्टं साधनं तत्र भूयिष्ठं ये तु तान् प्रति ॥२२॥
ततश्चानेकधा प्रायः पवनो यत्प्रकुप्यति ॥२३॥
अन्नपानौषधं तस्य युञ्जीतातोनुलोमनम् ॥२३॥

rogāḥ sarve 'pi jāyante vego-dīraṇa-dhāraṇaiḥ
nirdiṣṭaṁ sādhanaṁ tatra bhūyiṣṭham ye tu tān prati //22//
tataś-cānekadhā prāyaḥ pavano-yat-prakupyati
annapān-auṣadhaṁ tasya-yuñjītāto 'nulomanam //23//

dhāraṇīya vega (urges to be controlled)

धारयेत्तु सदा वेगान् हितैषी प्रेत्य चेह च ॥२४॥
लोभेर्ष्याद्वेषमात्सर्यरागादीनां जितेन्द्रियः ॥२४॥

dhārayettu sadā vegān hitaiṣī pretya ceha ca
lobh-erṣyā-dveṣa-mātsarya-rāgādīnāṁ jitendriyaḥ //24//

Importance of seasonal cleansing

यतेत च यथाकालं मलानां शोधनं प्रति ॥२५॥
अत्यर्थसञ्चितास्ते हि क्रुद्धाः स्युर्जीवितच्छिदः ॥२५॥
दोषाः कदाचित्कुप्यन्ति जिता लङ्घनपाचनैः ॥२६॥
ये तु संशोधनैः शुद्धा न तेषां पुनरुद्भवः ॥२६॥

yateta ca yathā kālaṁ malānāṁ śodhanaṁ prati
atyartha sañcitāste hy kruddhāḥ syur-jīvitacchidaḥ //25//
doṣāḥ kadācit-kupyanti jitā langhana pācanaiḥ
ye tu saṁśodhanaiḥ śuddhā na teṣāṁ punar-udbhavaḥ //26//

Rejuvenation and strengthening after cleansing

यथाक्रमं यथायोगमत ऊर्ध्वं प्रयोजयेत् ॥२७॥
रसायनानि सिद्धानि वृष्ययोगांश्च कालवित् ॥२७॥

yathā-kramam yathā-yogam ata-ūrdhvaṁ prayojayet
rasāyanāni siddhāni vṛṣya-yogāmśca kālavīt //27//

the sequence of purification, nourishment and rejuvenation

भेषजक्षपिते पथ्यमाहारैर्बृंहणं क्रमात् ॥२८॥
शालिषष्टिकगोधूममुद्गमांसघृतादिभिः ॥२८॥
हृद्यदीपनभैषज्यसंयोगाद्रुचिपक्तिदैः ॥२९॥
साभ्यङ्गोद्वर्तनस्नाननिरूहस्नेह वस्तिभिः ॥२९॥

तथा स लभते शर्म सर्वपावकपाटवम् ॥३०॥
धीवर्णेन्द्रियवैमल्यं वृषतां दैर्घ्यमायुषः ॥३०॥
bheṣaja-kṣapite pathyam-āhārai-bṛmhaṇaṁ kramāt
śāli-ṣaṣṭika-godhūma-mudga māmsa-ghṛtādibhiḥ //28//
hṛdya-dīpana bhaiṣajya saṁyogād-rucipaktidaiḥ
sābhyaṅgodvartana snāna nirūha-sneha-vastibhiḥ //29//
tathā sa labhate śarma sarva-pāvaka-pāṭavam
dhī-varṇendriya-vaimalyaṁ vṛṣatāṁ dairghyam-āyuṣaḥ //30//

āgantu rogaḥ: diseases due to external causes

ये भूतविषवाय्वग्निक्षतभङ्गादिसम्भवाः ॥३१॥
रागद्वेषभयाद्याश्च ते स्युरागन्तवो गदाः ॥३१॥
ye bhūta-viṣavāyvagni-kṣata-bhaṅgādi-sambhavāḥ
raga dveṣa[11]-bhayādyāśca te syur-āgantavo gadāḥ //31//

त्यागः प्रज्ञापराधानामिन्द्रियोपशमः स्मृतिः ॥३२॥
देशकालात्मविज्ञानं सद्वृत्तस्यानुवर्तनम् ॥३२॥
tyāgaḥ prajñāparādhānām-indriyopaśamaḥ smṛtiḥ
deśa-kālātma-vijñānaṁ sadvṛttasyānuvartanam //32//

अथर्वविहिता शान्तिः प्रतिकूलग्रहार्चनम् ॥३३॥
भूताद्यस्पर्शनोपायो निर्दिष्टश्च पृथक् पृथक् ॥३३॥
atharva-vihitā śāntiḥ pratikūla grahārcanam
bhūtādya sparśanopāyo nirdiṣṭaśca pṛthak pṛthak //33//

अनुत्पत्त्यै समासेन विधिरेषः प्रदर्शितः ॥३४॥
निजागन्तुविकाराणामुत्पन्नानां च शान्तये ॥३४॥
anutpatyai samāsena vidhireṣa pradarśitaḥ

---

[11] *kāma-krodha bhyādyāśca … - this is another variation of this verse*

nijāgantu-vikārāṇām-utpannānāṁ ca śāntaye //34//

Cleanse on time to avoid diseases originating due to season changes

शीतोद्भवं दोषचयं वसन्ते विशोधनं ग्रीष्मजमभ्रकाले ॥३५॥
घनात्यये वार्षिकमाशु सम्यक् प्राप्नोति रोगानृतुजान्न जातु ॥३५॥

śītodbhavaṁ doṣa-cayaṁ vasante
viśodhayan grīṣmajam-abhrakāle
ghanātyaye vārṣikam-āśu samyak
prāpnoti rogān-ṛtujān-na jātu //35//

Formula for freedom from all diseases

नित्यं हिताहारविहारसेवी समीक्ष्यकारी विषयेष्वसक्तः ॥३६॥
दाता समः सत्यपरः क्षमावानाप्तोपसेवी च भवत्यरोगः ॥३६॥

nityam hitāhāra-vihāra-sevī
samīkṣyakārī viṣayeṣv-asaktaḥ
dātā samaḥ satyaparaḥ kṣamāvān
āptopasevī ca bhavaty-arogaḥ //36//

इति श्रीवैद्यपतिसिंहगुप्तसूनुश्रीमद्वाग्टविरचितायामष्टाङ्गहृदयसंहितायां
सूत्रस्थाने रोगानुत्पादनीयो नाम चतुर्थोध्यायः ॥४॥

iti śrī-vaidyapati-simhaguptasūnu-vāgbhaṭa-viracitāyām
aṣṭāṅga-hṛdaya-samhitāyām sūtrasthāne
rogānutpādanīyo nāma caturthodhyāyaḥ

Index

N

S